Disorders of the Cardiovascular System

Disorders of the Cardiovascular System

DAVID PATTERSON, MD, FRCP

Consultant Physician and Cardiologist, Bloomsbury and
Islington Health Authority
Hon. Senior Lecturer in Medicine, University College and
Middlesex School of Medicine, London

and

TOM TREASURE, MD, MS, FRCS

Consultant Cardiothoracic Surgeon, St George's Hospital, London

Edward Arnold
A division of Hodder & Stoughton
LONDON BOSTON MELBOURNE AUCKLAND

© 1993 Edward Arnold

First published in Great Britain 1993
Distributed in the Americas by Little, Brown and Company
34 Beacon Street, Boston, MA 02108

British Library Cataloguing in Publication Data

A CIP catalogue record for this book
is available from the British Library

ISBN 0 340 53593 8

Whilst the advice and information in this book is believed to be true
and accurate at the date of going to press, neither the author nor the
publisher can accept any legal responsibility or liability for any errors
or omissions that may be made. In particular (but without limiting the
generality of the preceding disclaimer) every effort has been made to
check drug dosages; however, it is still possible that errors have been
missed. Furthermore, dosage schedules are constantly being revised
and new side effects recognised. For these reasons the reader is
strongly urged to consult the drug companies' printed instructions
before administering any of the drugs recommended in this book.

Typeset in Linotron Caledonia by Rowland Phototypesetting
Limited, Bury St Edmunds, Suffolk. Printed in Great Britain
for Edward Arnold, a division of Hodder and Stoughton Limited,
Mill Road, Dunton Green, Sevenoaks, Kent TN13 2YA by
Butler and Tanner Limited, Frome, Somerset.

PREFACE

We have aimed to write a short textbook of cardiology that will serve as an introduction to the subject for students and for junior doctors who have not yet entered higher specialist training. It was at times a worrying task because, as we wrote, we were impressed by how much has changed in the twenty years or so since we were clinical students ourselves, and we were aware that sometimes we have had to make statements that are unlikely to remain true for very long. Of course, we do not know which they are. But we spent little time in idle speculation. We believe that what we have written is well within the established body of current cardiological knowledge and practice.

This book is a clinical companion to the *Cardiovascular Physiology* by Fitzsimons and Barnes (Edward Arnold, 1993). An understanding of physiology and anatomy is an excellent basis for learning medicine and yet we are impressed by how often the student's attempts to work out what might or what 'ought' to happen, leads him or her to desperately wrong conclusions. A simple and commonly repeated example is the student's initial assumption that, because there is obstruction to flow at the aortic valve, all patients with aortic stenosis must have low blood pressure. Student and teacher might work on it a bit further and recall that systemic pressure is controlled in the arterial system, not in the ventricle, but the real lesson is that if clinical medicine could all be worked out from first principles, a logical mind in a darkened room would have solved it all long ago. The plain fact is that there is a body of knowledge, based on hard-earned experience, and it has to be learned if we are going to offer our patients the level of expertise that is expected from a doctor in this day and age.

Heart disease is still the biggest cause of death in the more developed countries. Even if we cannot cure or prevent a particular heart disease, we may modify its course. For some there is a discrete lesion that may be overcome by technical methods but for all there must be a holistic approach, applying what we know about the environment, dietary risk factors, hypertension, avoidable hazards such as smoking, the best available and, where possible, the least invasive investigations, and the best combination of therapy for each individual. This may include pharmacology, a direct technical attack on the lesion, advice on life style and, where appropriate, genetic counselling with the health of the next generation in mind. Sometimes even this broad approach is not enough and we as individuals or as a profession have to lobby our politicians, our food manufacturers or our industrialists in order to effect change that will benefit our patients.

We are a cardiologist and a cardiac surgeon and have brought together our shared experience as physician and surgeon in a discipline where the two are complementary. Between us our work includes the spectrum of heart disease from general medical 'take', through specialized investigation and management, to technically based medicine and surgery. We have not taken individual responsibility for different chapters. Although one man must mark the page first, every chapter is the work of both. We have exchanged draft manuscripts and computer discs, and peered at VDU screens together. We have risked being authoritative and didactic, but believe that what we recommend is mainstream practice at a standard that should be available as a routine.

D.L.H.P.
T.T.

Acknowledgements

We are indebted to Mr John Moseley for contributing Chapter 10.

We are also grateful to Dr Graham Leach for providing the echo and Doppler illustrations.

D.L.H.P.
T.T.

CONTENTS

1

CORONARY ARTERY DISEASE

Coronary anatomy

A basic knowledge of coronary anatomy is essential to an understanding of the various patterns of presentation with coronary artery disease. The extent, severity and combinations of coronary lesions also sort patients into groups of different degrees of hazard, and the anatomical sites of stenoses in an individual patient determine the risk of death from any subsequent myocardial infarction. Without an appreciation of the significance of particular anatomical sites of atherosclerotic obstruction, and the chances of relieving the obstruction, it is impossible to give rational advice about the degree of benefit that might be gained by an intervention. The anatomical knowledge need be no more detailed than this. Confusion can arise because while the aorta has two coronary orifices, we speak of 'triple vessel disease'. As elsewhere in the heart the words 'left' and 'right' are less than completely descriptive and the word 'dominance' does not carry the obvious implication.

The 'three vessels'

The left ventricle is supplied with arterial blood in approximate thirds for the majority (90 per cent) of people. These are anteroseptal, lateral and inferior territories (Fig. 1.1) and they correspond to the sites of major infarction that may follow occlusion of one of the three major vessels.

The left main stem is 1–2 cm long and is important because a stenosis or occlusion at this site puts two-thirds of the left ventricular myocardium at risk with one lesion.

The left anterior descending coronary artery

The 'LAD' is also known by anatomists as the anterior interventricular artery; it descends, as named, in the anterior interventricular groove, from its origin at the bifurcation of the left coronary artery to the apex of the heart (Fig. 1.2).

The diagonal branches of the LAD run laterally to supply the anterior surface of the left ventricle and it also gives a series of septal branches. The septum is an important functional part of the left ventricle, not just a partition. The first septal perforator is of particular importance in that a single coronary stenosis proximal to it puts at risk a large amount of muscle and, in some patients, the conducting system.

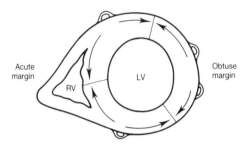

Fig. 1.1 A cross-section across the heart demonstrates how the septum forms a functional part of the left ventricle, contributing to its circular configuration of musculature. We can also see how the anteroseptal, lateral and inferior parts are supplied in approximate thirds. The acute and obtuse margins can also be appreciated.

The circumflex system

The other branch from the bifurcation of the left main stem is called the left circumflex coronary artery. The details of its anatomy are very variable and its branches are known as obtuse marginal or lateral circumflex branches (Fig. 1.2). It is the least dangerous site of coronary lesions and infarcts in this territory are rarely massive, probably because some of its several branches are usually spared.

The right coronary artery

Arising anteriorly is the right coronary artery, which runs round the heart, supplying the right atrium and ventricle (Fig. 1.3). In the majority (90 per cent) of hearts it is still a large vessel (>2 mm) when it reaches the inferior surface of the heart, where it branches to give a posterior descending (or inferior inter-ventricular) artery and one or more branches to the inferior surface of the left ventricle. The extent to which the circumflex and right coronary arteries supply the inferior surface is thus rather variable and other than when the right coronary does not contribute at all (i.e. the remaining 10 per cent), it is called, rather confusingly, a 'dominant' right system.

Pathology

The lesions of atherosclerosis occur mainly within the intima. They include the fatty streak, the fibrous plaque and the complicated plaque. In the more advanced lesions of atherosclerosis, secondary changes may be found in the media of the artery underlying the intimal lesion.

The process of atherosclerosis begins in childhood with the development of flat, lipid-rich lesions called fatty streaks (Fig. 1.4). These lesions consist of lipid-laden macrophages and smooth muscle cells. Fatty streaks can be found in the aorta shortly after birth and appear in increasing numbers during adolescence. The lesions are yellowish, cause no obstruction and have no clinical sequelae. The lesions occur even in populations that do not develop severe atherosclerosis.

In populations in which there is a high incidence of atherosclerosis and its complications, more advanced lesions begin to develop in the arteries of people

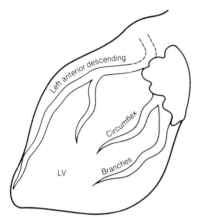

Fig. 1.2 A left anterior oblique view of the heart, showing the normal branches of the left coronary artery with, in this example, a normal (non-dominant) circumflex system.

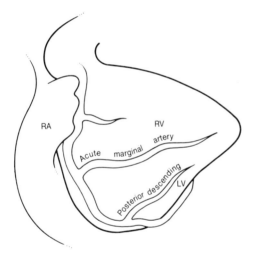

Fig. 1.3 A view of the heart from the right and slightly below, showing the commonest pattern of the dominant right coronary artery as found in 90 per cent of cases.

in their early 20s. The fibrous plaque is white in appearance. The suggestion that these fibrous plaques are derived from fatty streaks has not been proved. The plaque may become elevated and protrude into the lumen of the artery. At least four cell types participate in the formation of the plaque: the endothelial cell, the macrophage, the platelet and the smooth muscle cell. The endothelial cell is believed to be the site where formation of the plaque begins. There are several theories to explain the development of the atheromatous plaque; they are not mutually exclusive. An important step in the process is thought to be an alteration in the functional or structural barrier of the endothelial cell lining of the vessel wall. These alterations may be caused by an increased sheer stress from the flow of blood or may be induced by toxins or other injurious agents. These factors lead to changes in the permeability of the endothelial cells. Lipid-

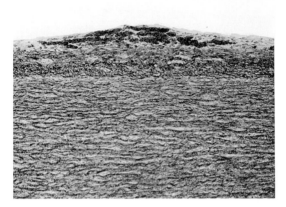

Fig. 1.4 Section of the aorta of a child, showing a fatty streak. (Frozen section: lipid stained black) ×20. (Reproduced, with permission, from R. M. N. MacSween and K. Whaley (Eds.), 1992, *Muir's Textbook of Pathology*, 13th edn, Edward Arnold, London.)

filled monocytes can pass normally into or out of the intima between endothelial cells. These monocytes may have a scavenging role and can remove low density lipoprotein (LDL) cholesterol. They can become macrophages in certain situations. It seems likely that these monocytes have the potential to alter the properties of the endothelial cell. This may induce the release of a growth factor from the endothelial cells and also from the platelets; this in turn may cause the proliferation and migration of smooth muscle cells, which then migrate up into the intima, to secrete a protein which becomes the collagen matrix.

An alternative hypothesis suggests that both the initiation and the progression of the lesion can be associated with elevated levels of plasma cholesterol or LDL. Increased amounts of LDL cholesterol infiltrate the intima and undergo oxidative modification. This modification stimulates the recruitment of circulating monocytes which undergo a change in form and function to become resident macrophages. These macrophages are then retained in the lesion due to the inhibitory effect of the oxidatively modified LDL. Many of the lipid-laden cells may become necrotic and release their lipid into the extracellular spaces. Some of the oxidized LDL is taken up by scavengers such as high density lipoprotein (HDL) which is then removed from the intima for degradation elsewhere. Other oxidized LDL is taken up to form foam cells within the fatty streak.

A third theory proposes that atherosclerotic plaques develop from a single precursor cell that proliferates like a tumour. Some triggering agent for the initiation of atheroma must be invoked, such as a virus, a chemical or a pre-existing genetic defect.

The complicated plaque (Fig. 1.5) is a degenerative lesion composed of fibrous tissue, fibrin, calcium, intracellular and extracellular lipid, and extravasated blood. The plaque is covered by a fibrous tissue cap. It can become vascularized from the lumen as well as from its underlying media. The atheromatous plaque bulges outwards towards the media, and not inwards as previously described in arteries that had been fixed and processed in the undistended state.

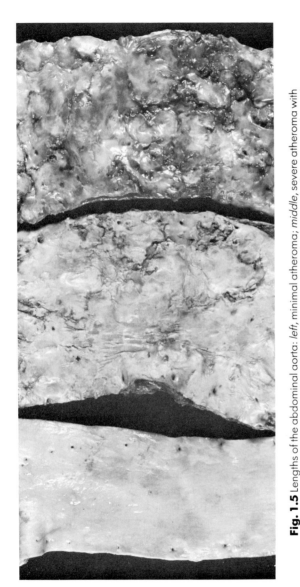

Fig. 1.5 Lengths of the abdominal aorta: *left,* minimal atheroma; *middle,* severe atheroma with cracking and early ulceration of patches; *right,* very severe atheroma with ulceration and mural thrombosis. Note also that the two atheromatous aortas have lost their elasticity and have stretched; this may be due to atrophy of the media beneath the extensive atheroma, but could also be the result of arteriosclerosis. (Reproduced, with permission, from J. R. Anderson (Ed.), 1985, *Muir's Textbook of Pathology,* 12th edn, Edward Arnold, London.)

Clinical manifestations of coronary artery disease

The five main clinical manifestations of coronary artery disease are:

1. Sudden death
2. Myocardial infarction
3. Unstable angina
4. Stable angina pectoris
5. Heart failure

A better understanding of the various mechanisms involved is beginning to emerge. Coronary artery thrombi are directly implicated in the pathophysiology of the first three manifestations of acute myocardial ischaemia: namely, sudden death, unstable angina and myocardial infarction (Fig. 1.6). Stable atheroma (A in Fig. 1.6) may exist for years without any manifestations and is part of the ageing process. The first event that may bring symptoms to the attention of the patient relates to the rupture of the fibrous cap. This allows blood from the lumen to dissect into the intima and into the lipid pool of the plaque. A thrombus, rich in platelets but also containing some red cells and fibrin, forms within the intima and leads to expansion of the plaque. Over the site of rupture, thrombus forms in the lumen (Fig. 1.6, B). This mass of luminal thrombus initially does not occlude the lumen, but waxes and wanes in size over hours or even days. Some patients may have a massive thrombotic response within the lumen with minimal fissuring. The intraluminal thrombus may grow to become totally occlusive (Fig. 1.6, C) or may become completely lysed and the plaque fissure resealed (Fig. 1.6, D). The earlier stages of plaque fissuring are found in patients with

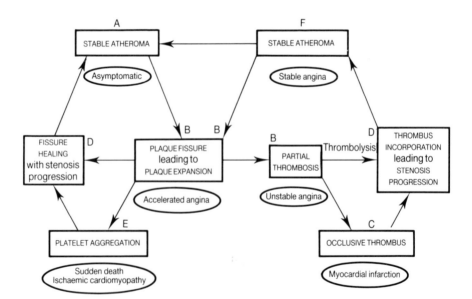

Fig. 1.6 How coronary artery thrombi can be directly implicated in the pathophysiology of sudden death, unstable angina and myocardial infarction.

unstable angina or those who suffer sudden ischaemic death. Patients who develop an established regional infarct (Fig. 1.6, C) are those in whom the thrombus has occluded the lumen at least for long enough to induce myocardial necrosis. This does not explain why some patients die suddenly before the arterial lesion is fully occlusive (Fig. 1.6, E). Sudden death may be caused by an arrhythmia caused by platelet emboli arising from the thrombus being 'washed downstream'; the mechanism is equivalent to that causing transient cerebral ischaemic attacks. Plaque fissuring can also invoke local arterial spasm.

By this concept the three presentations of acute cardiac ischaemia all have a common basis. Patients with a plaque fissure who escape one of these manifestations will be left with an atheromatous plaque larger than previously. This episodic plaque growth is an important factor in the development of stable angina (Fig. 1.6, F).

The speed at which thrombi evolve and regress over a relatively short period of time emphasizes the importance of the haemostatic and fibrinolytic systems, both as part of the acute or subacute complications of atheroma and also more chronically in the initial development of the atheromatous lesion. Many of these haemostatic factors can be rapidly modified by stressful stimuli.

It is worthwhile reviewing briefly the factors involved in platelet aggregation, thrombus formation and fibrinolysis. From the therapeutic standpoint, an understanding of these factors and how they interrelate is becoming more important.

The vascular endothelium

The vascular endothelium synthesizes prostacyclin, which is a potent vasodilator and has anti-aggregatory properties. The endothelium also activates or inactivates a number of vasoactive substances present in the blood, influences the amount of vasoactive substances reaching the deeper layers of the blood vessel wall and modifies the responsiveness of the vascular smooth muscle of the media.

Platelets

Platelets can produce a number of vasoactive substances which include serotonin, thromboxane, adenine nucleotides, vasopressin and platelet-activating substance. Each of these substances produces constriction of the smooth muscle of coronary arteries when there is a damaged endothelium. In the presence of an intact endothelium, relaxation occurs. How can these opposite effects be explained? It is postulated that the endothelium-derived relaxing factor (EDRF), or a component of it, plays an important part. If platelets begin to aggregate in a normal artery with an intact endothelium, the response of the smooth muscle to the substances released from the platelets is that of relaxation, mediated by EDRF. This relaxation is reinforced if the platelet aggregation sets the coagulation cascade in motion, causing the formation of thrombin. If the endothelium is damaged or not functioning properly, the response of the coronary vessels to the platelet products and thrombin is that of constriction – which further reduces the lumen and increases the obstruction to blood flow.

Platelet activation can be demonstrated during episodes of unstable or variant angina. In contrast, platelet activation is not demonstrable at rest nor during exercise-induced ischaemia in patients with stable angina.

Fibrinolysis

Fibrin is the natural substrate of the fibrinolytic system (Fig. 1.7). It is formed from circulating fibrinogen by the action of thrombin. Together with the interaction of the platelets, it forms the scaffolding of the intravascular thrombus or haemostatic plug. Fibrin also plays a decisive role in its own dissolution by accumulating various components of the fibrinolytic system into the thrombus. These accelerate the action of tissue-type plasminogen activator (t-PA) on plasminogen. Plasmin, formed by activation of plasminogen, is the key enzyme in the fibrinolytic system (Fig. 1.7, A). Its non-specific proteolytic activity in the circulation is controlled by protease inhibitors, the most important of which is α_2-antiplasmin (α_2-AP). The major role of α_2-AP is to neutralize plasmin in the circulation. It is also incorporated into growing fibrin clots where it is bound by the action of clotting factor XIII. Both plasminogen and α_2-AP are themselves modulated by several factors.

Plasminogen activation is the main regulatory process of the fibrinolytic system (Fig. 1.7, B). There are at least three different routes of activation that can be distinguished and quantified. Of the three, the pathway catalysed by the tissue-type plasminogen activator (t-PA) has received most attention (Fig. 1.7, C). t-PA is secreted by endothelial cells into the circulation and is itself modified

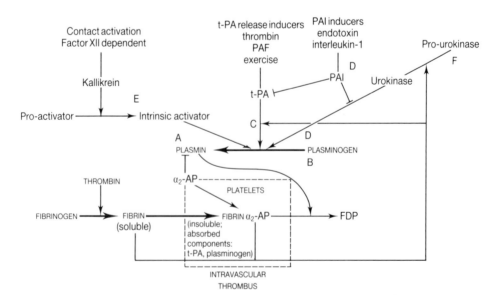

Fig. 1.7 Some of the factors involved in thrombus formation and in fibrinolysis. α_2-AP, α_2-antiplasmin; FDP, fibrin degradation products; t-PA, tissue type plasminogen activator; PAI, plasminogen activator inhibitor.

by the action of plasminogen activator inhibitor (PAI). The diurnal variation in fibrinolytic activity, the reduced t-PA after surgery or after a myocardial infarction, is due mainly to changes in PAI (Fig. 1.7, D). Two other main pathways influence plasminogen activation: the factor XII-dependent pathway (Fig. 1.7, E) and the factor XII-independent pathway (Fig. 1.7, F), which account for about half of the intrinsic activation system; the latter is also known as the urokinase-related pathway.

A number of essential interacting factors are selectively adsorbed onto the growing fibrin network; platelets contribute additional PAI and the vessel wall can react with the release of extra t-PA. Once fibrinolysis has started, the stimulatory effect of fibrin on plasminogen activation in the clot matrix may increase many times. Attempts at antithrombotic intervention have been based on one of two principles – either using anticoagulants to slow down the formation of thrombi or, alternatively, using drugs to speed up their dissolution. It has become clear from studies of patients with acute myocardial infarction that thrombolysis is achieved with a much smaller dose of the thrombolytic drug if it is introduced early in the development of thrombus.

Risk factors for coronary artery disease

The different incidence and prevalence of coronary artery disease between countries has stimulated the search for factors that might predict the development of the disease. These are now referred to as risk factors. They include not only the physicochemical characteristics of the individuals but also aspects of lifestyle such as diet, smoking and behaviour patterns. It was hoped that the discovery of such risk factors might help the effort to prevent coronary artery disease. It was recognized that the association of these variables with the disease did not establish any aetiological relationship. Unfortunately, a high proportion of patients who develop coronary artery disease do not have any treatable risk factor. Furthermore, a large proportion of patients with risk factors do not develop the disease. Most of the reversible risk factors are predictive of coronary artery disease only in relatively young people; this suggests that in older people the disease process is principally related to ageing itself rather than one of the avoidable risk factors.

Diet

Epidemiological studies have provided evidence that some diets may be associated with an increased risk of coronary artery disease. These studies fall into three main categories:

1. Between-country correlations of coronary artery disease rates and food intake
2. Prospective observation of subjects for whom individual diet histories are available
3. Associations between diet and various measures of lipid metabolism known to be associated with coronary artery disease

Epidemiological data support the suggestion that the incidence of coronary artery disease in a community is related to the saturated fat intake and, to a lesser extent, to the sucrose intake of that community. The evidence for a link between an individual's saturated fat intake and the frequency of coronary artery disease is less persuasive. The evidence to suggest that a high ratio of polyunsaturated/saturated fat intake is associated with a lower incidence of coronary artery disease is not very strong. Of the various measures of an individual's lipid metabolism, only serum cholesterol has been shown to bear any relationship to the diet. In the typical Western diet 40 per cent of energy is provided by fat. A serum cholesterol reduction of about 10–15 per cent can be achieved if the proportion is reduced to 30 per cent and the ratio of polyunsaturated/saturated fat is increased. A further factor influencing this relationship between coronary artery disease and an individual's lipid levels is the effect of certain long-chain polyunsaturated fatty acids such as linoleic acid and eicosapentaenoic acid. These fatty acids, which are found particularly in fish, also have an effect on the thrombotic tendency of the blood.

Abnormalities of lipid metabolism

The total serum cholesterol appears to be the most important determinant of the geographic distribution of coronary artery disease. Among individuals within populations the association is also strong. There is no cut-off point between a normal value, with no risk, and an abnormal value; the risk tends to increase throughout the range (Fig. 1.8). Whilst the absolute risk associated with any given cholesterol value varies between different parts of the world, within most population samples, the risk is greater in subjects with higher cholesterol values. The association of total cholesterol with coronary artery disease mortality relates almost entirely to the LDL fraction. The total fasting triglyceride and very low

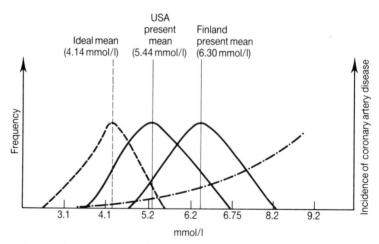

Fig. 1.8 The relationship between plasma cholesterol level and incidence of coronary artery disease superimposed on three plasma cholesterol distributions for middle-aged subjects.

density lipoprotein (VLDL) are probably not independent risk factors. The role of HDL as a protective factor has recently caused some interest. The mechanism by which it exerts its protective effect is not known; it may augment the removal of cholesterol from the interior of cells or influence the binding and absorption of LDL by the cells.

The metabolic disorder of familial hypercholesterolaemia has been shown to be due to a reduction in the number of, or effectiveness of, the receptors for LDL on the cell surface (Fig. 1.9). The homozygote form is fortunately rare and occurs in only about 1 in a million people; it occurs more frequently in communities in which consanguinity is common. Patients with this form have extreme hyper-cholesterolaemia and develop severe coronary artery disease in childhood. The heterozygote form occurs in a frequency of 1 in 500, which makes it one of the most common genetic disorders; patients with this form have moderate elevation of cholesterol and develop coronary artery disease in early or mid-adult life (Fig. 1.10). A polygenic form of inheritance can be demonstrated in other

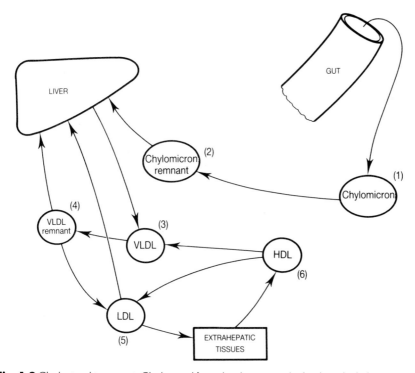

Fig. 1.9 Cholesterol transport. Cholesterol from the diet enters the body with chylomicrons (1). The triglycerides of the chylomicrons are hydrolysed, and residual particles called chylomicron remnants (2) are rapidly removed by the liver. The liver secretes triglyceride-rich lipoproteins called very low density lipoproteins (VLDLs). These are degraded into VLDL remnants (4) which can be converted into low density lipoprotein (LDL) (5) or removed by the liver. The major pathway for removal of LDL is via LDL receptors on liver cells but, to a less extent, LDL can be removed via LDL receptors on extrahepatic tissues. High density lipoprotein (HDL) (6) may accept cholesterol from extrahepatic tissue or other sources and transfer it to LDL or VLDL; the cholesterol carried on these lipoproteins can then be removed by the liver.

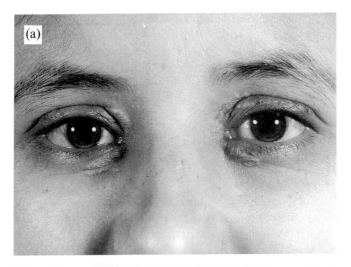

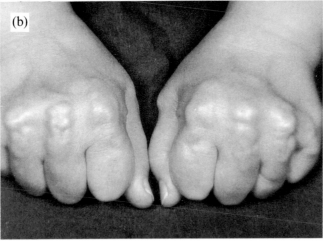

Fig. 1.10 Familial hypercholesterolaemia. (**a**) A 25-year-old female. Lipid deposits can be seen around the eyes (xanthelasma) and she also has an arcus. (**b**) A 35-year-old female. Tendon xanthomata are seen which are attached to and move with the extensor tendons.

patients. LDL receptor activity may be one of the factors that underlie the wide variation of plasma cholesterol within populations and between populations.

Figure 1.11 outlines the metabolism of cholesterol and the site of action of the various categories of drug used to treat an elevated level.

Glucose intolerance

Atheromatous coronary artery disease occurs more frequently in patients with diabetes. It is not clear whether this relationship is an independent one or a

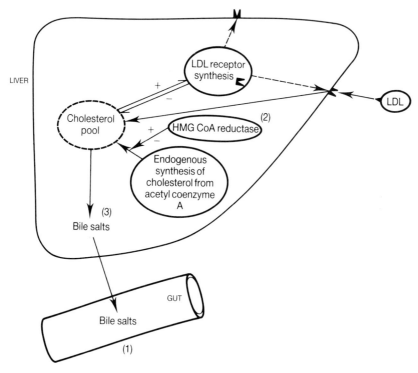

Fig. 1.11 Intracellular cholesterol regulation. The size of the cholesterol pool is stabilized by the regulation of the synthesis of LDL receptors and by the activity of the rate-limiting enzyme in the endogenous synthetic pathway for cholesterol, hydroxymethyl glutaryl coenzyme A (HMG CoA) reductase. These control mechanisms exist in most tissues of the body. In the liver the synthesis and excretion of bile salts are unique to it. These are secreted into the bile and then reabsorbed in the terminal ileum and recirculated. Drugs can act by: (1) preventing the reabsorption of bile salts; (2) inhibiting the HMG CoA reductase which stimulates synthesis of LDL receptors to maintain the intracellular cholesterol pool; (3) increasing the production of cholesterol-containing bile salts.

consequence of the association between abnormal glucose or insulin levels and hyperlipidaemia.

Obesity

The association of obesity with coronary artery disease is almost certainly mediated by association with other risk factors such as hypertension or lipid abnormality. In some communities obesity is not associated with an increased risk.

Blood pressure

Prospective follow-up studies have demonstrated an almost linear relationship between increasing levels of blood pressure and an increasing risk of subsequent development of coronary artery disease. The systolic blood pressure is as good a predictor of risk as the diastolic blood pressure.

Haemostatic factors

The dominance of the lipid hypothesis for atheroma has tended to obscure the role of both platelets and the coagulation system. Fibrinogen is a co-factor in platelet aggregation and the fibrinogen level is one of the main determinants of platelet aggregation. Raised levels of fibrinogen increase blood viscosity and the risk of coronary artery disease. The fibrinogen level is rapidly increased by stressful stimuli and by smoking and reduced by a high intake of fish oils.

High concentrations of factor VII are associated with an increased risk of death from coronary artery disease; high concentrations are found with oral contraceptive usage, after the menopause, with obesity, in patients with diabetes and with increasing age.

Smoking

Several longitudinal studies in many countries have demonstrated that people who smoke have a higher incidence of, and risk of dying from, coronary artery disease than non-smokers.

Alcohol

Heavy drinkers of alcohol have an excess mortality from coronary artery disease. It was thought that non-drinkers had a slightly higher mortality from coronary artery disease than people who consumed a moderate amount of alcohol; it appears attractive and possible that a moderate intake of alcohol is protective against coronary artery disease perhaps by raising the level of plasma HDL cholesterol.

Psychosocial factors

Coronary artery disease is more common in wealthy countries than in poor countries. Paradoxically, it is the poorer groups who are most at risk in the wealthy countries.

A possible explanation is that relatively poor intrauterine nutrition, followed by ample feeding in adult life may predispose to coronary disease. Two approaches have been taken to assess the psychosocial factors. The first is to identify potentially stressful situations that may increase the risk of coronary artery disease; the second is to identify a particular behaviour pattern. This is discussed in more detail in Chapter 13.

Age

Increasing age is associated with an increasing risk of coronary artery disease.

First degree relatives

Relatives of the patient presenting with the premature onset of arterial disease have been shown to have an increased risk of death from coronary artery disease. The genetic factors can be difficult to separate from the effects of the common family environment; however, it is possible to mount and sustain the argument that genetic factors are the more important.

Physical inactivity

Although there is some evidence that men who engage in physical activity have a reduced likelihood of developing coronary artery disease, it is uncertain whether the exercise is beneficial or whether the findings merely reflect the healthier constitution among those who take exercise.

Geographical factors

The mortality from coronary artery disease varies with the seasons. It is consistently higher in the winter months. Throughout the year there is an inverse relationship between the temperature and mortality. This association is independent of other factors. The reason for the association is unclear. There is also a negative association between water hardness and mortality from coronary artery disease. This negative correlation has been demonstrated in many countries but there is no very satisfactory explanation.

Prevention

The prevention of a disease whose aetiology is unknown presents major problems. Prevention is somewhat arbitrarily divided into primary and secondary prevention; primary prevention is concerned with preventing the development of the disease, whilst secondary prevention is concerned with preventing further manifestations of the disease in someone who has already developed the disease. There have been two main approaches to test the feasibility of preventing the development of premature coronary artery disease. Initially, studies were established that were designed to modify only one risk factor. More recently, attempts have been made to modify several risk factors simultaneously.

Single factor intervention

Cholesterol

The results of several studies suggest that the reduction in plasma cholesterol levels by drug treatment reduces coronary events; however, total mortality has not been changed in these studies. The evidence of benefit from reducing the cholesterol level by dietary measures alone is not very persuasive. It is important to emphasize the difference between a healthy level of plasma cholesterol in a community and the 'normal' values. The upper limit of normal is difficult to define. European and American authorities recommend a level of 5.2 mmol/l

(200 mg/dl). It can also be appreciated that to try to shift the cholesterol distribution curve enough to the left will require a huge investment of time, effort and money.

Blood pressure

Numerous trials have shown the beneficial effect of treating moderate and severe hypertension. The benefit has been the reduction in the incidence of strokes, renal failure and heart failure; it has not made any impact on the incidence of coronary artery disease.

Smoking

Although there is demonstrable benefit in giving up smoking, this benefit is slow to appear and may be less than was thought. Smoking increases the individual's risk of coronary artery disease threefold compared with those who do not smoke. After cessation of smoking the risk reduces over three years but may still be demonstrated some 20 years later.

Multiple factor intervention

Several reports suggest that multiple factor intervention does reduce the risk of coronary artery disease. These interventions can be applied to individuals, to groups such as factory workers or to a larger community.

There are two main approaches to multiple factor intervention and it is very important that they are seen to be complementary; there is no merit in trying to determine which is the better. The first is the population approach which aims to educate the public about a healthy way of life. In order to be successful the resources of many professional groups need to be harnessed; these will include not only the health care professionals but also local government departments such as social services, housing and recreation, the education authorities, the mass media and central government departments. The tobacco, food and alcohol industries also need to be involved. The relevant measures to be taken will include advice about a healthy diet, the dangers of smoking and the benefits of a healthy life style.

The complementary approach is to identify high risk individuals. Once identified they will need advice, appropriate treatment and follow-up. General practitioners are best suited to effect this since they will see 75–85 per cent of their patients in any one year. The practice nurse can help in this identification; the routine taking of the blood pressure should now be common practice and can be complemented with details of the family history, smoking habits and other relevant details. A profile of risk can thus be available to the general practitioner.

Angina

Although a great deal has been learned since 1884 when von Leyden first drew attention to the different manifestations of coronary artery disease, we are still a long way from determining the ideal management of individual patients or from preventing the disease. To be able to prevent the disease in the first place is the ideal; in the meantime treatment is developed to help alleviate the patient's symptoms and, if possible, to modify the natural history of the disease process.

Definition of angina

Angina is a symptom and not a disease. Heberden, in his classic description of the symptom in 1772, wrote of a '. . . most disagreeable sensation in the heart. . . '. It is worthy of emphasis that although the term 'pain' is often used to describe the symptom, the term used by Heberden is often more accurate. The Latin word 'angere' means to choke, and the symptom is more completely called angina pectoris, a choking sensation in the chest, to distinguish it from the now rare infective conditions of the throat such as Vincent's angina and Ludwig's angina. Other descriptive words that are used include discomfort, tightness and pressure. Patients' use of language is enormously variable and we have found the body language employed – a clenched fist held on the chest or some other gesture, and the characteristic radiation into the left arm or the neck – to be more helpful in leading to the diagnosis than being over-fussy about semantics.

There have been many descriptions of the symptoms of angina, but there have been few definitions suggested. Most clinicians accept that angina:

1. Is a discomfort located in the chest or adjacent area
2. Is associated with a disturbance of myocardial function
3. Is not associated with myocardial necrosis

Other conditions that give rise to angina, because they too result in myocardial ischaemia, such as valvular heart disease, congenital coronary artery anomalies, cardiomyopathy and coronary artery vasculitis, will not be considered further in this chapter but must be included in the differential diagnosis of the symptom.

Myocardial ischaemia can occur without producing angina but it will still cause a disturbance of myocardial function causing, for example, acute left ventricular failure or arrhythmias and the patient will then present with tiredness, fatigue, shortness of breath or palpitation. Ischaemia influences both biochemical and mechanical events. The most important biochemical effects are depletion of tissue adenosine triphosphate (ATP), the activation of glycolysis and the mobilization of tissue catecholamines. The first mechanical or haemodynamic change during exercise-induced ischaemia is the slowing of isovolumic relaxation and contraction. This is followed by an increase in the end-diastolic pressure due to impaired contraction and increased wall stiffness of the ischaemic ventricular wall segment. The ST segment depression follows these changes. Angina is usually the last event to occur but may be absent. During recovery the sequence occurs in reverse.

There are three suggested mechanisms for the production of myocardial ischaemia: the increase in myocardial need in the presence of coronary artery obstructions, transient dynamic stenoses and alteration in regional myocardial function or metabolism. They may all be relevant in the same patient at different

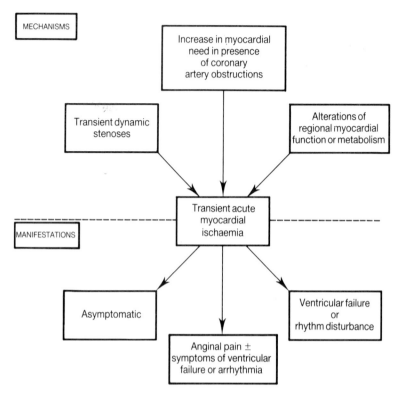

Fig. 1.12 Mechanisms and manifestations of transient acute myocardial ischaemia.

times or at the same time (Fig. 1.12). There is some merit in considering them as separate pathogenic mechanisms of transient acute myocardial ischaemia.

Myocardial oxygen requirements and coronary blood flow

In the normal heart myocardial oxygen requirement and coronary blood flow are finely adjusted. It is clear that the control lies in the heart itself and the adjustments are brought about by alterations in arteriolar calibre. There may also be local release of vasodilator metabolites which are increased when myocardial Po_2 falls; this leads to the production of adenosine, a most potent metabolic vasodilator. There are additional modulatory factors such as hydrogen ions which, by displacing calcium from the contractile apparatus of smooth muscle cells, are able to induce smooth muscle relaxation and long-term vasodilation. Stimulation of α-adrenoceptors and β_2-adrenoceptors in coronary vascular smooth muscle cells plays a subsidiary role in the regulation of the coronary circulation.

Coronary blood flow accounts for about 4 per cent of the cardiac output. Oxygen extraction by the myocardium is almost at a maximum level at rest; this produces a wide and constant arteriovenous oxygen difference between the coronary arteries and the coronary sinus. Any increase in oxygen consumption and demand has to be met by a proportional increase in coronary blood flow. The greater part of this flow is to the left ventricle, of which at least two-thirds occurs during diastole because of the throttling effect that systole has on myocardial perfusion. The main coronary arteries are on the epicardial surface of the heart. Because of this and the hindrance to coronary flow during systole, the subendo-cardial region of the left ventricle is more vulnerable than the outer two-thirds of the muscle wall.

Collateral vessels are formed where coronary artery narrowings produce a pressure gradient between two neighbouring coronary beds. Collateral vessels can appear during spasms of coronary arteries without the presence of obstruc-tive coronary atherosclerosis. These collateral vessels do not necessarily prevent ischaemia of the myocardium but may prevent infarction. Collateral flow stops immediately the antegrade perfusion of the vessel is re-established and re-appears when antegrade flow is reduced. It is not clear whether collaterals have the ability to dilate and contract or are merely inert tubes. Unfortunately, during exercise-induced ischaemia, the collateral blood flow decreases and probably even stops in some patients.

Increase in myocardial need in the presence of coronary artery obstructions

In patients with typical angina of effort due to severe coronary artery disease, the coronary artery is narrowed by 70 per cent or more. This applies particularly in the proximal left anterior descending and left circumflex branches, but in the right coronary artery 50 per cent narrowing can lead to ischaemia. This degree of obstruction is in the same range as that provoking ischaemia in animals. Most of the research concerning the relationship between flow and the degree of obstruction has been performed in animals. In dogs it has been demonstrated that coronary artery flow on exercise starts to decline at a degree of stenosis of approximately 50 per cent and is completely abolished when the stenosis reaches approximately 95 per cent. Coronary flow can be maintained during increased oxygen demand by coronary arteriolar dilation, leading to a compensatory decrease in peripheral coronary resistance. With progressive increase in the degree of stenosis there is initially no change in flow, followed by a linear decrease in flow with a rising degree of obstruction; finally, in high degree obstruction the relationship becomes an exponential one. This explains why at a severe level of obstruction very small changes in diameter can lead to con-siderable changes in flow.

It is not only the degree of stenosis but also its length that influence coronary blood flow. Obstruction in series also adversely influences the coronary reserve. In proximal obstructions with a 75 per cent stenosis, distal obstructions begin to reduce coronary flow when these stenoses reach 60 per cent. This underlines the importance of serial obstructions in major coronary arteries and the necessity to encompass them if revascularization is performed. The extent to which the results of these studies in animals can be applied to the situation in man remains in question.

Transient dynamic stenosis

In 1910 Osler suggested that some of the symptoms of myocardial ischaemia might be caused by increased contractile tone of the coronary arteries. In 1959 Prinzmetal reported a group of patients whose angina occurred at rest and was associated with transient ST segment elevation. This was called 'variant angina' and was thought to be related to a temporary occlusion of a large diseased artery due to an increase in the tone of the vessel. The phenomenon of coronary arterial spasm is now well described angiographically, clinically and experimentally. The pathophysiological basis is still poorly understood. In people with angina the predominant mechanism ranges from classic exercise-related angina pectoris in patients with mainly fixed atheromatous lesions, to unstable angina where both fixed and dynamic stenoses are important, to variant angina where the predominant mechanism is spasm.

Spontaneous rhythmic activity has been recorded in many arterial segments, including human coronary arteries. Enhancement of this activity is seen with a number of substances, which include noradrenaline, acetylcholine, histamine, some prostaglandins, vasopressin, serotonin, ergonovine and potassium. Substances such as nitroglycerine, lignocaine and calcium blocking drugs inhibit this rhythmic motion. It is noteworthy that α- and β-adrenergic blocking drugs and histamine blocking drugs have no effect. This rhythmicity is probably related to transmembrane calcium movement.

Coronary artery spasm can be induced by oesophageal stimuli. The means by which a change in the acidity, temperature or pressure in the oesophagus can produce smooth muscle contraction in the coronary arteries is not known.

The relationship of hyperventilation to coronary artery spasm has introduced a new interest in its basis. Hyperventilation, which was first described and documented 60 years ago, is known to cause ST segment depression and flattening or inversion of the T wave. The clinical presentation is usually described as a manifestation of, and secondary to, an underlying anxiety state. However, hyperventilation is often the primary disorder and the anxiety symptoms are the result of the severe and often alarming symptoms that result from it. With frequent repetition the response takes on some of the characteristics of a conditioned reflex. The physiological disturbance of chronic anxiety and hyperventilation are inextricably mixed and it can be difficult to separate the cause from the effect. Therapeutically it is very important to treat the cause rather than the effect.

Alteration of regional myocardial function or metabolism

The large epicardial coronary arteries as well as the intramural vessels are affected by local myocardial metabolites. These metabolic 'mediators' help match coronary flow to myocardial consumption. The partial pressures of oxygen and carbon dioxide and the concentration of hydrogen ion, lactic acid, potassium, adenine nucleotide and adenosine have all been shown to affect epicardial vessels in dogs. This epicardial vessel dilation in response to a stimulus, such as increased myocardial oxygen consumption, occurs prior to any change in proximal perfusion pressure.

It is possible that the typical circadian variations in ischaemic pain patterns are effected by the myocardial metabolites. Differing metabolic rates during the 24 hours will result in different hydrogen ion concentrations. This may influence the degree of calcium ion blockade caused by the hydrogen ion and thus influence the vasomotor tone in the susceptible individual. Hyperventilation and a buffer infusion may produce coronary artery spasm through a similar mechanism.

The transient narrowing of epicardial coronary arteries with the resultant decrement in coronary flow can cause myocardial ischaemia. There is no single trigger to the spasm. There appears to be a circadian variation to the responsiveness: at night and in the early morning the tone of the coronary artery is high and the vessel diameter smaller than later in the day. Under conditions of high tone, even a slight degree of sympathetic discharge may provoke coronary artery spasm. This is a possible mechanism to explain the association of rapid eye movement sleep with variant angina. It may also partially explain the diurnal variation in the frequency of angina which is often independent of the amount of exertion undertaken.

Medical management of the patient with stable angina

Medical management of the patient presenting with angina must take account of the fact that the condition is a dynamic process. An example of a life history of a patient with angina is shown in Fig. 1.13. It illustrates a possible natural history with some interventions and treatments.

Mechanisms and precipitating factors

It is important to identify the mechanisms causing the angina in order to ensure optimal medical treatment. Therapy must be given appropriate to the mechanism and also to the timing of the symptoms. Aggravating or precipitating factors such as hypertension, anaemia, heart failure or arrhythmias should be treated. Other possible causes of angina such as aortic valve disease, cardiomyopathy or a vasculitis will need to be considered and treated appropriately.

Patient understanding

The variable nature of the symptoms of coronary artery disease make it essential for the clinician to give the patient an understanding of the condition. Information booklets in addition to the careful explanation by the clinician are of considerable help. Quite apart from the issue of the right of patients to have some information about the disease causing their symptoms, there are a number of advantages to giving the patient an understanding of the problem. It is possible, although unproven, that an understanding of the underlying disease and the factors that produce symptoms may modify the cardiovascular reactivity in an individual patient and modify the prognosis.

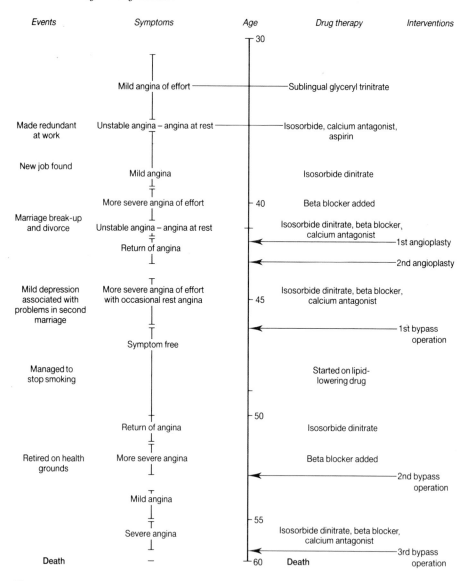

Fig. 1.13 Example of a life history of a patient with angina.

Patients presenting with stable angina should be encouraged to achieve and maintain a normal body weight. They should also be encouraged to be as active as they can within the constraints of the angina. The concept of the angina being 'a built-in warning device' rather than something to be feared is one to be encouraged. They will be able to continue driving a private car but must be advised to stop driving a heavy goods vehicle or public service vehicle. They will not be able to continue being a pilot of a plane.

The patient will need to be given the confidence to be able to approach the clinician whenever the angina becomes more frequent or more severe. Furthermore, the physical barriers that exist between the patient and doctor will need to be circumvented; these include the delays inherent in any appointments system. The consultation with a different doctor at each visit is detrimental to the establishment of the doctor–patient relationship and to the confidence that is so vital in the management of a patient with angina.

The topic of sexual activity will need to be raised by the clinician as patients may be too shy to raise the matter themselves. This subject is considered in more detail later in this chapter under 'Myocardial infarction'.

Drug treatment of stable angina

It is clear from the discussion on the pathophysiological basis of angina that, to produce symptomatic improvement, a drug must increase the blood supply to the myocardium, improve the metabolic state of the myocardial cells and/or reduce oxygen demand.

Nitrates

The nitrates have been the mainstay of treatment of angina pectoris for many decades. Amyl nitrite was first used in 1867 to 'lessen the arterial tension' in a patient with nocturnal angina. In 1933 Sir Thomas Lewis suggested that its effect was mainly due to its dilatation of the coronary arteries. This conflict has been resolved since we now know that both coronary and peripheral effects are important.

Chemistry and mode of action
The nitrates used in the treatment of angina are simple nitric acid esters of polyalcohols. The basic pharmacological effect of the nitrates is the widespread and non-specific relaxation of smooth muscle. The effect of the venodilatation is to reduce the filling pressure of the heart; the effect of the arteriolar dilatation is to reduce the afterload of the heart. There is thus a decrease in ventricular volume and systolic pressure. This decreases ventricular wall tension which is a major determinant of myocardial oxygen requirements. Nitrates produce a reflex increase in heart rate which tends to increase myocardial oxygen demand but this is overshadowed by the reduction in ventricular wall tension.

Coronary dilatation also occurs in certain clinical situations. In contrast to agents such as serotonin, the nitrates do not need an intact endothelium to produce vasodilatation. In angina with fixed coronary artery stenoses, nitrates probably do not increase total coronary blood flow although they cause some coronary artery dilatation. There is improved regional blood flow to ischaemic areas, which may be important in some patients; this is effected through the collateral and subendocardial vessels. However, in patients with coronary artery spasm coronary artery dilatation accounts for most of the therapeutic benefit.

Pharmacokinetics
The use of organic nitrates is influenced by the presence of a hepatic organic nitrate reductase which inactivates the drug when given orally. The bio-availability of most orally administered organic nitrates is very low. If therapeutic levels of the drug are required rapidly, the sublingual or intravenous route is preferred. Both glyceryl trinitrate and isosorbide dinitrate are absorbed efficiently by the sublingual route and achieve therapeutic plasma levels within a few minutes. If sufficient doses of oral, buccal and possibly dermal nitrate preparations are used, adequate plasma concentrations can be achieved despite the extensive first-pass hepatic metabolism.

There is also a mononitrate form. This has the theoretical advantage that it does not require first-pass metabolism and so blood levels are more predictable and prolonged. Whether this renders it more effective in the relief of symptoms of patients with angina is yet to be determined.

Adverse effects
The major adverse effects of the organic nitrates relate to their vasodilatory properties. Orthostatic hypotension, tachycardia and throbbing headaches are frequent adverse effects, often made worse when combined with other vaso-dilators such as alcohol. The nitrates should not be used in the presence of raised intracranial pressure. There is no evidence of physical dependence on therapeutic doses of organic nitrates.

Tolerance to nitrates can be demonstrated by the attenuation of its effect on the systemic blood pressure. There is a continued effect on exercise tolerance and angina frequency when nitrates are given on a twice or thrice daily basis but not when the slow-release or the transdermal preparations are used. The rate of change of nitrate levels appears to be more important than the absolute level. An appropriate drug-free interval in the evening and night ensures the continued effect of the drug the following day.

Choices of nitrate
The various preparations are displayed in Table 1.1.

Sublingual glyceryl trinitrate has been used with good effect for many decades and typically produces relief within 1–3 minutes. The tablet needs to be crushed between the teeth and actively sucked to obtain a rapid effect. Protection lasts for only 10–20 minutes but does enable the tablet to be used in anticipation of exertion. It is not well tolerated by some patients because of the headaches it can cause; taking a fragment rather than the whole tablet can sometimes solve this problem. The use of glyceryl trinitrate needs to be carefully explained to the patient; it is often not taken because the patient believes that it may be addictive.

Glyceryl trinitrate tablets have the disadvantage of slowly losing their potency

Table 1.1   The various nitrate preparations available for the treatment of angina

Compound	Route	Duration of action
Glyceryl trinitrate (trinitrin, GTN)	Sublingual	1.5 min to 1 h
	Spray	1.5 min to 1 h
	Transdermal patches	Up to 24 h
	Oral, sustained-release	Up to 8–10 h
	Intravenous	During infusion and 30 min after
Isosorbide dinitrate	Sublingual	5 min to 1 h
	Oral	Up to 6–8 h
	Chewable	Up to 2 h
	Slow release	Up to 6 h
	Intravenous	During infusion and 30 min after
Isosorbide mononitrate	Oral	Up to 6–10 h
	Slow release	Up to 24 h

while on the shelf. The aerosol spray has the advantage of having a shelf life of 3 years and appears to be very effective, albeit more expensive.

Long and short acting nitrates can be combined. Patients already receiving isosorbide mono- or dinitrate can benefit from the addition of sublingual glyceryl trinitrate.

β-Adrenoceptor blocking drugs

It is now over 20 years since propranolol was first introduced into clinical practice in the UK. Since then many other β-adrenoceptor blocking drugs have been developed. They dramatically changed the management of angina. Their introduction into the UK some years before the USA was probably a major factor in causing the discrepancy in the bypass operation rates in the two countries.

Mode of action
The β-receptors are divided into the β_1-receptors found in heart muscle and the β_2-receptors found in the bronchial and vascular smooth muscle. It is now known that there are β_2-receptors in the myocardium. Situated on the cell membrane, the β-receptor is probably part of the adenylate cyclase system which, when stimulated, produces cyclic AMP from ATP. Cyclic AMP is the intracellular messenger for beta stimulation. β-Adrenoceptor blocking drugs compete for the receptor sites. They therefore slow the heart rate, particularly the heart rate on exertion, reduce myocardial contractility and lower the systemic blood pressure. The net effect is to reduce myocardial oxygen consumption. Occasionally the decreased myocardial contractility can lead to enlargement of the heart and increased oxygen consumption.

Pharmacokinetics
Most drugs are well absorbed after oral administration, with peak concentrations about 1–3 hours after ingestion. Sustained-released preparations are available.

Oral bioavailability is variable, mainly due to variations in first-pass metabolism. The drugs are rapidly distributed. The clinical effects of these drugs are often prolonged well beyond the time predicted from the half-life data.

Adverse effects
A variety of adverse effects occur. Central nervous effects include sedation, sleep disturbance and depression. The major adverse effects are predictable and relate to the worsening of obstructive airways disease or asthma. Severe cardiac failure can be provoked in susceptible individuals. However, in the ischaemic heart the introduction of a β-adrenoceptor blocker can improve heart function. Raynaud's phenomenon or claudication are sometimes, but not always, made worse. Care has to be exercised in the use of the drug in diabetic patients using insulin, as the symptom of hypoglycaemia can be masked.

Choice of drug
There is a variety of β-adrenoceptor blocking compounds available which are equally effective in the treatment of angina pectoris provided the doses of the drug are equipotent. It is doubtful whether intrinsic sympathomimetic activity (ISA) or cardioselectivity confers any real advantage.

Although β-adrenergic blockade is a competitive phenomenon, physicians use the term 'fully beta-blocked' to determine the point at which there is no additional symptomatic gain in increasing the dosage. This point is probably reached when the heart rate after mild exertion does not increase by more than 10 beats per minute. A resting heart rate of 50–60 beats per minute is, on its own, a poor guide because the resting heart rate is determined by vagal activity and varies widely between individuals. The resting heart rate cannot be used alone as a measure of β-blockade with drugs that have intrinsic sympathomimetic activity.

Calcium antagonists

This group of drugs has many important effects on the cardiovascular system. They have been available in Britain for over 20 years. There are many new drugs now being developed. 'Calcium entry blockers' is a more correct term than 'calcium antagonists' as these substances block calcium influx in the slow calcium channel without interacting specifically with calcium. This effect interferes with the action of calcium-dependent ATPase which is required for the energy needs of myocardial contractility and smooth muscle contraction. As a result there is a reduction in myocardial contractility and dilation of vascular smooth muscle. The vasodilating properties are not confined to systemic arteries but also affect the coronary arteries. Other effects of these drugs may also be important: verapamil has been shown to inhibit the formation of platelet clusters; nifedipine has been shown to increase red cell deformability.

Pharmacokinetics
Oral absorption is rapid and complete. Because of extensive first-pass hepatic metabolism, bioavailability is relatively low. Although these drugs have a

common mode of action, they differ significantly with respect to their relative effect on myocardial contractility, systemic vascular resistance, coronary vasodilatation and antiarrhythmic activity (Table 1.2).

Table 1.2 Different properties of various calcium antagonists

Compound	Negative inotropic activity	Delayed AV conduction	Smooth muscle relaxation
Nifedipine	++	–	+++
Verapamil	+++	++	++
Diltiazem	+	++	++
Nicardipine	–	–	++

Adverse effects

Drugs in this group can produce peripheral oedema and a feeling of heaviness in the legs, particularly in hot weather.

Combination therapy

The benefits of each of the three classes of drugs have been clearly demonstrated in numerous studies. Whether one category of drug is superior to another in a different class is far from clear. Methodological problems have made it difficult to compare drugs under identical circumstances.

β-Adrenoceptor blockers are often combined with nitrates. There is some advantage of the combination, as the β-adrenoceptor blocker will tend to cancel the reflex tachycardia of the nitrates. The net effect will be to reduce cardiac work whilst increasing coronary blood flow. The combination of a β-adrenoceptor blocking drug with a calcium antagonist has also been shown to produce an improvement in symptoms or exercise tolerance. This combination is quite safe so long as they are both given orally; extreme bradycardia and death have been reported in patients given the drugs intravenously soon after one another. It is unwise to give an intravenous calcium blocking drug to anyone receiving β-adrenoceptor blockers orally. Calcium antagonists can be combined with nitrates.

The combination of nitrates, a β-adrenoceptor blocker and a calcium antagonist is now widely used. The addition of a third drug in many patients can be extremely helpful; in a few patients the exercise tolerance is actually made worse.

Other drugs

Apart from the specific antianginal drugs considered above, there are numerous other drugs that can help in the management of the patient with angina. The patient who presents with angina as a result of stress can be helped by tranquillizers or sedatives. However, sympathetic listening to the problems as perceived by the patient and appropriate counselling can sometimes be far more effective than any drug therapy. Indeed, if the emotional aspects are not adequately handled, a lot of the potential benefit of drug therapy is lost.

Antianginal drugs will provide symptomatic relief for most patients. There is no convincing evidence yet that they have any beneficial effect on the underlying disease process in humans.

Should the symptoms of angina persist despite good medical therapy, an exercise electrocardiogram test can be very helpful in assessing the adequacy of treatment. The relative importance of the symptoms, the ST segment shifts and the blood pressure response during exercise are dealt with below. If the patient is able to perform more exercise than anticipated, it may suggest either that coronary artery spasm is playing a more important part than was hitherto realized, or that a false impression of the exercise tolerance has been gained. It will allow a reassessment of the therapy.

If the symptoms remain unacceptable to the patient, consideration should be given to coronary arteriography with a view to assessment for angioplasty or coronary bypass surgery.

Resting electrocardiogram

The resting electrocardiogram is normal in 50–70 per cent of patients with stable angina. There may be abnormalities in the QRS complexes, ST segments and T waves if there has been myocardial damage.

Exercise testing

The test can be used for a number of different reasons: it can help detect the presence of the disease; it can help determine the severity and extent of the disease; and it can also help determine the likelihood of future coronary events and death.

The diagnosis of angina due to coronary artery disease in a given patient is a probability judgement that is based on the clinician's interpretation of the symptoms and signs. Probability estimates of coronary artery disease based on simple clinical criteria exert a marked effect on the diagnostic yield of non-invasive investigations. All these investigations are less than perfect. Some patients with coronary artery disease will have negative tests and, conversely, some with normal coronary arteries will have positive tests. The test result is no more than a statement of probability. This probability will be determined by three main elements:

1. The sensitivity of the test: the ability to detect the disease when it is present
2. The specificity of the test: the ability to detect coronary artery disease and no other
3. The incidence of the disease in the population under study

In any given population there is a trade-off between increasing the specificity by using more extreme criteria and thereby decreasing the sensitivity, or vice versa. In a hospital population the incidence of the disease is high enough to allow confident statements about the probability of the disease in the patient being tested. However, it is more difficult to be so confident when it is used as a screening investigation in a population with a low incidence of the disease. Bayes' theorem states that the predictive value of an investigation is variable and depends on the probability of the disease in the population under study. Thus a test that is positive for myocardial ischaemia has the greatest predictive value when the pretest likelihood, or probability, of coronary artery disease is high. In contrast, a negative test result has the greatest predictive value when the pretest probability is low (Fig. 1.14). This theorem has important implications for the non-invasive diagnosis of coronary artery disease. A positive result in a patient with a classic history, who smokes and has a family history of premature vascular disease is strongly predictive. However, it contributes little new diagnostic information although it may give some estimate about the extent of the disease.

Submaximal exercise tests can be used in which the test is terminated if the patient reaches a predetermined heart rate. The predictive value of a stress test is increased when maximal tests are used. These are terminated by symptoms, very marked ST segment depression, ventricular arrhythmias or a fall in blood pressure. The risk of maximal tests is greater than submaximal but still very low; mortality is about 1 in 20000 and infarction occurs in 1 in 3000 tests. The test should always be performed with full resuscitation equipment readily available and a doctor nearby.

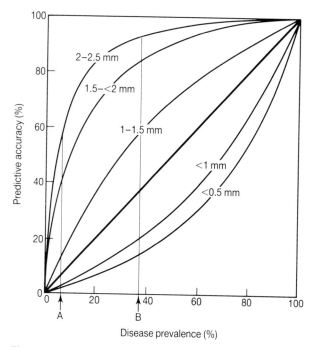

Fig. 1.14 Relationship between predictive accuracy and disease prevalence according to the amount of ST segment depression. It can be appreciated that at A, where the disease has a low prevalence, even using 2–2.5 mm ST segment depression, predictive accuracy is less than 60 per cent. At B, with a disease prevalence of 38 per cent, there is a 90 per cent predictive accuracy using 2–2.5 mm ST segment depression or a 60 per cent accuracy using 1–1.5 mm.

Prediction of the presence of coronary artery disease

ST segment depression of 1 mm or more is one of the criteria of an abnormal test. If more stringent criteria are used, the specificity rises at the expense of the sensitivity. Severe disease, and therefore a less good prognosis, is suggested by a low exercise tolerance, a fall or a failure of the blood pressure to rise with exertion, marked and persistent and widespread ST segment depression and an end-point of angina. The most valuable function of the maximal stress test is to identify patients who have severe disease and a poor prognosis. The prognosis of patients with coronary artery disease is largely determined by the symptoms, the severity of the underlying disease and the severity of left ventricular dysfunction. Exercise testing is a non-invasive means of making an assessment of these variables (Fig. 1.15).

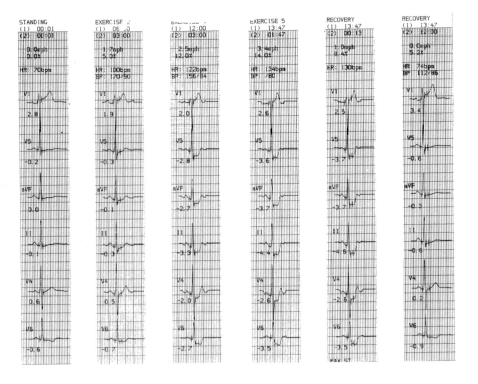

Fig. 1.15 Selected ECG leads are shown of a patient undergoing an exercise stress test on a treadmill. The patient had to stop at stage 4 of the protocol because of chest pain and also because the blood pressure failed to rise. The recording shows marked ST segment depression occurring with exertion in leads II, aVF, V4 and V6. The number under each lead is the ST segment depression measured 80 ms after the J point. The numbers under each stage of the test indicate (1) the duration of exercise and (2) the duration of each phase of the protocol.

Nuclear cardiology

The techniques of nuclear imaging can be subdivided into three main categories. The first involves assessment of cardiac performance; these require radioactive tracers that remain in the cardiovascular space during the period of study. The second involves assessment of myocardial perfusion, viability and metabolism; these require radioactive tracers that pass through the capillary network and are accumulated intracellularly. The third involves the use of radiolabelled bio-logically active materials such as red cells, antibodies and metabolites; the use of these positron-labelled substances has provided the means of studying regional myocardial metabolism in a non-invasive way.

Cardiac performance
Cardiac performance can be assessed in one of two ways, one of which is the first-pass technique in which the radiolabelled isotope is rapidly injected intra-venously and its passage through the heart recorded. Alternatively, the equilibrium-gated blood pool technique can be used. In this technique the ECG is used as the reference point to enable the gating of the data into 16, 32 or 64 frames or pixels per cycle. The data are collected over multiple heart beats until there is sufficient to allow analysis. Direct assessment can be made of transit times, ventricular ejection fractions, ventricular volumes and regional wall motion. The changes in spatial information during the cardiac cycle can be used to generate colour-encoded images representing the amplitude and phase of regional wall motion; this is called parametric imaging and can demonstrate any discoordinate or dyskinetic zones. Multiple studies can be performed over several hours (Fig. 1.16).

Myocardial perfusion
Myocardial imaging with ionic tracers provides information concerning relative regional myocardial perfusion, regional viability and qualitative anatomical information about left ventricular cavity size and wall thickness. Thallium is usually used as the radionuclide tracer. Comparison of images obtained imme-diately after exercise with those taken some 2–4 hours later allows assessment of the reversible relative hypoperfusion that characterizes transient ischaemia (Fig. 1.17).

Positron emission tomography
The ultimate clinical application of positron tomography remains to be defined. The information that could possibly be obtained includes the definition of altered myocardial metabolism in a variety of conditions. It may then be possible to relate this metabolic information with the structure and function knowledge that is currently available.

In most patients with angina a good history, physical examination and, if appropriate, a left heart catheter will give the clinician enough information to enable appropriate decisions to be made about the management; whether radionuclide tests give extra information that is relevant to the decision-making process is open to doubt.

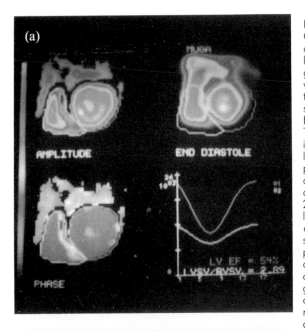

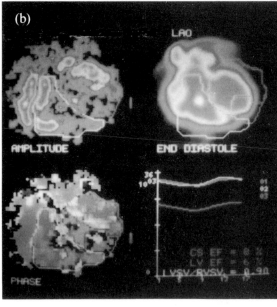

Fig. 1.16 MUGA (MUltiple Gated Acquisition) scans of (**a**) a patient with good left ventricular function who has aortic regurgitation and (**b**) a patient with poor left ventricular function. The principle of the MUGA scan is to use the R wave of the ECG as the triggering signal. The radionuclide data from the injected radioisotope are collected and segregated temporally into 16–28 equal divisions, or pixels, depending on the heart rate. Studies require 2–10 minutes for completion. A left and right ventricular time–activity curve is based on analysis of the left anterior oblique position. By constructing volume curves throughout the cardiac cycle from each pixel of the gated blood pool scan, [colour-coded] images of amplitude of regional wall motion and phase of wall motion can be generated. In the normal patient (**a**), the normal phase image shows that both ventricles contract uniformly and in synchrony; the atria are 180 degrees out of phase. The amplitude image shows vigorous contraction of the left ventricle. The markedly different stroke volumes of the ventricle are caused by the aortic regurgitation. The scan in (**b**) shows general very poor ventricular function. The amplitude image shows poor amplitude of left ventricular wall motion. The phase image is extremely fragmented, demonstrating discoordinate ventricular contraction. The ejection fraction of each ventricle is of the order of 6–8 per cent. If an operation were being contemplated, the chances of getting the patient off the operating table alive would be very slim.

24-Hour ambulatory monitoring

A large amount of objective information can be collected by ambulatory monitoring during a patient's unrestricted activities (Fig. 1.18). The investigation was introduced in the 1960s and was initially used to study arrhythmias. Technical improvements in the recording apparatus has enabled accurate reproduction of

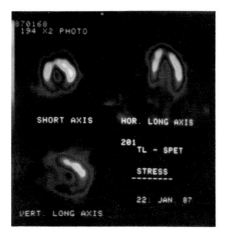 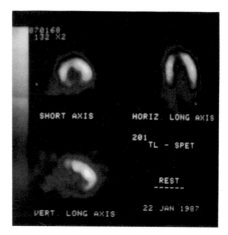

Fig. 1.17 Thallium myocardial images of a patient with angina of effort, taken (**a**) immediately after exercise and (**b**) at rest 3 hours later. Three projections are shown in each: the vertical long axis, the horizontal long axis and the short axis. After exercise the anteroseptal aspect of the left ventricle is poorly perfused; this is seen best on the long axis views. It reperfuses slightly at rest. These changes are seen more clearly with colour representation.

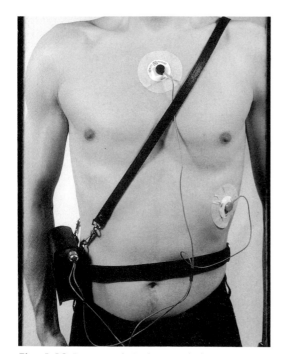

Fig. 1.18 Patient with 24-hour ambulatory monitoring apparatus; only one lead is being recorded. There is a facility for the patient to insert an electrical signal onto the recording tape; this enables subsequent correlation to be made of the rhythm at the time of symptoms. The recorded information is played back at 60 times real speed. The analysis is performed with the help of a computer.

the ST segment. Patients with coronary artery disease may have transient ST segment depression throughout the 24 hours. These changes are similar to the ST segment changes seen with exercise testing. They can be demonstrated with exertion, at rest and at night, and are often not accompanied by any pain. The ST segment change in a patient with angina is associated with myocardial ischaemia. ST segment elevation and depression also occurs in about 30 per cent of normal

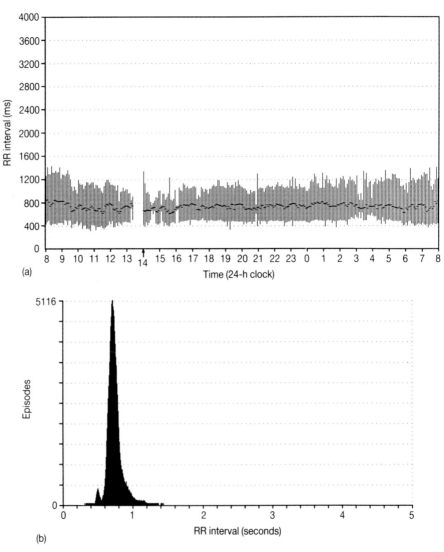

Fig. 1.19 Data from 24-hour ambulatory monitoring can be displayed in a variety of ways. (**a**) The RR interval is plotted at 20-minute intervals over the 24 hours; the mean and range of the RR interval are shown for each interval. (**b**) The RR interval is plotted in the form of a histogram. (**c**) The rhythm in real time; the patient has numerous ventricular premature beats and a run of ventricular tachycardia. (**d**) The ST segment changes over the 24 hours.

subjects, and with change in posture, with hyperventilation, with gastroscopy, with neurocirculatory asthenia and during a sauna. Care must therefore be exercised when interpreting these changes (Fig. 1.19).

Echocardiography

The two-dimensional echocardiogram can, by detecting abnormalities in left ventricular wall motion, be used for detecting coronary artery disease. This technique is considered in more detail in Chapter 6.

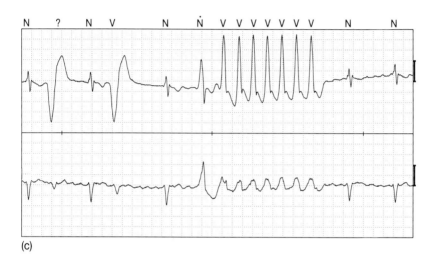

(c)

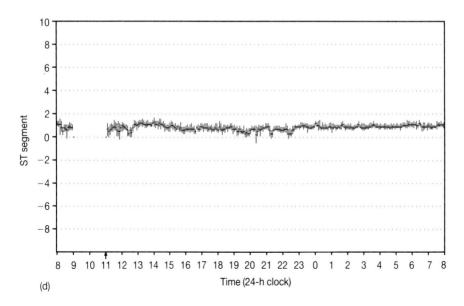

(d)

Cardiac catheterization

Selective coronary arteriography was first developed in the late 1950s. The procedure of left heart catheterization, left ventricular angiography and coronary angiography is mildly unpleasant for the patient, as it is performed under local anaesthetic. It is a procedure that usually takes no more than 30 minutes to perform. The mortality from the investigation is about 0.5 per cent. Most deaths occur in patients with severe multivessel disease or with impaired left ventricular function. Peripheral arterial injury, thromboembolic complications and myocardial infarction occur very rarely. Minor allergic reactions to contrast material occur occasionally but anaphylactic reactions are exceedingly rare. The investigation gives accurate information about the resting ventricular function and about the site and degree of narrowing of the coronary arteries (Fig. 1.20).

A number of provocative tests have been used with coronary arteriography in order to assess the importance of alterations in vasomotor tone in the pathogenesis of symptoms in patients with cardiac pain. These provocations include sustained handgrip, hyperventilation and exposure to cold or the use of a drug such as ergometrine. The complication rate is higher with provocative tests than with routine investigations, and they are therefore not routinely performed.

Medical management of the patient with unstable angina

Unstable angina is a term that was adopted to try to describe conditions which are neither stable angina pectoris nor myocardial infarction. Other terms include preinfarction angina, acute coronary insufficiency, intermediate coronary syndrome, crescendo angina and threatening infarction.

Natural history

The syndrome of unstable angina is a transient phenomenon which, if successfully managed in the acute phase, allows the majority of patients to return to their previous stable angina or become asymptomatic. The pathophysiology of unstable angina is complex and has been covered at the beginning of the chapter.

Management of unstable angina

Unstable angina is a serious condition which requires immediate attention. Identification of any provocative factor is important. A vigorous effort must be undertaken to diagnose medical conditions that cause a transient increase in myocardial oxygen demands; these include tachyarrhythmias, thyrotoxicosis, exacerbation of pre-existing heart failure and anaemia. Treatment of these problems will abolish or diminish episodes of rest pain in some patients.

Evidence of stress, related to 'life events', should be specifically sought. The recognition and discussion of this with the patient may be sufficient to alleviate the discomfort. In some circumstances mild sedation or removal from the emotionally taxing situation may be required.

A number of drugs have been used in the treatment of the patient with

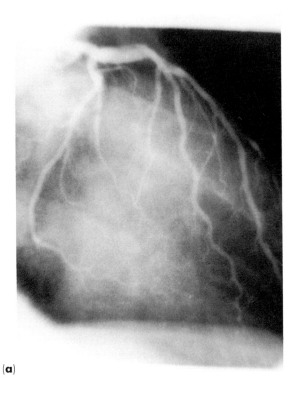

(a)

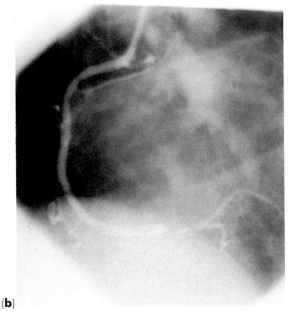

(b)

Fig. 1.20 Views of the coronary arteriogram (**a**) of the left coronary artery in the right anterior oblique projection and (**b**) of the right coronary artery in the left anterior oblique projection. The left coronary artery is normal; the right coronary artery has a tight stenosis just before the origins of the posterior descending and posterior left ventricular branches.

unstable angina. The use of nitrates, β-adrenergic blocking drugs and calcium antagonists have been discussed earlier in the chapter. Aspirin decreases the incidence of death and acute myocardial infarction in patients with unstable angina. Problems may occur with bleeding if surgery is performed; the drug will need to be stopped some days before a bypass operation.

There is some good evidence of benefit with intravenous heparin. Fibrinolytic drug therapy is not of any value in unstable angina.

Other forms of treatment

Intra-aortic balloon counter-pulsation
Patients in whom medical management has failed may be helped by intra-aortic balloon counter-pulsation. It often results in the prompt relief of chest pain. This technique is useful only because it allows the safe performance of coronary arteriography.

Percutaneous transluminal coronary angioplasty
Good results have been reported in some patients with unstable angina who have one-vessel disease with discrete proximal lesions.

Coronary artery bypass grafting
This form of treatment has been shown to eliminate or markedly decrease anginal pain in patients with unstable angina. There is no clear evidence that surgery decreases mortality or the incidence of acute myocardial infarction in patients presenting with unstable angina. The criteria for early surgery are still not clear; surgery undoubtedly has a place for patients who fail to respond to adequate medical treatment or, having initially responded, deteriorate in the succeeding weeks or months.

Laser angioplasty
This therapeutic technique is still at a very early stage of development. Its place in the management of patients has yet to be determined.

The vast majority of patients will settle with the appropriate medical treatment. They can be subsequently assessed after some weeks or months in a manner similar to that of patients with stable angina.

Differential diagnosis

Oesophageal pain can be confused with the pain or discomfort of myocardial ischaemia. Heartburn, caused by incompetence of the lower oesophageal sphincter, produces symptoms in a position similar to that of angina. Diffuse oesophageal spasm may also present with pain in this position and it may also be relieved by glyceryl trinitrate. It may also be helped by calcium antagonists. Furthermore, ergometrine provocation can produce oesophageal pain. In patients who have recently gained weight, chest pain of oesophageal origin can be provoked by exertion.

Oesophageal pain and myocardial ischaemia are both common symptoms and may occur in the same patient. The coexistence of the two conditions causing the symptoms appears too frequently to be due to chance. The interrelationships between the two has recently attracted interest. Both conditions need to be recognized and treated if full symptomatic relief is to be obtained.

The threshold of exertional angina is modified by oesophageal stimulation with acid. Angina occurs on walking a shorter distance after acid is instilled into the oesophagus than when normal saline is instilled. This effect is more marked in those patients who experience oesophageal symptoms on a regular basis. The mechanism by which the angina threshold is reduced is not known; it is possible that a viscerocardiac reflex might cause a reduction in the calibre of the coronary arteries.

Surgical management of the patient with angina

In the 1930s and 1940s a number of procedures were used to try to restore the blood supply to an ischaemic left ventricular muscle. Attempts to establish a collateral flow to the heart through pericardial adhesions failed because the adhesions, created by the application of asbestos powder or talc, were avascular. In 1950 Vineberg mobilized the internal mammary artery from the chest wall and swung it across to bury it in a tunnel of left ventricular muscle. The technique depended upon anastomoses developing between the artery and the micro-circulation of the heart. It was unpredictable in its effect. This technique was developed before the first cardiopulmonary bypass and a decade before angiographic visualization of the coronary arteries.

During the 1960s coronary angiography and then saphenous vein bypass grafting were pioneered at the Cleveland Clinic in the USA. In this operation the long saphenous vein is dissected from the leg. With the patient on cardio-pulmonary bypass and the heart kept still either by elective ventricular fibrillation or potassium cardioplegic arrest, the vein is meticulously anastomosed to the coronary artery beyond the obstructing atheroma; the other end is anastomosed to the ascending aorta. Various combinations of end-to-side and side-to-side anastomoses are made so that as many as possible of the obstructing lesions are bypassed. The internal mammary artery is a highly successful alternative to the vein, with significantly better patency rates at and beyond 10 years.

As operative techniques improved and the mortality fell to quite low levels, indications for surgery were modified and extended. The number of operations performed steadily increased until, in the mid-1980s, it reached 750 per million population in the USA and over 400 per million in Australia; in the UK it was only 100 per million. This marked discrepancy in the rates between countries is starting to decrease as the rate in the USA has begun to decline and the rate in the UK is still increasing. There are still very different rates in different parts of the country within the UK.

Surgery for symptoms

There is little doubt about the efficacy of a successful operation in controlling the symptom of angina. The grafts deliver blood to the myocardium beyond the demonstrable and obvious obstructions. The benefit becomes obvious to the patient within days of the operation and the majority can return to levels of physical activity that have been denied them perhaps for years. The relief of angina is related to the number, the quality and, as time passes, to the continuing patency of grafts. Unfortunately there is a slow but progressive increase in the proportion of patients who get a return of symptoms of angina. With the improvement in surgical techniques this trend has improved but about 40 per cent of patients will have a return of some angina at 5 years. Although reoperation is possible, the mortality risk is higher and the symptomatic benefit not so good as with the first operation. Nevertheless, some years of angina-free life may be extremely important to the patient.

Surgery for improvement in survival

As well as causing angina, coronary atheroma is a common cause of death. If bypass grafts prevent angina by the restoration of blood supply to the ischaemic myocardium, it would seem likely that there might be an improval in survival. This has been remarkably difficult to demonstrate conclusively.

Who should be operated upon?

Two potential areas of benefit must be considered: the relief of angina and the possibility of prolonging life. In reaching a conclusion about the best way to manage an individual patient, the likelihood of achieving either or both these objectives and the likely duration of improvement must be weighed against the disadvantage of surgery.

The risk of death with surgery is low, and is less than 3 per cent in good units. In advising the individual, the next question is, does he resemble the patients who do well or does he have a more-than-average risk of perioperative death? A number of factors increase the risk of death:

1. Age is an incremental risk factor: in the 20 000 patients operated on at the Texas Heart Institute the risk for the age group 30–39 was 1.6 per cent, for the group 50–59 it was 2.5 per cent and for the group 60–69 it was 4.1 per cent. The quality and duration of benefit also are adversely influenced by age.
2. Gender is an important factor: women have twice the risk of men.
3. Left ventricular function is an important factor. With the improvement in operative techniques, so it has been possible to operate successfully on patients with impaired left ventricular function. Furthermore, this group of patients do badly with medical treatment; surgery has a good margin of benefit and so, in spite of the operative risk, poor left ventricular function is an argument in favour of operative management.
4. Emergency surgery carries an increased risk.

The risk of death without surgery is largely influenced by three factors: the severity of the symptoms of angina; the site, distribution and severity of the atheromatous narrowings; and the left ventricular function. There is good evidence to suggest that patients with significant narrowing of their left main-stem coronary artery, with three-vessel disease and impaired left ventricular function and perhaps those with a proximal lesion in their anterior descending, have a higher risk of dying without surgery than with.

The morbidity associated with cardiac surgery is low. A small minority of patients suffer clinically detectable, focal, central nervous system damage during surgery. Some recover completely. Cardiopulmonary bypass itself is associated with diffuse cerebral malfunction characterized by non-specific neurological signs and impaired performance on neuropsychological testing. This usually recovers fully.

Percutaneous transluminal coronary angioplasty

This technique was first performed in man in 1977. It involves guiding a deflated balloon, which has been introduced percutaneously into the femoral or brachial artery, across the narrowing in the coronary artery. The balloon is then inflated for short intervals to a pressure of 5–10 atmospheres. This results in a reduction of the stenosis and an improvement in the symptoms. The risks are now low and the restenosis rate is improving.

This technique is attractive in a number of respects: for the patient it should mean a short hospital stay, no surgery and a quick return to normal activities; for the clinician it means that an increased number of patients can be successfully treated; and for the economist it should produce an attractive cost–benefit analysis compared with other remedies. However, it is too early to determine its exact place in the management of patients with coronary artery disease. Randomized trials are now being established to compare the results of this technique with surgery and with medical treatment.

Laser angioplasty and coronary atherectomy are still at the stage of research and their place in clinical practice is yet to be determined.

Myocardial infarction

Of the people who experience a heart attack, approximately half die within 20 days of the onset. Half of these deaths occur within 2 hours of the onset of symptoms (Fig. 1.21). Many patients thus fail to reach medical care and succumb to potentially reversible ventricular fibrillation. Between 5 and 15 per cent will die in hospital and a further 5 per cent in the first month after discharge.

Hospital or home treatment

The decision about whether the patient is best managed at home or in hospital will depend on a number of factors. These include the medical condition of the patient, the length of time from the onset of symptoms, the suitability of the home circumstances and the distance from hospital. An experienced doctor can

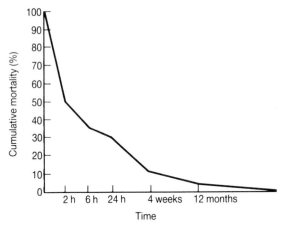

Fig. 1.21 Percentage cumulative mortality over time in patients who die from a myocardial infarction. The community mortality is about 50 per cent at 20 days.

identify those patients for whom hospital admission offers little advantage over home care. These include patients whose infarct was more than 12 hours previously and who are no longer in pain or whose pain is easily controlled.

The problem of delay before the patient comes under effective medical care is one to which there is no easy answer. Education of the public will encourage earlier reporting of symptoms. The patient will sometimes put up with symptoms for up to 6 hours before reporting them; women tend to put up with symptoms for longer than men. Mobile coronary care and the training of ambulance staff to perform advanced life support bring the care to the patient. Attempts have also been made with a programme of public education to raise the level of knowledge and practical skills about basic life support. This is considered in more detail in Chapter 12.

Clinical presentation

Acute myocardial infarction may be the first manifestation of coronary artery disease. Only about 50 per cent of patients admitted with a myocardial infarct have a past history of vascular disease. Many patients give a preceding history of fatigue and rather non-specific other symptoms.

Chest or epigastric pain or discomfort is the presenting symptom in more than 80 per cent of patients. The pain or discomfort may radiate to the throat, jaw, arm or fingers. It will last longer and be more severe than any preceding angina. It is described as being pressing, squeezing or crushing in character. Sweating and shortness of breath are usually associated although they may not be dominant symptoms. The association of the pain or discomfort with nausea, and sometimes belching, may reinforce the belief that it is dyspepsia and thus delay the summoning of medical help. A proportion of patients, particularly in the older age groups will sustain a painless and symptomless myocardial infarction which is discovered only by a change in the cardiogram or an altered exercise tolerance.

Physical examination

The appearance of the patient is determined mainly by the severity of the pain and the degree of fear and anxiety. There may be overactivity of the sympathetic nervous system due to either of these factors. The findings on examination will depend on the extent of myocardial injury: if this is severe, there will be evidence of ventricular failure with crackles at the bases, an elevated jugular venous pressure and a gallop rhythm. Because of the acute onset and even though the ventricular failure is severe, the lung fields may initially be clear and the venous pressure normal. An atrial or fourth heart sound is invariably present in the acute stages of an infarction and may also be palpable. When there is extensive myocardial damage a third heart sound is also audible and may be associated with evidence of a dyskinetic movement of the damaged left ventricular wall; this will be manifest by a systolic movement visible and palpable over the third and fourth left interspaces. The abnormal precordial movement becomes less obvious as the patient's condition improves. Fever may develop some 24 hours after infarction. Its elevation and duration will reflect the size of the infarction. Pericarditis is a common complication; a pericardical friction rub is frequently heard between the second and fourth days. Pericarditis may be associated with further chest pain; it is important clinically to differentiate this pain from that of further myocardial ischaemia.

Investigations

Electrocardiography

The ECG may sometimes be normal at the time of initial presentation. The initial diagnosis is therefore clinical and can be made irrespective of the ECG.

A full-thickness, or Q wave, infarction suggests a myocardial infarction involving the epicardium; however, the correlation with pathological evidence of a full-thickness infarction is not good. The initial ECG manifestation of an acute infarction is ST segment elevation, the 'current of injury pattern'. The elevated ST segment is usually convex upwards and associated with reciprocal ST segment depression in the electrodes situated at an angle of 180 degrees (Fig. 1.22). Sometimes the initial ECG shows excessive peaking of the T waves with some ST segment elevation; these are called hyperacute changes. The duration of ST segment elevation is variable but usually resolves within 24–48 hours. The T wave then gradually becomes inverted, assuming a symmetrical appearance (Fig. 1.23). The T wave inversion usually persists for many months and may remain a permanent feature. Persistent elevation of the ST segment was once regarded as suggestive of a cardiac aneurysm; it actually suggests the presence of an extensive area of akinetic or dyskinetic myocardium.

The reason for the ST segment elevation is controversial. One hypothesis is based on the existence of a diastolic current of injury. At the onset of injury the resting intracellular potential decreases from about $-90\,\text{mV}$ to $-70\,\text{mV}$. Because injured cells leak negative ions, their exterior becomes relatively negative compared with the normal cells. A current of injury thus flows between the negative injured cell and the positive or normal region. This produces a negative

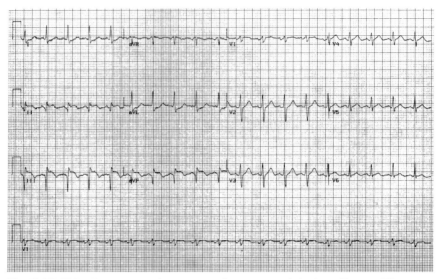

Fig. 1.22 ECG of a patient with an acute inferior myocardial infarct. There is ST segment elevation which is convex upwards, and which is maximal in leads II, III and aVF. There is reciprocal ST segment depression in the leads at 180 degrees; i.e. I and aVL.

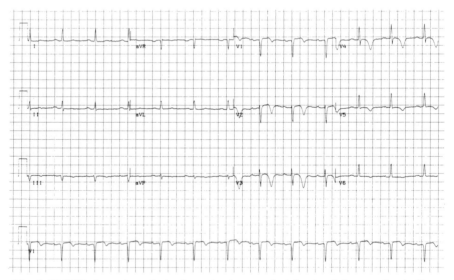

Fig. 1.23 ECG of a patient who had sustained an anterior infarction 6 days previously. There are symmetrically inverted T waves in the anterior leads.

displacement of the surface ECG baseline in the leads facing the injured area.

The production and significance of the Q wave is also controversial. It used to be thought that Q waves occurred only with transmural infarctions. The depth of the Q wave is roughly proportional to the thickness of the wall damage; it is quite possible therefore to have Q waves in a partial-thickness infarction if the damage is extensive although not full-thickness. It is now apparent that the Q wave can be a transient phenomenon. Whenever the degree of injury is severe enough to produce hypopolarization to about −60 mV, the cells become electrically inexcitable even though they are not irreversibly damaged; hence Q waves occur. However, if acute intervention is successful the Q waves disappear.

Laboratory investigations

The death or ischaemia of myocardial cells results in the release of intracellular enzymes. The detection of these enzymes may help substantiate the diagnosis. Several enzymes have been used in this way and they vary in their time relationship; the isoenzyme of creatine phosphokinase (CPK-MB) rises within a few hours of the infarction and remains elevated for 24–48 hours. Unlike creatine phosphokinase it is not released from skeletal muscle damage such as occurs with an intramuscular injection. Aspartate transaminase levels usually rise within 12–24 hours after infarction and return to normal approximately 48–72 hours later. The enzyme is present in other tissues, including liver and lungs; pulmonary infarction and hepatic congestion will therefore also cause a rise. Hydroxybuty-rate dehydrogenase (HBD) starts to rise 48 hours after an infarct and will return to normal some 72 hours later. The characteristic pattern of enzyme elevation is that of a sequential rise and fall (Fig. 1.24). The neutrophil count and, later, the erythrocyte sedimentation rate (ESR) both rise in response to the presence of dead myocardial tissue. Impaired glucose tolerance is a common finding after myocardial infarction; severe and uncorrected impairment is associated with a poor prognosis.

Knowledge of the serum potassium level is particularly important in the patient's early course; a low level is associated with arrhythmias and needs to be corrected promptly.

Differential diagnosis

This will need to include aortic dissection, pulmonary embolus, spontaneous pneumothorax, pericarditis, pancreatitis and oesophageal rupture. A particular

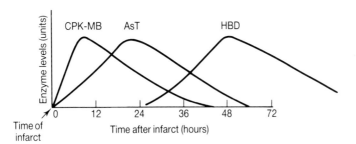

Fig. 1.24 Sequential rise and fall of three enzymes after a myocardial infarction. The creatine phosphokinase myocardial isoenzyme (CPK-MB) rises within a few hours. The aspartate transaminase (AsT) reaches its peak at about 24 hours after the infarction and the hydroxybutyric dehydrogenase (HBD) reaches its peak after about 48 hours.

and important differential is that of 'the cafe coronary'. In this condition the patient is typically a man in a restaurant eating meat and having had some alcohol to drink. He aspirates his food, clutches his chest or throat and is unable to breathe. He then becomes cyanosed and dies. Prompt recognition of the aspiration of meat and appropriate action will save his life. This condition is considered more fully in Chapter 12.

Clinical management

Early management

Analgesia
In the early stages of myocardial infarction rapid and effective analgesia is the main requirement. The drugs of choice are morphine or diamorphine and initially are best given by slow intravenous injection. The emetic effects of the drug may be circumvented by the intravenous administration of cyclizine. Further intravenous injections may be required if the pain is not relieved or if it returns. These potent analgesics may produce some degree of respiratory depression. They will also cause venodilatation which, by reducing the filling pressure of the ventricle, may cause hypotension. This may need to be treated with elevation of the bottom of the bed or, in severe cases, with intravenous fluids.

Oxygen
It is common practice to administer oxygen routinely during the acute stages of myocardial infarction; 100% oxygen is used although effectively only 60% is delivered. Only in those patients who have severe respiratory disease and who depend on their hypoxic drive is a high concentration of oxygen contraindicated. Oxygen is continued for the first few hours of admission to treat the hypoxaemia that is commonly encountered.

Aspirin
There is good evidence that aspirin, given soon after a myocardial infarction, will reduce the mortality. This is additive to the benefit with a fibrinolytic agent. The patient should therefore be asked to chew an aspirin as soon as the diagnosis is made. It can alternatively be given intravenously. A daily oral aspirin should then be continued indefinitely.

Fibrinolysis
There is good evidence that fibrinolysis will reduce the mortality and the size of the infarct if the patient is treated soon after the onset of symptoms. There is also an improved longer term prognosis. Thrombolytic drugs enhance the body's own thrombolytic mechanisms. The thrombolysis is facilitated by the use of intravenous streptokinase, recombinant human tissue-type plasminogen activator (t-PA), recombinant pro-urokinase, or anisoylated plasminogen streptokinase activator complex (APSAC) (see Fig. 1.7). The t-PA is more 'clot specific'; of particular note is the fact that there are no allergic manifestations even if given a

second time. These drugs are most beneficial when given early after the onset of symptoms. There is considerable benefit if given within 6 hours but some benefit is still present up to 12 hours. In future, general practitioners may need to carry the drug for use in the patient's home or place of work. Perhaps in due course high risk patients might carry their own supply?

Rhythm monitoring
The patient is attached to a monitor in order to monitor continuously the rhythm over the ensuing 24–36 hours. It is no longer thought to be possible to predict the likelihood of ventricular fibrillation by the identification of warning arrhythmias. Nevertheless, the knowledge of the rhythm is very valuable in this period, particularly if the patient is, or becomes, haemodynamically compromised. A low serum potassium level will make arrhythmias more likely.

Bedrest
There has been a progressive reduction in the period of recommended immobilization after myocardial infarction. Most patients are free of pain 24–48 hours after the infarction and can then begin to be mobilized. Patients without evidence of left ventricular failure or of further chest pain can be discharged from hospital to a suitable home environment within a few days of admission. Patients whose course is complicated by rhythm abnormalities, by continuing chest discomfort or whose home circumstances are not ideal will need to stay in hospital for a longer period.

Anticoagulation
There is some evidence that anticoagulants have some beneficial effect in preventing both systemic and pulmonary thromboembolic problems, particularly in those patients who have extensive myocardial injury and severe heart failure. It is unlikely that there will be additional benefit if the patient has already been given a thrombolytic drug on admission.

β-Adrenoceptor blocking drugs
These drugs have been used in the acute phase of an infarction in order to try to reduce infarct size. The results have been equivocal.

Arrhythmias and their management
Ventricular tachyarrhythmias Ventricular fibrillation is encountered in approximately 10 per cent of all patients presenting to hospital with acute myocardial infarct. The incidence of the arrhythmia is highest within the first 2 hours of the onset of symptoms; any circumstance that facilitates early admission to hospital results in a relatively high incidence of ventricular fibrillation. Conversely, delay in the admission of a patient results in a low hospital incidence. In the absence of ventricular failure, ventricular fibrillation is nearly always correctible if treated immediately; it does not adversely affect the prognosis. For many years it was thought possible to anticipate the onset of ventricular fibrillation by recognizing certain warning arrhythmias; this has now been shown to be incorrect, and prophylactic drug treatment is rarely used

because of the lack of evidence of its efficacy. Treatment of ventricular fibrillation depends on immediate defibrillation. The greater the delay from the onset of the cardiac arrest to the DC cardioversion, the poorer the chances of a successful outcome. The details of cardiopulmonary resuscitation are dealt with in Chapter 12. Although there is no very good evidence that antiarrhythmic drugs prevent further episodes of ventricular fibrillation, it is common practice to use an infusion of lignocaine for 24 hours after an episode of ventricular fibrillation. It is not necessary thereafter to treat with an antiarrhythmic drug.

Ventricular tachycardia is a more serious arrhythmia in the context of a myocardial infarct than in other circumstances (Fig. 1.25). It can progress to ventricular fibrillation and needs to be treated either with DC cardioversion or with intravenous lignocaine.

Ventricular premature beats and short runs of ventricular complexes (Fig. 1.26) do not require any treatment unless there is any associated haemodynamic disturbance.

Supraventricular tachycardias   Sinus tachycardia (Fig. 1.27) is often a manifestation of anxiety or pain in the early stages of infarction and need not be specifically treated. It may also reflect the presence of left ventricular failure and represents an attempt to maintain an adequate cardiac output.

Atrial fibrillation is quite a common arrhythmia after myocardial infarction (Fig. 1.28). Its management depends upon the ventricular rate and whether the rate is well tolerated by the patient. Digoxin is a useful drug because of its action on atrioventricular nodal conduction, which will reduce the ventricular rate. Intravenous amiodarone is a useful alternative. Intravenous verapamil is best avoided because of its negative inotropic action.

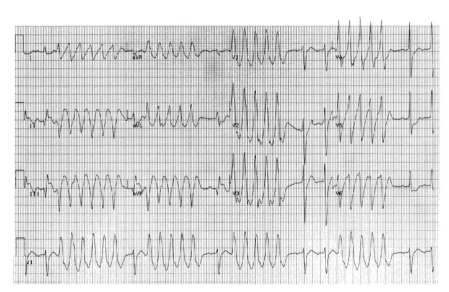

Fig. 1.25 ECG of a patient who has sustained an acute inferior infarction. There is a run of ventricular tachycardia that terminates spontaneously.

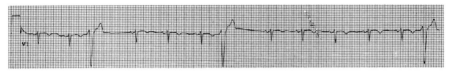

Fig. 1.26 Rhythm strip of V₁, showing sinus rhythm with some ventricular premature beats.

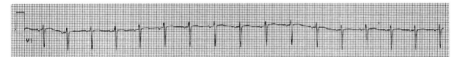

Fig. 1.27 Rhythm strip of V₁, showing a sinus tachycardia.

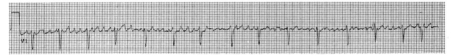

Fig. 1.28 Rhythm strip of V₁, showing atrial fibrillation with a normal ventricular rate.

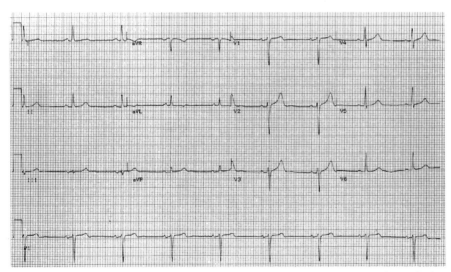

Fig. 1.29 A normal ECG apart from a sinus bradycardia, which is best seen in the V₁ rhythm strip.

Atrial tachycardia is not a common arrhythmia after myocardial infarction. It may respond to measures that increase vagal tone, such as carotid sinus pressure or the induction of retching or the Valsalva manoeuvre. Occasionally, drugs such as digoxin need to be used.

Atrial flutter is not a common arrhythmia after myocardial infarction. It responds in a similar manner to an increased vagal tone.

Bradycardias Sinus bradycardia (Fig. 1.29) is frequently encountered after an inferior myocardial infarction. It is usually well tolerated and resolves spontaneously. However, if it is associated with evidence of poor peripheral perfusion, it may need treatment with intravenous atropine.

Atrioventricular block is not uncommon after myocardial infarction. The atrioventricular node is supplied by the right coronary artery in about 80 per cent of people and by the circumflex coronary artery in the other 20 per cent. Patients with an inferior infarct may develop atrioventricular conduction problems without sustaining extensive myocardial destruction. For an anterior infarction to produce complete atrioventricular block the amount of myocardium destroyed must be considerable or, alternatively, there must be extensive coronary artery disease. Patients with an inferior myocardial infarction may progress gradually through the various degrees of block. First degree atrioventricular block is characterized by a prolonged PR interval (Fig. 1.30). Second degree, Wenckebach or Mobitz type I block may then develop. Complete atrioventricular block may ensue (Fig. 1.31). In an anterior myocardial infarct the progression

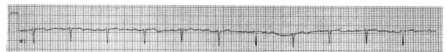

Fig. 1.30 Rhythm strip of V_1, showing sinus rhythm with a prolonged PR interval (first degree atrioventricular block).

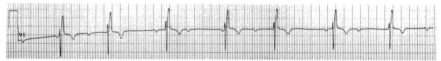

Fig. 1.31 ECG of a patient with complete atrioventricular block. There is no relationship between the P waves and the QRS complexes.

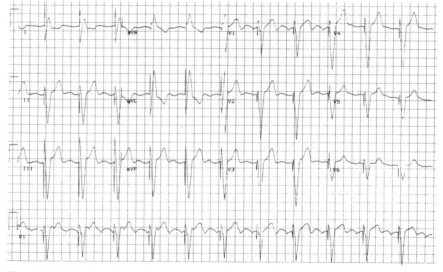

Fig. 1.32 ECG of a patient with a temporary pacemaker. The pacemaker artefact can be seen as a vertical line just before each QRS complex.

through these degrees of block may not be seen. Transvenous pacing is necessary if the ventricular rate is inadequate. A bipolar pacing electrode is introduced percutaneously into a vein such as the subclavian. It is then advanced to the apex of the right ventricle under fluoroscopic control. A pacing rate of between 60 and 70 beats per minute is then set (Fig. 1.32). Patients are paced until there is a return to normal conduction. This usually occurs within 24–48 hours.

Complications of myocardial infarction

Pulmonary oedema
The principles of treatment of pulmonary oedema due to left ventricular failure are similar to those described in Chapter 3. There is an important distinction to be made between mild heart failure associated with a few crackles at the bases and the more severe form. There is often no need to treat the former, which occurs in most patients after an infarct; to do so may reduce the filling pressure of the left ventricle and thereby reduce the cardiac output. The more severe form does require careful treatment; the most useful drugs in the initial management are intravenous diuretics, opiates and vasodilators; the beneficial effects of the opiates include their venodilatory properties.

Cardiogenic shock
It is important to be specific in the use of this term. The patient who looks 'shocked' is not necessarily in cardiogenic shock. The term should be restricted for patients who are peripherally vasoconstricted, have oliguria producing less than 20 ml/hour for longer than a few hours and have a systolic blood pressure of less than 90 mmHg. Mental confusion is often present. 'Cardiogenic shock' should be used only to describe patients in whom this clinical picture occurs in the absence of a correctable arrhythmia or unrelieved severe pain. Occasionally a patient presents this way because of a low left ventricular filling pressure in spite of a normal, or even a raised, jugular venous pressure. This often occurs as a result of excessive diuretic therapy; they dramatically improve when the circulating volume is restored. The vast majority of patients have cardiogenic shock because of severe and extensive myocardial destruction. The treatment of this condition is considered in Chapter 3. The outcome of treatment of patients with cardiogenic shock is extremely disappointing, with mortality rates in excess of 80 per cent.

Myocardial rupture
This accounts for about 18 per cent of the deaths due to infarction that occur in hospital. There are three presentations.

Cardiac rupture   This condition is more common than rupture of the interventricular septum and accounts for approximately 14 per cent of all deaths from myocardial infarction in hospital. The usual site of rupture is the free wall of the left ventricle. It usually occurs between 6 and 8 days after infarction but may be as late as 3 weeks.

Rupture of the interventricular septum   This most commonly occurs between the fourth and sixth day after myocardial infarction and is accompanied by sudden haemodynamic deterioration. Typically a long systolic murmur develops over the precordium and may be accompanied by a thrill. Surgical repair of the rupture can be attempted. An acceptable survival rate is obtained so long as the remaining cardiac function is reasonable.

Mitral regurgitation due to papillary muscle injury   The severity of this complication varies from that of mild papillary muscle ischaemia, producing minimal mitral regurgitation, to that of papillary muscle rupture, producing gross pulmonary oedema. Clinical management depends on the severity of the mitral regurgitation. Surgical repair can be performed as long as the remaining ventricular function is reasonable.

Systemic embolization
This complication is unusual and occurs in less than 2 per cent of patients admitted with a myocardial infarct. Sometimes it is possible to demonstrate the presence of a thrombus within the cavity of the left ventricle with echocardiography. There is no relationship between the presence of the demonstrable thrombus and the occurrence of systemic embolization.

Pulmonary embolism
The practice of early mobilization has reduced the incidence of pulmonary embolization and deep venous thrombosis. Nevertheless, in patients with a complicated infarct who need to remain in bed for a long period, the incidence is higher. Frequent leg exercises reduce the risk, as does prophylactic subcutaneous heparin. If the patient has already received a fibrinolytic drug, the incidence is likely to be very small indeed.

Dressler's syndrome
This occurs between 2 weeks and several months after the event. It is usually a self-limiting febrile illness accompanied by pericardial and/or pleural pain together with evidence of inflammation of serosal surfaces. It responds to indomethacin or aspirin, although occasionally steroids are needed. This syndrome has characteristics of an immunological condition and is triggered by myocardial damage; it can also occur after heart surgery or following blunt trauma to the heart.

Later management

Once the patient has recovered from the acute event it is necessary to consider the further management. This can be divided into two main parts. Firstly it is important to help the patient deal with the return to a normal life. Secondly there is the need to consider how the risk of further vascular episodes or death can be reduced.

The return to a normal life
The insult of a heart attack needs to be put into some sort of context for the patient to be able to cope positively with the future. There are a number of

information booklets available which can usefully be given to the patient; these are of value not only to the patient but also to the relatives who can easily be forgotten in the rehabilitation process. The booklets are not used in isolation; they are used as an adjunct to the careful explanations by the clinicians.

At the time of discharge from hospital the patient will already have been fairly mobile and will have gained some confidence thereby. However, the move to the home environment can be stressful and the patient will need the support of family or friends together with the known availability of the GP or hospital staff. Over the course of the next few days this anxiety will usually subside although there are likely to be a number of symptoms that may be focused on the heart and for which appropriate reassurance will be needed.

The patient should be encouraged to take regular physical exercise. Care must be taken in advising patients about the amount and type of exercise undertaken, as excessively vigorous exercise can be hazardous. Formal rehabilitation with a structured supervised exercise programme is advocated by some. Most patients can be helped to appreciate their own body signals that hitherto they may have ignored; they should be encouraged to continue exercising at their own rate so long as they feel they have the energy. They should be dissuaded from exercising at an imposed rate and need to be helped to develop the confidence to stop or slow down when they feel it is appropriate. Regular physical exercise may improve psychosocial functioning, reduce fear and dependency, and increase self-confidence and self-esteem. It can reduce the risk of subsequent death by 24–32 per cent.

It is important to both encourage and enable patients to give up smoking. It will reduce mortality and morbidity by about 30–40 per cent. Some patients will need little help to give up; the insult of the heart attack is quite enough! Others will need help perhaps in the form of group therapy, acupuncture or hypnosis.

A healthy diet should be encouraged which will reduce cholesterol levels. There is some emerging evidence that aggressive lipid lowering may cause coronary artery lesions to regress or to progress at a slower rate; these angiographic changes are associated with a reduced incidence of further coronary events and an improved survival rate. The numbers of patients in these trials are relatively small but the results look very encouraging.

The proper control of the blood pressure is important because of its cerebrovascular and renal complications; its control has little effect on the coronary artery complications.

The topic of sexual activity will need to be raised by the clinician. Patients may be too shy to raise the matter themselves. They will often be concerned lest coitus might provoke an infarct or cause death; in fact, within a stable relationship this risk is low and reassurance needs to be given. Sexual intercourse is not the only aspect of sexual relations that needs to be discussed with the patient. The linking of physical activity with sexual intercourse serves to deny the existence of a vast area of sexual contact which may be very important to the patient and may also be therapeutic. Some patients are able to use the insult of a myocardial infarct as an opportunity to rebuild their sexual life with the partner they love. It may enable them to concentrate more on those aspects that they previously rushed through on the way to the relief of their sexual frustration. The rediscovery of the sensual pleasures associated with cuddling, touching, caressing, stroking, licking, kissing and looking may not only enhance the relationship and give mutual pleasure but may also enable patients to learn more about their own bodies and the response to stimuli. It may enable the spouse of the patient to become more involved in helping in a constructive way. There is often a deterioration in the emotional relationships of those who do not resume sexual activities after myocardial infarction.

Most patients will be able to return to their previous work. They can usually return within a few weeks of the infarct; there is little to be gained in keeping patients away from work for months. It is important that they achieve the correct balance between work and leisure. The opportunity must not be missed to encourage them to reassess their previous pattern. There are some jobs that are not appropriate; a very heavy manual job may need to be modified if this is possible in the present employment circumstances. A patient who used to drive a public service vehicle, such as a bus, or a heavy goods vehicle, will need to report the fact of the heart attack to the relevant licensing authority, who will usually withdraw the licence. The patient can start driving a private car after about 6 weeks.

The reduction of further vascular deaths

The overall community mortality following myocardial infarction is approximately 50 per cent at 20 days. Deaths attributable to ventricular fibrillation are at their peak within the first few hours of infarction. Depending on the interval between onset of symptoms and arrival in hospital and the age group of the patients, the hospital mortality will be in the order of 10–15 per cent. It may prove possible to reduce this to 5–10 per cent with the advent of aspirin and fibrinolytic drugs.

On discharge from hospital the main factor determining the prognosis is the age of the patient. The next most important factor is the extent of myocardial damage. A poor prognosis is therefore associated with increasing age, previous infarction, evidence of heart failure, evidence of a large infarction and failure to raise the blood pressure or heart rate during exercise stress testing. The annual mortality will be in the order of 3 per cent for patients with satisfactory ventricular function and 20 per cent for patients with impaired function.

Exercise stress tests have been used a few days after myocardial infarction to try to define a high risk group. The results from such studies have been mixed. There is some doubt as to whether, knowing all the clinical risk factors, the exercise test gives extra information. There is no good evidence yet that any measures will alter the prognosis of the high risk group so identified.

Drugs   A number of drugs have been used to attempt to reduce the risk of further vascular events:

1. β-Adrenoceptor blocking drugs. When introduced 7, 14 or 21 days after the infarction, there is evidence that the risk of both death and further vascular events can be reduced. Unfortunately, these drugs can be associated with a feeling of lethargy and they also affect sexual performance.
2. Aspirin. Pooled data from a number of studies have shown that the risk of

death can be reduced by 15 per cent and further vascular events by 30 per cent. The ideal dosage is not clear; 300 mg on alternate days seems to be a reasonable compromise. There is an increased risk of gastric bleeding with larger doses.
3. Anticoagulants. Pooled data from several studies show a slight benefit.

Surgery   There is no evidence to suggest that bypass surgery after myocardial infarction is likely to be beneficial. In an important American study, the Coronary Artery Surgery Study (CASS) there was no survival benefit to those patients who were asymptomatic or had mild angina after myocardial infarction.

Angioplasty   There is no evidence that angioplasty is of value after myocardial infarction.

Further reading

Opie, L. H. (Ed.) (1991) *Drugs for the Heart*. W. B. Saunders, Philadelphia.

2

THE ELECTROCARDIOGRAM AND ARRHYTHMIAS

The electrocardiogram (ECG)

The string galvanometer, the original electrocardiograph, was first employed in humans by Willem Einthoven (1860–1927) in 1903. The first electrical recording of the human heart was reported by Augustus Waller (1856–1922) in 1887; the capillary electrometer he used for the recordings presented a lot of technical difficulties. It was because of these difficulties that Einthoven used the galvanometer, which had been invented by Johannes Schweigger of the University of Halle (1779–1857).

In 1913 Einthoven, Fahr and de Waart developed a method of studying the electrical activity of the heart by representing it graphically in an equilateral triangle. Although this representation is not mathematically true, it has provided the clinician with a practical working model which, in spite of many objections, has stood the test of time. Electrocardiography has developed empirically since then.

The basic electrocardiographic waveform

The waveforms of the ECG were arbitrarily labelled by Einthoven P, Q, R, S, T since he did not know the origin of the waves and did not want to impart any interpretation by the labels.

The contraction of any muscle is associated with electrical change, called depolarization. These changes can be detected by electrodes attached to the skin. The contraction of heart muscle will only be clearly identified if the patient is fully relaxed and there is no skeletal muscle contracting.

The P wave of the ECG is caused by atrial contraction. Because the muscle mass of the atria is small the electrical change accompanying their contraction is also small. The muscle mass of the ventricles is large and they produce a substantial deflection, called the QRS complex. The return of the ventricular mass to its resting electrical state is called repolarization and produces the T wave.

The different parts of the QRS complex are arbitrarily labelled. The first negative, or downward, deflection is called a Q wave. A positive, or upward, deflection is called an R wave; this may, or may not, be preceded by a Q wave. Any deflection below the baseline following an R wave is called an S wave. The presence and relative size of the waves can be indicated by a convention using combinations of either a capital letter, signifying a large deflection, or a small letter, indicating a minor deflection (Fig. 2.1).

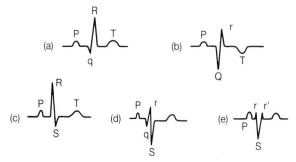

Fig. 2.1 The labelling of the PQRST complexes. The use of a capital or small letter for the QRS complex indicates the relative size of the deflection: (**a**) a qR complex; (**b**) a Qr complex; (**c**) an Rs complex; (**d**) shows a qrS complex; and (**e**) an rSr' complex; the r' or R' indicates a second R wave.

Initiation and propagation of the heart beat

Certain tissues of the heart are concerned with the initiation and propagation of the heart beat. The cells in these tissues can discharge spontaneously and initiate action potentials, thus acting as pacemaker tissue for the rest of the heart. They thereby ensure that the stimulation of the chambers of the heart proceeds in an orderly sequence. The tissues are the sinoatrial node, the atrioventricular junction, the bundle of His and the Purkinje network of fibres.

The sinoatrial node, described by Keith and Flack in 1907, is situated in the lateral wall of the right atrium close to the entry of the superior vena cava. It consists of fibres that are much smaller than the surrounding atrial musculature with which they fuse. It is a right-sided structure embryologically and receives its parasympathetic supply mainly from the right vagus. It has the fastest spontaneous discharge rate of all the conducting tissues and therefore initiates the heart beat. It conducts very slowly (Table 2.1). Depolarization spreads from this node to both the atria along three bundles of Purkinje-type atrial fibres to reach the atrioventricular (AV) node. These three pathways are called the anterior, middle and posterior internodal tracts.

The AV node, described by Tawara in 1906, consists of fibres that are similar in appearance to those of the sinoatrial (SA) node. The AV node is on the posterior and right border of the interatrial septum, close to the mouth of the coronary sinus. It is a left-sided structure embryologically, receiving its parasympathetic supply from the left vagus. A substantial part of the AV node is not capable of pacemaker activity. The fibres in this node conduct slowly and can protect the

Table 2.1 Conduction velocity in conducting tissue and heart muscle

	Conduction velocity (m/s)
Sinoatrial node	0.05
Atrial muscle	1.00
Atrioventricular node	0.10
Bundle branches	2.00
Purkinje fibres	1.00
Ventricular muscle	0.40

ventricles from excessively fast atrial stimuli such as occurs in atrial tachyar-rhythmias.

The bundle of His, described by Wilhelm His in 1893, is composed of Purkinje fibres that are histologically and electrophysiologically different from cardiac muscle fibres. It is of particular importance because it is the only conducting pathway between the atria and the ventricles. It passes through the fibrous skeleton of the heart which physically separates them. The bundle of His passes down from the AV node to the anterior part of the muscular interventricular septum just below the membranous part and between the right and non-coronary aortic valve cusps (Fig. 2.2). Over a distance of 5–15 mm, fibres of the left bundle depart from the main bundle and fan out widely within the subendo-cardium of the left side of the ventricular septum. About halfway to the apex, the left bundle separates into two major divisions, the anterior–superior and the posterior–inferior fascicles, which continue to the bases of the papillary muscles and the adjacent myocardium. The right bundle starts from the distal end of the common bundle as a thin bundle. It passes towards the right ventricular apex with branches passing through the moderator band to the anterior papillary muscle of the right ventricle while other branches innervate other areas of the apex of the ventricle. The final spread of electrical activity within the ventricular wall is through the gap junctions of the intercalated discs.

Electrical and mechanical events

The characteristic feature of the co-ordinated cardiac activity is a regularly repeated sequence of events, the cardiac cycle. The electrical events of the heart that have been described above trigger contraction of cardiac muscle through a process known as excitation–contraction coupling. The means by which the electrical signal is converted into a mechanical event is considered in detail in the companion book *The Physiology of the Heart and Circulation*. The cardiac cycle is initiated and ordered by these electrical events. The mechanical consequences can be divided into five phases:

1. Atrial systole
2. Isovolumic or isovolumetric ventricular contraction
3. Ventricular ejection

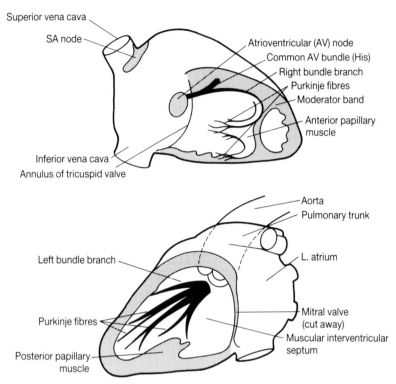

Superior vena cava
SA node
Atrioventricular (AV) node
Common AV bundle (His)
Right bundle branch
Purkinje fibres
Moderator band
Anterior papillary muscle
Inferior vena cava
Annulus of tricuspid valve

Aorta
Pulmonary trunk
Left bundle branch
L. atrium
Purkinje fibres
Mitral valve (cut away)
Muscular interventricular septum
Posterior papillary muscle

Fig. 2.2 The conducting system of the heart and its relationship to other structures during its course.

4. Isovolumic or isovolumetric ventricular relaxation
5. Rapid ventricular filling

Ventricular systole, manifest electrically by the QRS complex on the ECG, starts in phase 2 and finishes towards the end of phase 3. Phases 4 and 5 constitute ventricular diastole. Atrial systole, manifest electrically by the P wave on the ECG, occurs during the latter part of ventricular diastole (Fig. 2.3). The events on the two sides of the heart are similar although the pressures are very different.

Atrial systole, initiated by an impulse arising in the sinoatrial node, adds an additional 20–30 per cent to ventricular filling. Atrial systole generates an A wave which can be seen as a venous pulsation in the neck, or it can be recorded. The X descent is caused by a combination of atrial relaxation and the downward movement of the AV valve ring at the beginning of ventricular systole. The C wave is also caused by this descent of the valve ring as the ventricle creates more space by contracting and emptying.

The start of ventricular systole is signalled by the atrioventricular valves closing. The ventricle becomes a 'closed chamber'. No blood can enter nor can any flow out. This phase is termed isovolumic, or isovolumetric, ventricular contraction (Fig. 2.3). When the intraventricular pressure reaches the declining aortic diastolic pressure, the aortic valve opens and the phase of rapid ventricular ejection starts. From this point onwards until the aortic valve closes, the ventricular and aortic pressures rise together (Fig. 2.3). About 50 per cent of emptying occurs in the first 25 per cent of the ejection phase, and emptying is complete by 75 per cent of the way through this phase.

The rapid fall in intraventricular pressure that occurs as the muscle relaxes results in a backflow of blood from the aorta towards the ventricles, causing the aortic valve to snap shut (Fig. 2.3). The end of systole or the beginning of diastole is usually taken as the time at which the semilunar valves close, although the ventricles have actually started to relax before this.

The phase from the closure of the aortic and pulmonary valves until the opening of the AV valves is called isovolumic, or isovolumetric, relaxation; the ventricle is again 'closed' until its pressure drops below that of the atrium. The V wave of the atrial trace, which occurs during ventricular systole, is caused by the continuing arrival of blood to the atria at a time when the AV valves are closed, thus creating the pressure wave. The Y descent occurs as the ventricular pressure falls below the atrial, the AV valves open and blood is actively sucked into the ventricular cavities; this is called the phase of rapid ventricular filling. It is followed by a phase of slow ventricular filling; the change from one phase to the other can, in the young heart, be identified by the generation of the third heart sound. The increase in ventricular volume is maximal in early diastole, with 70 per cent of filling taking place in the first third of diastole. Ventricular diastole

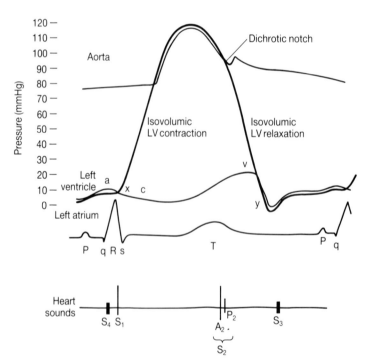

Fig. 2.3 The cardiac cycle, showing the pressure curves of the left side of the heart, the heart sounds and the ECG.

can therefore be shortened considerably before there is a decrease in stroke volume. With increasing heart rates it is diastole that shortens proportionally more than systole (Table 2.2). In adults with normal hearts, ventricular filling remains adequate up to heart rates of about 180/min. Rates of 200/min or more, which can occur with some paroxysmal tachycardias, may therefore be associated with dizziness, breathlessness or chest pain. Patients with abnormal hearts or diseased valves may be affected at slower rates.

Table 2.2   Duration of ventricular systole and diastole at two different heart rates

	Heart rate	
	75/min	200/min
Duration of cardiac cycle	0.8 s	0.3 s
Duration of ventricular systole	0.3 s	0.16 s
Duration of ventricular diastole	0.5 s	0.14 s

The ECG recording

ECG machines run at a standard rate and use paper that has standard squares. Each large square is equivalent to 0.2 s. Each small square is equivalent to 0.04 s and there are five of these for each large square. There are five large squares per second, or 300 per minute. The ventricular rate can be calculated easily from the ECG by measuring the RR interval: if it is 0.2 s or one large square, the rate is 300/min; if it is 0.4 s or two large squares, the rate is 150/min and so on. This quick method assumes a regular RR interval.

The distance between the various components of the PQRST complexes shows the time taken for conduction to spread through the different parts of the heart. The PR interval is measured from the beginning of the P wave to the beginning of the first deflection of the QRS complex whether it is a Q wave or an R wave (Fig. 2.4). It represents the time taken for excitation to spread from the SA node, travel through the atrial muscle, through the AV node, down the bundle of His

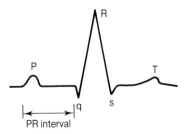

Fig. 2.4 The PR interval, which is measured from the beginning of the P wave to the beginning of the first deflection of the QRS complex whether it be a q(Q) wave or an R(r) wave.

and into the ventricular myocardium. The normal PR interval varies with the ventricular rate: it will be longer with slow heart rates and shorter with faster rates. It is normally between 0.12 and 0.2 s. If it is shorter, it suggests that the atria have been depolarized by a pacemaker sited closer to the AV node or, alternatively, that there is some abnormality of conduction from the atria to the ventricles such as an accessory conducting bundle.

The duration of the QRS complex shows how long excitation takes to spread through the ventricles. The normal duration is 0.11–0.12 s. Any abnormality of conduction will cause this to be increased. The QT interval is measured from the first deflection of the QRS complex until the end of the T wave. This interval varies with the heart rate and has to be corrected to a rate of 60/min (QT_c). The QT interval is a measure of the repolarization time of the ventricles.

Recording an ECG

In order to take an ECG the patient must be connected to the recording machine by means of leads which are attached to the four limbs and to the chest. These electrical leads are physically attached to the skin by means of an electrode held in position by suction or a strap. Good electrical contact is obtained by rubbing electrode jelly into the skin or by using wet pads. If the patient has a hairy chest, it is sometimes necessary to shave some parts of it in order to gain good contacts.

The ECG compares the electrical events detected in the different electrodes. There are two types of recording: the bipolar lead records between two points on the body, and the unipolar between a single surface electrode and an indifferent electrode. The indifferent electrode is obtained by connecting together the leads of the arms and the left leg. The unipolar lead is used to record the chest or precordial leads termed V_1 to V_6. The bipolar leads are the standard leads I, II, III and aVL, aVR and aVF (Fig. 2.5).

The ECG recorder must be correctly calibrated in order for information to be deduced from the height of the PQRST complexes. A signal of 1 mV should move the stylus 1 cm, or two large squares, upwards. This calibration signal should be included on every recording. The significance of an increased voltage, or height, of the various parts of the complexes is considered later.

The 12-lead ECG

Twelve ECG leads are usually recorded. Six of these are the standard bipolar leads and six are the unipolar or chest leads. Each lead 'looks at the heart' from a different direction. The interpretation of the ECG is relatively easy if it is remembered from which vantage point the lead views the heart.

The six standard leads can be considered to be looking at the heart in the frontal or vertical plane. Leads I, II and aVL look at the left lateral surface of the heart, III and aVF look at the inferior aspect and aVR views the right atrium.

A V lead is attached to the chest wall by means of a suction electrode. Six recordings are made from positions in the fourth and fifth intercostal spaces. Leads V_{1-2}, recorded in the fourth interspace on either side of the sternum, look at the right ventricle. Lead V_3 is recorded from between V_2 and V_4. Leads V_{3-4}

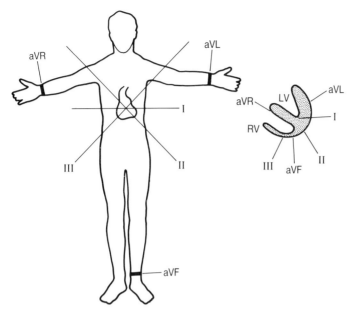

Fig. 2.5 The bipolar leads and their relationship to the heart.

look at the interventricular septum. Leads V_{4-6} are recorded in the fifth intercostal space; leads V_{5-6} look at the left ventricle (Fig. 2.6).

When an ECG recording is made with a single-channel recorder the following steps are followed:

1. The patient must be lying down, relaxed, comfortable and warm
2. The electrodes are connected, ensuring correct lead attachment and good skin contact
3. The recorder is calibrated
4. The standard leads are recorded; four to six complexes of each is sufficient
5. The individual chest or precordial leads are recorded

With the advent of more sophisticated recorders, a number of the above steps are amalgamated. The ECG machine simultaneously records all the leads and may interpret them also! However, steps 1 and 2 still remain crucially important.

The QRS complex

Depolarization spreads through the heart in many directions simultaneously; the deflection of the QRS complex shows the average direction in which the depolarization is spreading. If the depolarization is spreading towards an electrode it will cause an upward or positive deflection; if it is moving away, it will cause a negative or downward deflection. If the depolarization wave is travelling at right angles to the electrode, it will cause equal R and S waves or an equiphasic complex.

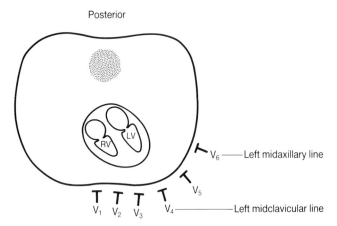

Fig. 2.6 The positions of the precordial leads. V_1 and V_2, recorded in the fourth intercostal space on either side of the sternum, look at the right ventricle. Leads V_3 and V_4 look at the interventricular septum. Leads V_5 and V_6, recorded in the fifth intercostal space, look at the left ventricle.

The QRS axis

The electrical axis can be defined as a vector originating in the centre of Einthoven's equilateral triangle. A vector is a mathematical value expressed in the form of an arrow which has direction and magnitude. The average direction of spread of the depolarization wave in the frontal plane is called the QRS axis. The axis can be simply assessed from the frontal leads I, II and III. There are more accurate means of calculating the axis using all the frontal leads (Fig. 2.7). The

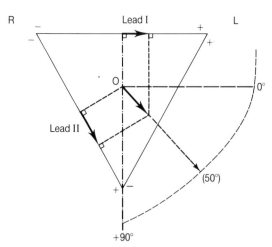

Fig. 2.7 Any two standard leads can be used to derive the QRS axis. A line is drawn to scale from the mid-point of each lead, representing the direction and magnitude (in mm) of the QRS deflection. Perpendiculars are then drawn; the points of intersection are the zero and maximal points of electrical axis. Joining the points of intersection produces the QRS vector, the direction and amplitude of which represent the direction and amplitude of the electrical axis of the heart.

normal axis will produce a predominately positive deflection in all three leads (Fig. 2.8).The deflection will be greatest in the lead towards which the main vector flows. The normal QRS axis is between −30 and +110 degrees.

In right axis deviation the main QRS vector will cause a predominately negative deflection in I and a positive one in III. This may occur with pulmonary conditions that put a strain on the right side of the heart. It may also occur with diseases of the conducting system (Fig. 2.9).

In left axis deviation the main QRS vector produces a predominately negative deflection in III and a positive deflection in I. The predominant deflection in II will also be negative (Fig. 2.10). This is seen in conduction tissue disease or in some congenital heart disease. Minor degrees of axis deviation are not in themselves very significant since they can occur in people who are rather thin or

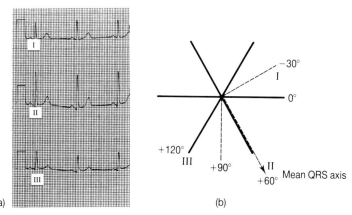

(a)   (b)

Fig. 2.8 An example of a normal QRS axis. Three frontal leads are shown on the left; there are predominantly positive deflections in all three leads. The mean QRS axis is in the direction of the lead in which there is the maximum deflection; in this instance the mean QRS axis is +60 degrees.

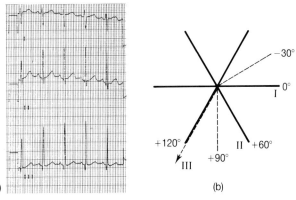

(a)   (b)

Fig. 2.9 An example of right axis deviation. Three frontal leads are shown on the left; there is a predominantly negative deflection in I and a positive deflection in III. The deflections are 'reaching' for each other; thus right axis deviation. Compare with Fig. 2.10 in which these leads are 'leaving' each other. In this instance the mean QRS axis is +120 degrees.

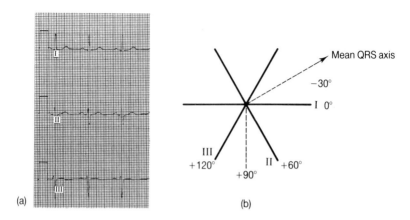

(a)   (b)

Fig. 2.10 An example of left axis deviation. Three frontal leads are shown on the left; there is a predominantly negative deflection in III and a positive deflection in I. The deflections are 'leaving' each other; thus left axis deviation. Compare with Fig. 2.9, in which these leads are 'reaching' for each other. In this example the mean QRS axis is −40 degrees.

fat. However, it should alert the clinician to the possibility of other abnormalities in the ECG.

The QRS complex in the chest leads

The shape of the QRS complexes in the chest leads is determined by the pattern of depolarization of the interventricular septum and the fact that the left ventricle

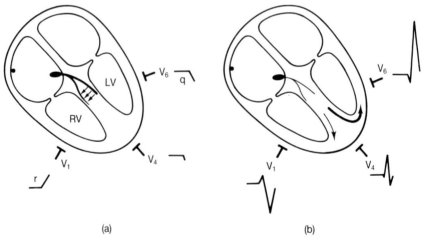

(a)   (b)

Fig. 2.11 Normal depolarization of the ventricles as viewed by the precordial leads. The interventricular septum is depolarized first and, because of the characteristics of the left bundle, is depolarized from left to right. The initial deflections are shown in (**a**); because the V_1 lead is looking towards the oncoming vector, the deflection is positive. In V_6 the initial deflection is negative because the vector is leaving it. As the main mass of the ventricle then depolarizes (**b**) the main deflection in V_6 becomes positive and in V_1 negative. Lead V_4 will be biphasic.

has a large mass compared with the right. The interventricular septum is depolarized first and the wave spreads across the septum from left to right (Fig. 2.11a). Thus in V_6, which 'looks' at the left ventricle, the initial deflection is negative and a small Q wave results. In V_1, looking at the right ventricle, the initial wave is positive and an r wave results. As the main mass of the left ventricle now depolarizes, the main deflection in V_6 is positive, and in V_1 negative. Leads V_{3-4} will be intermediate between these two and biphasic complexes will result (Fig. 2.11b). The position of the septum is identified by the positive and negative deflections being similar.

Vectorcardiography

Vector analysis of the cardiac electrical forces was first used by Einthoven. The vectorcardiogram is recorded in three planes of the body – horizontal, vertical and sagittal – using combinations of three scalar leads at right angles to each other (Fig. 2.12). This technique can sometimes offer help where the ECG is confusing or misleading.

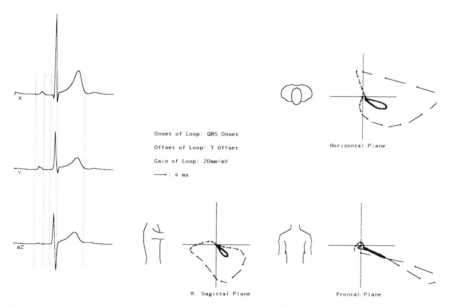

Onset of Loop: QRS Onset

Offset of Loop: T Offset

Gain of Loop: 20mm/mV

⟶● : 4 ms

Horizontal Plane

R. Sagittal Plane

Frontal Plane

Fig. 2.12 A vectorcardiogram showing the three planes of recording: horizontal, vertical and sagittal. The marker ⟶● (centre) represents 4 ms and also indicates the direction of the vector.

Abnormalities of the P, QRS and T waves

Abnormalities of the P wave

Apart from the alteration in the shape of the P wave associated with rhythm changes, there are two important abnormalities. Right atrial enlargement will cause the P wave to become peaked, the so-called 'P pulmonale' (Fig. 2.13). Left atrial hypertrophy will cause a 'P mitrale' in which the wave is broader than normal and bifid (Fig. 2.14). In lead V₁ the negative deflection becomes larger than the positive; this can happen rapidly and be an index of the changing left atrial pressure (Fig. 2.15).

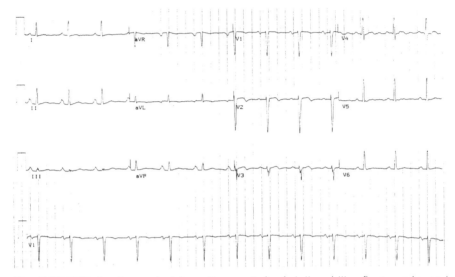

Fig. 2.13 ECG showing peaked, large P waves in leads I, II and III, reflecting right atrial hypertrophy.

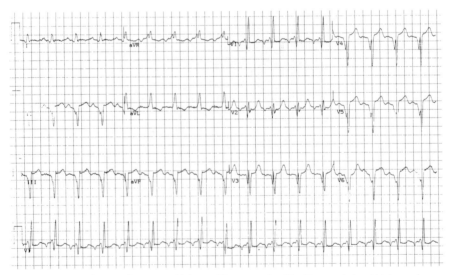

Fig. 2.14 ECG showing features of left atrial hypertrophy. The P wave in lead V₁ has a larger negative deflection than positive. The duration of the P wave in lead II exceeds 120 ms. The ECG also shows right bundle branch block and an old anterior and inferior infarction. (See also Fig. 2.15.)

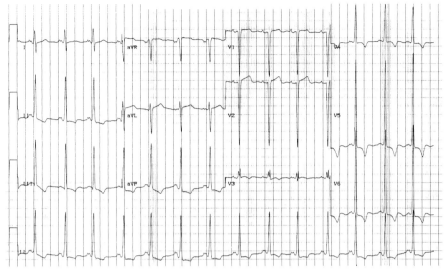

Fig. 2.15 ECG showing the criteria of left ventricular hypertrophy: (i) the sum of the R waves in V_6 and the S in V_1 is >35 mm; (ii) the largest R or S wave in the standard leads is >20 mm; (iii) the height of the tallest R wave in the precordial lead is >27 mm. The presence of ST segment and T wave abnormalities over the left precordial leads increases the specificity. There is also evidence of left atrial hypertrophy (P mitrale).

Abnormalities of the QRS complex

The normal QRS complex can be characterized by:

1. A duration of no greater than 0.12 s
2. In V_5 or V_6 the height of the R wave is less than 25 mm
3. In V_1 or V_2 the S wave is greater than the R wave
4. In V_5 or V_6 the Q wave should be less than 1 mm duration and less than 2 mm deep.

Abnormal width of QRS complex

In the presence of bundle branch block the QRS duration is prolonged (Figs. 2.16 and 2.17). A ventricular extrasystole may also produce a widened QRS complex.

Abnormal height of QRS complex

In the presence of hypertrophy of either ventricle the height of the QRS complex may be increased. Evidence of right ventricular hypertrophy is best seen in the right ventricular leads (Fig. 2.18). The height of the R wave in V_1 will exceed the s wave; there will also be a deep s wave in V_6.

Left ventricular hypertrophy produces a large R wave in the left chest leads. Unfortunately, this criterion alone is not very satisfactory for the diagnosis. By

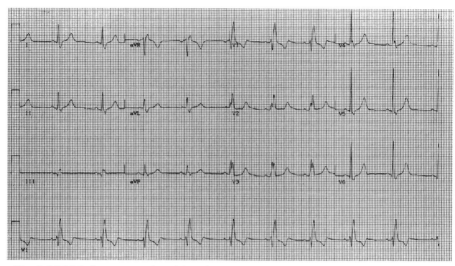

Fig. 2.16 ECG showing a widened QRS duration of 156 ms. Because the initial part of the QRS complex is normal and the latter part abnormal, this is a right bundle branch block.

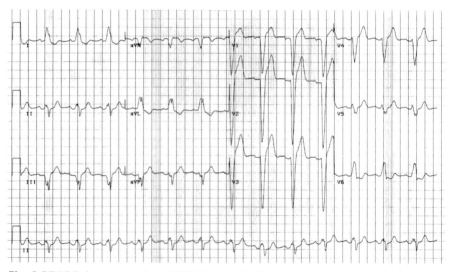

Fig. 2.17 ECG showing a widened QRS duration of 160 ms. Because the initial and subsequent parts of the QRS complex are abnormal, this is a left bundle branch block.

including other features and scoring them, the sensitivity and specificity are improved; these other features include the ST segment and T wave changes, and the QRS axis (see Fig. 2.15). Information from echocardiography or, in due course, magnetic resonance imaging, will give much better information about the presence of hypertrophy.

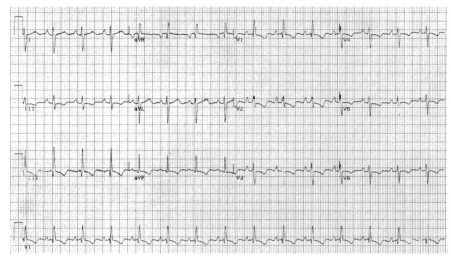

Fig. 2.18 ECG showing sinus rhythm. There is an R wave in lead V_1 that is larger than the S wave, and there are deep S waves in V_6. The QRS axis is difficult to determine and is orientated posteriorly as well as to the right. This ECG shows the features of right ventricular hypertrophy and also right atrial enlargement.

Abnormal shape of the QRS complexes

The ECG changes of acute right heart strain are considered under pulmonary embolism in Chapter 1. The ECG changes associated with myocardial infarction are also considered in Chapter 1.

Abnormalities of the ST segment

The normal ST segment lies between the QRS complex and the T wave and should be isoelectric. This means that it is at the same level as the segment between the T wave and the next P wave.

Elevation of the ST segment

Elevation of the ST segment occurs in four conditions and it should be possible to distinguish them by the shape of the elevated segment. In acute myocardial infarction the ST segment is elevated in those leads reflecting the acutely ischaemic myocardium; the ST segment is concave upwards (Fig. 2.19). There is also reciprocal ST segment depression and there may be Q waves. In acute pericarditis the ST segment elevation is convex upwards; there is no reciprocal ST segment depression (Fig. 2.20) and no Q waves. There is also a normal variant of ST segment elevation which is sometimes called a racial variant. With the increasing use of electrocardiograms it has become apparent that this variant can occur in all races but is usually restricted to men. There is a 'high take-off' of the ST segment. This ST segment elevation becomes isoelectric with exercise or a

72   *The electrocardiogram and arrhythmias*

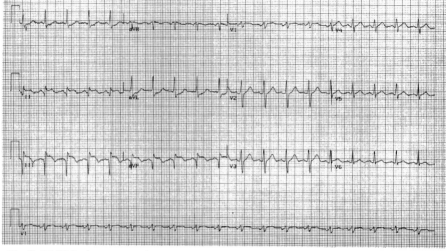

Fig. 2.19 ECG of a patient with an acute inferior myocardial infarction, showing the ST segment elevation in the inferior leads and reciprocal ST segment depression in leads I and aVL. The shape of the ST segment elevation is concave upwards. There are also deep Q waves in II, III and aVF. The PR interval is prolonged.

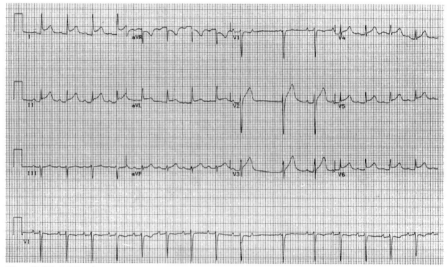

Fig. 2.20 ECG of patient with viral pericarditis. There is ST segment elevation that is most marked in lead II and the lateral chest leads. The shape of the ST segment is convex upwards and there is no reciprocal ST segment depression. There is also an atrial arrhythmia.

small dose of intravenous atropine. In hypothermia a very unusual J wave occurs (Fig. 2.21) in association with other abnormalities.

Depression of the ST segment

Depression of the ST segment is considered in Chapter 1.

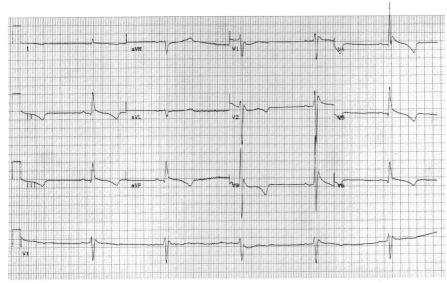

Fig. 2.21 ECG of a patient with hypothermia (26°C). There is a characteristic J wave present. This occurs at the junction of the QRS complex and where one might expect the ST segment to start. There are also other features of hypothermia present: the heart rate is slow and there is a long QT interval. The patient is too cold for shiver waves to appear.

Abnormalities of the T wave

The T wave is normally inverted in aVR and in V_1; it may sometimes be inverted in V_2 and occasionally in V_3. In a bundle branch block the abnormal depolarization is usually associated with abnormal repolarization; the inverted T waves have no significance of themselves in this circumstance. Left ventricular hypertrophy can cause flat or inverted T waves in the left ventricular leads; right ventricular hypertrophy will cause T wave changes in V_2 or V_3. Digoxin therapy will cause a characteristic tick-like shape to the ST segment and T wave; this is evidence of a digoxin effect and should not be mistaken for a sign of toxicity (Fig. 2.22). The T wave changes that are associated with myocardial infarction are discussed in Chapter 1.

Abnormally peaked T waves are associated with acute hyperkalaemia (Fig. 2.23); the T wave has a very narrow base. As the degree of hyperkalaemia increases so the QRS complex widens, the PR interval becomes prolonged and the P wave diminishes in size. If left untreated, death will usually ensue due to ventricular asystole or fibrillation.

There are numerous causes of ST segment and T wave flattening; they include anxiety, hypokalaemia which is often associated with a U wave (Fig. 2.24), hyperventilation or swallowing cold liquids. Often no cause can be found and the abnormality does not merit further investigation.

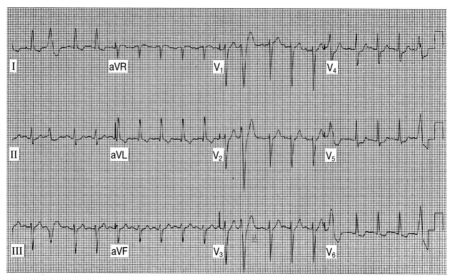

Fig. 2.22 ECG showing a sinus tachycardia with frequent ventricular premature beats. The ST segments in I, aVL and V₆ have a tick shape suggestive of a digoxin effect.

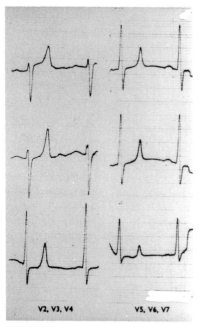

V2, V3, V4   V5, V6, V7

Fig. 2.23 Chest leads of a patient with a sudden rise of the serum potassium to 8.2 mmol/l. The T waves are typical of hyperkalaemia and are peaked with a narrow base.

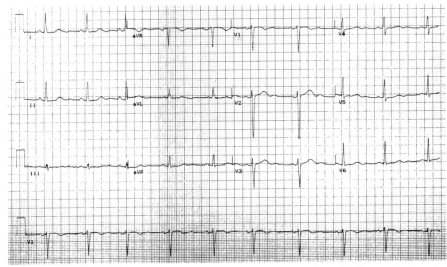

Fig. 2.24 ECG of a patient with hypertension being treated with a beta blocker and a thiazide diuretic. His serum potassium was 2.2 mmol/l. The ECG shows a sinus bradycardia. There are some non-specific ST segments and T wave abnormalities together with a U wave; this wave follows the T wave and is often associated with hypokalaemia.

Abnormalities of the QT interval

The QT interval normally shortens with an increasing heart rate. The normal corrected QT interval (QT$_c$) is 0.42 s. A lengthened QT interval is associated with a tendency to develop ventricular tachycardia. The QT interval can be lengthened by certain drugs such as the phenothiazines. Congenital prolongation of the QT interval can also occur.

Conduction problems

Sinus node

Sinoatrial block is recognized by the absence of an expected P wave. Since there is no atrial depolarization, ventricular depolarization does not take place and there is complete absence of a PQRST complex (Fig. 2.25). In most instances sinoatrial block is due to structural disease or drug toxicity; the drugs incriminated are digoxin, quinidine and salicylates.

Atrioventricular node and bundle of His

The time taken for the spread of depolarization from the sinoatrial node to the ventricular muscle is displayed by the PR interval. This is normally less than 0.2 s. If each wave of depolarization starting from the SA node is delayed, this will result in a longer than normal PR interval and the condition of first degree atrioventricular block (Fig. 2.26); this is often abbreviated to 'first degree block',

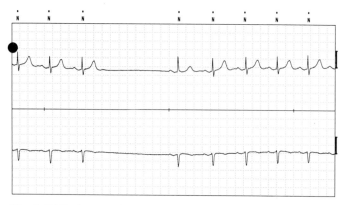

Fig. 2.25 Rhythm strip (V₅ above and V₁ below) of a patient with sinoatrial block. The first three complexes are conducted normally although there is a first degree atrioventricular block. There is then a pause without any atrial or ventricular activity before the sinus node initiates an impulse again.

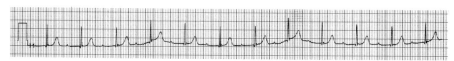

Fig. 2.26 Rhythm strip of a sinus bradycardia with a prolonged PR interval of 320 ms. First degree atrioventricular block is present.

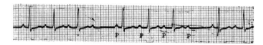

Fig. 2.27 Rhythm strip demonstrating a Mobitz type I block or Wenckebach phenomenon. There is progressive lengthening of the PR interval followed by a failure of conduction; this is followed by a conducted beat with a short PR interval and the cycle is repeated.

which is convenient if a little non-specific since sinoatrial block also occurs. First degree block may merely demonstrate a high vagal tone at rest in a fit person. Alternatively, it can be caused by one of the conditions listed in Table 2.3.

Second degree AV block exists when a normal impulse from the sinoatrial node fails to pass through the AV node or bundle of His. There are three varieties of second degree block:

1. Progressive lengthening of the PR interval is followed by a failure of conduction; this is followed by a conducted beat with a short PR interval and the cycle is repeated (Fig. 2.27). This is called the Wenckebach phenomenon or a Mobitz type 1 block. It is of interest that Wenckebach described the various degrees of AV block before the advent of electrocardiography!

2. Most beats are conducted with a constant PR interval but occasionally there is a P wave that is not conducted (Fig. 2.28). This is called a Mobitz type II block.

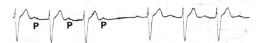

Fig. 2.28 Rhythm strip demonstrating a Mobitz type II atrioventricular block. Most beats are conducted with a constant PR interval but occasionally a P wave is not conducted. (Courtesy of Dr A. Hollman.)

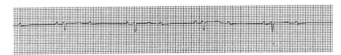

Fig. 2.29 Rhythm strip of lead V₁ in a patient with second degree atrioventricular block. Every second P wave is conducted to the ventricles and is then called 2:1 atrioventricular block.

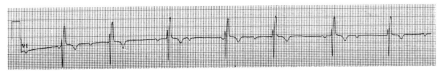

Fig. 2.30 Rhythm strip of a patient with third degree, or complete, atrioventricular block due to sarcoid. Atrial depolarization is normal but no P waves are conducted to the ventricles. There is no relationship between the atrial rate and the ventricular rate.

Table 2.3 Causes of atrioventricular block

Idiopathic fibrosis of bundle branches
Myocardial infarction
Digoxin toxicity
Aortic valve disease
Congenital
Cardiac surgery
Infiltrations: tumour, calcification
Inflammation: sarcoid, endocarditis, Chagas' disease, scleroderma
Rheumatic fever
Diphtheria
Dystrophia myotonica

3. A ratio exists between the conducted beats and the non-conducted ones; the PR interval of the conducted beats is constant (Fig. 2.29). The ratio may be 2:1 or 3:1 or more and may vary with time. Sometimes the non-conducted P wave is hidden in the T wave and difficult to spot.

Third degree AV block is also called complete heart block. It occurs when atrial contraction is normal but no P waves are conducted to the ventricles. The ventricle has its own pacemaker but this is at a very slow rate of 30–45/min (Fig. 2.30). It can occur as a congenital condition, when the ventricular rate tends to be faster. As an acquired condition it may be associated with asystole or ventricular fibrillation; this may result in death or, in the more fortunate patient, a syncopal episode; this latter symptom is called a Stokes–Adams attack. Although this term was originally used to describe syncope occurring in the context of complete heart block, it tends now to be used to describe syncope due to any cardiac arrhythmia.

Bundle branch blocks

Conduction blocks may occur in the right or left bundle branches. If the depolarization wave reaches the interventricular septum normally, the PR interval will be quite normal. However, due to a block in one or other bundle branches, there will be a delay in depolarization of part of the ventricular muscle; this will cause a lengthening of the QRS complex beyond the normal 0.12 s. Widening of the QRS complex also occurs when the initiation of the ventricular beat occurs within the ventricle such as in a ventricular tachycardia. In sinus rhythm and bundle branch block there is a P wave preceding each widened QRS complex (see Figs. 2.16 and 2.17).

The characteristics of left and right bundle branch block can be remembered easily if the normal pattern of depolarization of the interventricular septum is recalled (see Fig. 2.11). In a right bundle branch block (RBBB) the initial depolarization is quite normal (Fig. 2.31a) and the first part of the QRS complex is normal. The next phase of depolarization is also normal (Fig. 2.31b). The final

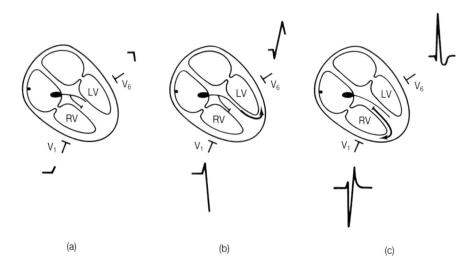

(a)   (b)   (c)

Fig. 2.31 ECG of right bundle branch block. The initial depolarization of the interventricular septum (**a**) is quite normal because the left bundle, which initiates the left to right depolarization, is normal. The next phase also is normal (**b**) and dominated by left ventricular depolarization. The final phase (**c**) is abnormal and causes the prolongation of the QRS complex because it takes so long for the depolarization wave to reach the right ventricle. This final depolarization occurs after the main depolarization of the left ventricle and causes the final positive deflection in lead V_1, an rSr′ pattern, and the S wave in V_6, the qRs pattern.

phase is abnormal because it takes so long for the depolarization wave to reach the right ventricle; there is thus a second R wave (R or r!) in V_1 and a slurred s or S wave in V_6 (Fig. 2.31c). In a left bundle branch block (LBBB) the pattern of depolarization is very different. The initial depolarization of the interventricular septum cannot occur from left to right and instead occurs right to left (Fig. 2.32a). This produces a Q wave in V_1 and an R wave in V_6. The right ventricle is depolarized before the left and, in spite of its smaller mass, is able to generate an upward deflection in V_6 and a downward deflection in V_1 (Fig. 2.32b). The later depolarization of the left ventricle then causes a further S wave in V_1 and an R wave in V_6 (Fig. 2.32c).

The presence of left bundle branch block indicates heart disease that is usually affecting the left side. Right bundle branch block indicates problems with the right side of the heart but may be found sometimes in normal people.

Distal conduction tissue disease

When there is disease affecting the anterior fascicle of the left bundle the ventricle has to be depolarized from the posterior fascicle. This causes a shift in the QRS axis towards the left (Fig. 2.33). Left axis deviation is therefore caused by left anterior fascicular block or left anterior hemiblock. If the posterior fascicle is diseased, the axis swings to the right due to the left posterior hemiblock; this is not a common condition. With a right bundle branch block the axis usually remains normal because the depolarization of the left ventricle remain normal. However, if there is a right bundle branch block (RBBB) and a left anterior hemiblock, the ECG will show a RBBB pattern with left axis deviation (Fig. 2.34). If there is a lengthening of the PR interval also, this may imply some impairment of conduction in the remaining posterior fascicle and may presage the development of complete heart block.

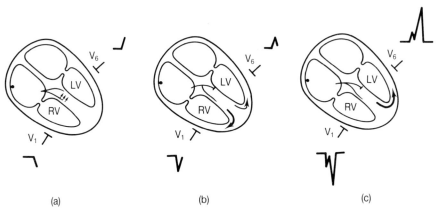

(a)   (b)   (c)

Fig. 2.32 ECG of left bundle branch block. The initial depolarization of the interventricular septum is abnormal and occurs in the opposite direction to normal because of the blocked left bundle (**a**). The right ventricle is then depolarized before the left (**b**), causing the notch in leads V_1 and V_6 before the later depolarization of the left ventricle (**c**) causes a further S wave in V_1 and an R wave in V_6.

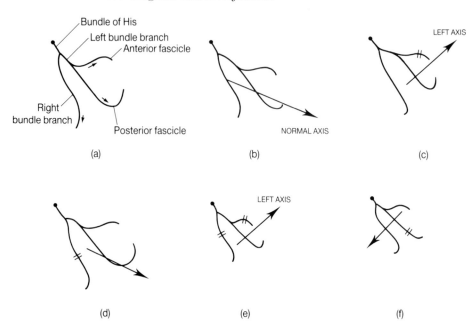

Fig. 2.33 Distal conduction tissue disease. (**a**) The conducting system of the ventricles. (**b**) The normal QRS axis. (**c**) The anterior fascicle is blocked and so the left ventricle has to be depolarized through the posterior fascicle, producing a left axis deviation. (**d**) The right bundle is blocked but this will not alter the axis because there is normal depolarization of the left ventricle. (**e**) Both the right bundle and the left anterior fascicle are blocked, producing a right bundle branch block pattern and left axis deviation. (**f**) The left posterior fascicle is blocked, which swings the axis to the right.

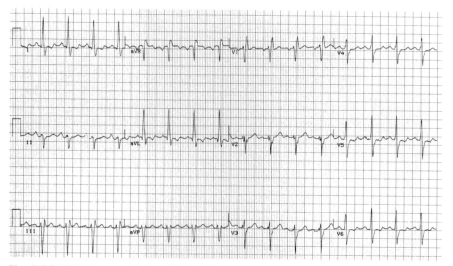

Fig. 2.34 ECG showing right bundle branch block and left axis deviation. This is due to a block in both the right bundle branch and the left anterior fascicle. (See also Fig. 2.33.)

Arrhythmias

An arrhythmia is defined as any heart rhythm other than sinus rhythm. The term 'dysrhythmia' is sometimes used instead but is etymologically incorrect.

Most parts of the heart have potential pacemaker activity and can discharge spontaneously and rhythmically. The actual rate of contraction of the ventricles will be determined by the part of the heart that is depolarizing most frequently. It is usually the sinoatrial node that has the highest rate of discharge. The development of dynamic 24-hour ambulatory monitoring has enabled us to determine the prevalence of arrhythmias in normal populations and, perhaps more importantly, helped us to realize the range of normal and healthy rhythms. The variation in sinus rhythm in young people was not appreciated before the introduction of ambulatory monitoring. The range between the fastest and slowest rates is remarkably wide and remains so into adult life (Table 2.4).

Table 2.4 Range of sinus rates in normal populations

Population	Maximum (awake)	Minimum (asleep)
Healthy children (7–11 years)	195	37
Healthy boys (10–13 years)	200	30
Male medical students	180	37
Young women (22–28 years)	189	40
Healthy runners	200	35

The frequency of arrhythmias was also found to be more common than was hitherto realized. Ventricular, AV junctional and atrial extrasystoles are commonly found in healthy individuals. Even episodes of ventricular tachycardia can occur. First degree and Mobitz type I AV block is found not infrequently, as are sinus pauses of up to 1.8 s. An appreciation of the frequency of the various rhythm disturbances that occur under normal circumstances will enable a more rational approach to be taken when assessing the patient presenting with cardiac problems.

Arrhythmias can be divided into disorders of impulse formation and disorders of conduction. Some of the conduction problems have already been discussed. Disordered impulse formation can be due to an abnormal origin of the impulse, to an abnormal rate of discharge or to both.

Mechanisms of arrhythmias

Normal automaticity

The most important factors determining the rate of firing of automatic cells are the slope of diastolic depolarization and the difference between the maximum diastolic potential and the threshold potential. The normal hierarchy of pacemaker dominance in the heart reflects the gradual decrease of the slope of phase IV depolarization as one moves down the conducting system (Fig. 2.35). The

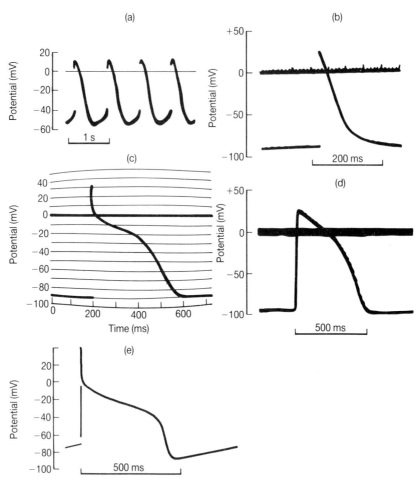

Fig. 2.35 The action potential has a different configuration in different parts of the heart. The sinoatrial node has the fastest phase IV depolarization and the greatest difference between the maximum diastolic potential and the threshold potential (**a**). The atrium (**b**) has a higher resting potential and a triangular shaped action potential. Purkinje fibres are sometimes quiescent (**c**) and sometimes show pacemaker activity (**e**). The ventricular fibres (**d**) have a much higher plateau and show no pacemaker activity. (Reproduced, with permission, from Noble.)

sinus node is under the influence of the vagus, which can influence its automaticity. The vagus has minimal effects on the automaticity of the latent pacemakers in the atrium or the His–Purkinje system.

Abnormal automaticity

Under certain conditions, ordinary atrial and ventricular cells, as well as specialized conducting tissue, may become capable of spontaneous impulse formation by phase IV depolarization. Thus in disease, the potential for impulse generation outside the sinoatrial node is increased.

Triggered activity

Cells exhibiting this mechanism may be quiescent in the absence of a stimulus. Once excited they give rise to two or more action potentials. This results in either early or late afterdepolarization or afterpotentials. The role of this mechanism in the genesis of arrhythmias in humans is not yet known.

Impulse conduction

Arrhythmias are more commonly caused by abnormalities of impulse propagation and conduction than impulse formation. Changes in local properties along the conduction pathway can result in decremental conduction. If a normal action potential encounters a region of myocardium with a slow conducting velocity, the amplitude of the propagating impulse gradually attenuates. Together with this loss of amplitude the impulse becomes a less adequate stimulus to unexcited tissues in its path. Severe decremental conduction will result in block.

The phenomenon of re-entry occurs when an impulse passes back through a region of the heart, re-exciting it. It is illustrated in Fig. 2.36. An impulse passing down through the muscle reaches a branching point with two divergent pathways, α and β. At some point further down the conducting pathway the two branches rejoin. Normally the impulse will pass down both the α and the β branches and reunite in the distal common pathway (Fig. 2.36a). In Fig. 2.36b a premature extrasystole passes down to the bifurcation to encounter pathways with different properties; the β pathway has a unidirectional block and so the impulse continues down the α pathway only. When it reaches the distal common pathway it is able to conduct down the common pathway; it is also able to conduct retrogradely up the β pathway (Fig. 2.36c). By the time the impulse reaches the proximal common pathway, it is able to conduct up it and also down the α pathway again (Fig. 2.36d). Thus repetitive re-entry can occur. This mechanism of re-entry can occur within the conducting system or anywhere within the

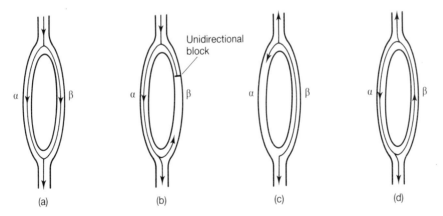

Fig. 2.36 Diagrammatic representation of re-entry. For description, see text.

myocardium. Sometimes a re-entry loop of this nature will fire repetitively and will supplant the normal pacemaker activity. In order for this phenomenon to occur, it is necessary for the time of conduction around the loop to be greater than the refractory time of the muscle. Thus conditions that produce slow conduction times or that shorten refractory times will predispose to re-entry arrhythmias.

Disorders of impulse formation

Sinus rhythm

In adults normal sinus rhythm is defined as a sinus node rate of 60–100/min. On the basis that conduction is normal, each P wave should be followed by a QRS complex (Fig. 2.37).

Sinus bradycardia

This is a slow sinus rhythm with a rate below 60/min (Fig. 2.38). It may be physiological, as in athletes or during sleep. It may be secondary to an acute infarct or to the sick sinus syndrome or to drugs such as β-adrenoceptor blockers. It may also be due to other medical conditions such as hypothyroidism, hypothermia or jaundice.

Sinus tachycardia

This is a fast sinus rhythm with a rate above 100/min. It may be a normal response to exercise, anxiety, fever or haemorrhage. It can occur in hyperthyroidism or other high output states.

Sinus arrhythmia

Gradual changes in rate associated with respiration are normally seen in young people. The rate usually increases with inspiration and is caused by changes in vagal tone.

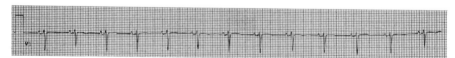

Fig. 2.37 Lead V$_1$, rhythm strip of a patient in sinus rhythm. Each P wave is followed by a QRS complex. The heart rate is 79/min.

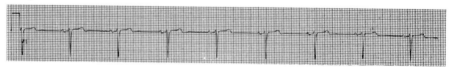

Fig. 2.38 Lead V$_1$, rhythm strip of a patient with a sinus bradycardia that was physiological. The heart rate is 52/min.

Extrasystole

An extrasystole is an impulse arising from the atria, the AV junction or the ventricles and which occurs prematurely in the cardiac cycle. Because the extrasystole is premature, the interval between it and the preceding beat (the coupling interval) is shorter than the cycle length of the dominant rhythm. Extrasystoles that arise from the same focus will tend to have the same coupling interval and the same configuration (Fig. 2.39). Other terms that are used synonymously include ectopic beats and premature contractions.

Atrial extrasystole

These are recognized by the occurrence of a premature P wave. Since the source and therefore the direction of atrial activation will be different from that during sinus rhythm, the P wave will be of abnormal shape (Fig. 2.40). Since they are premature, the P wave of the atrial premature beat may be hidden in the preceding T wave; these P waves can often be best seen in lead V_1 of the ECG. Most atrial extrasystoles are conducted to the ventricles in a manner similar to a normal sinus beat. Sometimes the atrial extrasystole, particularly if it is very

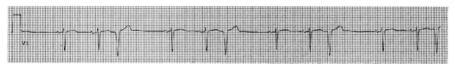

Fig. 2.39 Rhythm strip of lead V_1, showing sinus rhythm with premature contractions. The premature contractions have the same coupling interval (interval from preceding R wave of normal complex) and can therefore be assumed to be arising from the same focus. A P wave can be seen deforming the T wave of the premature beat; this P wave is occurring on time with the previous P–P interval. The premature contraction is followed by a full compensatory pause because the sinus node has been unaffected by the premature beat.

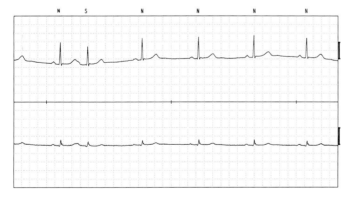

Fig. 2.40 Rhythm strip of simultaneously recorded leads V_5 and V_1 in a patient with a sinus bradycardia and an atrial premature beat. The first beat is a normal sinus beat which is followed by an atrial premature beat; the P wave of the premature beat is partially hidden in the T wave. The PR interval of the atrial premature beat is prolonged because the impulse encountered the atrioventricular node in a relatively refractory state.

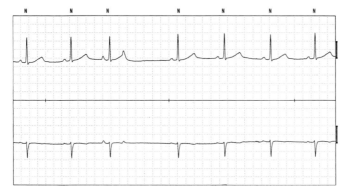

Fig. 2.41 Rhythm strips of leads V₅ and V₁ recorded simultaneously. The T wave of the third complex contains an atrial premature beat. This premature beat occurs so early that it encounters the atrioventricular node when it is absolutely refractory and no conduction occurs.

premature, may encounter the AV node or the bundle branches in a relative or absolute refractory state. If the AV node is absolutely refractory to the atrial extrasystole, no conduction takes place (Fig. 2.41) and it is blocked. If, on the other hand, the AV node is relatively refractory, the extrasystole is conducted but with a prolonged PR interval (see Fig. 2.40). Similarly, the bundle branches may be refractory at the time and lead to impairment of conduction in one or other branch. Since the right bundle branch has a longer refractory period, it is more common to get a right bundle branch block (RBBB) pattern with the extrasystole.

AV junctional extrasystoles

These used to be called nodal extrasystoles; it is now appreciated that a substantial part of the AV node is not capable of pacemaker activity. Moreover, it is not possible to distinguish between impulses arising from the bundle of His and the lower part of the AV node. The term junctional is therefore more satisfactory. The AV junctional extrasystole will produce a premature QRS complex that is similar in appearance to the normal sinus beat. The atria as well as the ventricles may be activated by the premature beat; there may be an inverted P wave in leads II and aVF, which may precede, follow or be buried within the QRS complex depending on the relative speeds of conduction from the AV junction to the atria and to the ventricles.

Ventricular extrasystoles

In contrast to atrial extrasystoles, there is no preceding P wave and the QRS complex is broad (usually >0.12 s) and bizarre in shape (Fig. 2.42). The shape and duration reflect the abnormal course of activation and the consequent slowing of ventricular activation. There is also an altered pattern of recovery which accounts for the abnormal ST segments and T waves.

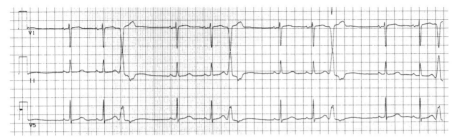

Fig. 2.42 Rhythm strip of simultaneously recorded leads V_1, II and V_5, showing sinus rhythm with premature ventricular complexes. The T wave of the premature complex is deformed by a P wave reflecting retrograde conduction through the AV node.

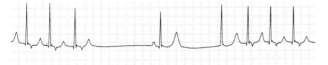

Fig. 2.43 A lead V_5 rhythm strip from a patient suffering from palpitation. The first three complexes are a junctional rhythm; the inverted P waves can be seen after each QRS complex. The fourth complex is a normal sinus beat. There is then a pause which is terminated by a QRS complex without a preceding P wave. This complex is a junctional escape beat which has a coupling interval that is greater than the dominant normal sinus rhythm. The junctional escape beat is then followed by a return of the junctional tachycardia.

Ventricular extrasystoles that occur very early may be superimposed on the T wave of the preceding complex; these are termed 'R on T' ventricular extra-systoles. It was once thought that this form of ventricular extrasystole was, particularly in an acutely ischaemic myocardium, likely to initiate a ventricular tachycardia or ventricular fibrillation. These rhythms have now been shown to be initiated as frequently by late extrasystoles.

The length of a pause after a ventricular extrasystole depends on whether the impulse is transmitted by the AV junction back to the atria. If there is no retrograde AV conduction the sinus node will be unaffected and there will be a full compensatory pause; the length of the cycles (RR interval) before and after the extrasystole will equal twice the sinus cycle length (Fig. 2.42). If the ventricular extrasystoles occur after each sinus beat the term 'ventricular bigemini' is used. If there is an extrasystole after every second sinus beat it is called 'ventricular trigemini'. If two ventricular extrasystoles occur together they are termed a couplet and if there are four or more it is termed ventricular tachycardia (see Fig. 2.56).

Escape beats

Escape beats arise from a subsidiary pacemaker when the dominant pacemaker fails to discharge. In direct contrast to extrasystoles or premature beats, they are late; the coupling interval is greater than that of the dominant rhythm (Fig. 2.43).

Escape beats can arise from the atria, the AV junction or the ventricles. Their site of origin can be determined by their configuration.

Tachycardias

The tachycardias can be considered under three main headings:

1. Supraventricular
2. Pre-excitation syndromes
3. Ventricular

Supraventricular tachycardia

A number of different tachycardias originate from the atria or AV junction (Table 2.5). Because they all arise from above the bundle branches, they all usually conduct normally, resulting in normal, narrow QRS complexes. Within this group there are major differences in the mechanisms of the arrhythmia, the ECG characteristics and the treatment.

Table 2.5 Tachycardias of supraventricular origin

Atrial tachycardia
Atrial flutter
Atrial fibrillation
Junctional tachycardia
AV re-entrant tachycardia

In atrial tachycardia the atrial rate is between 120 and 250/min. There may be a degree of AV block, which effectively protects the ventricles from being forced to adopt a very fast rate. The P waves are often best demonstrated in lead V_1 (Fig. 2.44). This condition is distinguished from atrial flutter by the atrial rate and the ECG evidence of a flat baseline between the P waves.

In atrial flutter the atria discharge at a rate of 250–350/min. In most instances a degree of AV block develops. The extremely fast atrial activity is reflected by flutter waves on the ECG (Fig. 2.45). There is usually no isoelectric line between them, so the baseline has a saw-tooth appearance.

Atrial fibrillation is characterized by an atrial discharge rate of 350–600/min. This chaotic activity is caused by individual atrial muscle fibres contracting independently; this is in contrast to the other supraventricular tachycardias where synchronous contraction occurs, albeit at an abnormal rate. There are no P waves and the ventricular response is irregular although the QRS complexes are usually normal in shape and duration (Fig. 2.46).

A junctional focus may activate both the ventricles and the atria. The QRS complexes may be preceded by or succeeded by an inverted P wave (Fig. 2.47). The P wave may, alternatively, be lost within the normal shaped QRS complex.

The main basic mechanism in the above arrhythmias is related to enhanced automaticity of atrial ectopic foci or of an AV junctional focus.

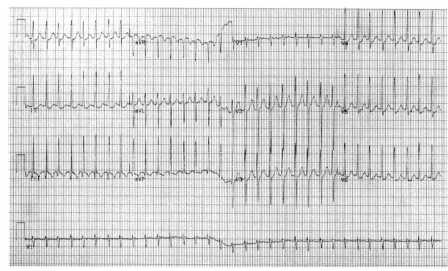

Fig. 2.44 ECG showing an atrial tachycardia with a rate of 200/min. There is a flat baseline between the P waves which, together with the rate, distinguish it from atrial flutter.

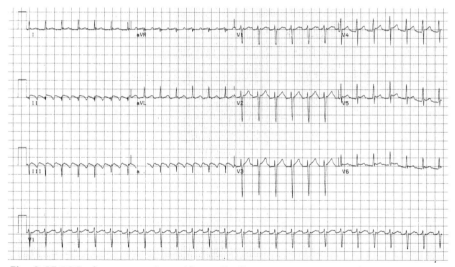

Fig. 2.45 ECG of a patient with atrial flutter. The flutter rate is approximately 300/min and the ventricular rate 150/min. The saw-toothed appearance is seen best in leads III and aVf, and there is no isoelectric line between the waves.

The mechanism of an AV re-entrant tachycardia is the repeated circulation of an impulse between atria and ventricles. The impulse is usually conducted from atria to ventricles by normal AV conduction and then re-enters the atria via an additional pathway; this additional pathway may lie within the AV node although it is functionally separate. It may, alternatively, be an anatomically distinct

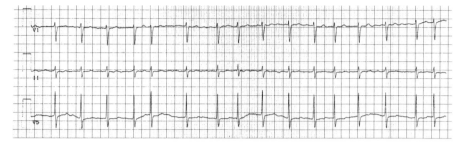

Fig. 2.46 Rhythm strip of leads V_1, II and V_5, showing atrial fibrillation. The atrial discharge rate is difficult to discern but is in the region of 350–600/min. There are no P waves and the ventricular rhythm is irregularly irregular.

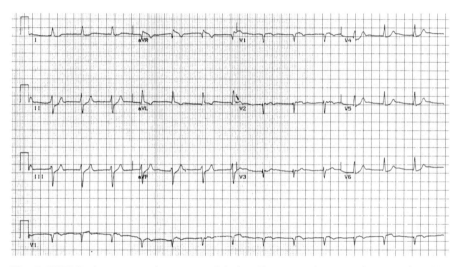

Fig. 2.47 ECG of a patient with a junctional rhythm. The ventricular rate in this example is 82/min. There are no P waves preceding the QRS complexes. The P waves can be seen best in lead V_2, where they are seen as a ripple in each succeeding T wave.

pathway between the atria and ventricles which is described below. The ECG characteristics are those of a regular tachycardia with usually normal duration and shape of QRS complexes; a right bundle branch block may develop at fast rates. The ventricular rate is usually 130–250/min. Since the circulating impulse re-enters the atria after ventricular activation there will always be a 1:1 relationship between atrial and ventricular activity (Fig. 2.48). Several terms are used to describe these arrhythmias; they include AV junctional re-entrant, reciprocating atrial or reciprocating junctional tachycardia. The term used should indicate the mechanism involved; for instance, the use of the term 'atrial tachycardia' for this particular arrhythmia is incorrect, since this is used to describe a tachycardia due to enhanced automaticity.

Pre-excitation syndromes

In a normal heart the atrial impulse can be conducted to the ventricles only via the AV node and bundle of His which pass through the fibrous skeleton. In the pre-excitation syndromes there is an additional connection between the atria and ventricles. This accessory bundle does not delay the conduction like the AV node. An atrial impulse can therefore be transmitted rapidly down this accessory bundle and will initiate ventricular activation before the impulse has passed through the AV node. Pre-excitation is said to be present when some part of the ventricular myocardium is activated earlier than would be expected if the impulse reached the ventricles by way of the normal specialized conducting system.

The AV node has a shorter refractory period than the accessory bundle; thus an appropriately timed premature beat is likely to be conducted anterogradely through the AV node at a time when the accessory pathway is in a refractory state. When the impulse has passed through the AV node, the accessory bundle will have recovered and is then able to pass the impulse retrogradely back up to the atria, thus precipitating the re-entry tachycardia (see Fig. 2.36).

In the Wolff–Parkinson–White (WPW) syndrome the accessory bundle is composed of ordinary myocardium and is called a bundle of Kent. This bundle may be situated anywhere in the AV groove. Because the bundle of Kent is not connected to specialized conducting tissue in the ventricular septum, early ventricular activation is relatively slow; this accounts for the characteristic ECG changes of a short PR interval and the delta wave (Fig. 2.49). Once the atrial impulse has traversed the AV node it fuses with the aberrant impulse and the subsequent conduction proceeds normally. Since the septum is activated in this abnormal manner, Q waves are produced which can be mistaken for a myocardial infarction. Two arrhythmias can occur in this condition. Atrial fibrillation is relatively uncommon but potentially dangerous because of the risk of ventricular fibrillation ensuing; in this instance the anterograde conduction may be down the accessory bundle. The more common arrhythmia is an AV re-entrant tachycardia in which conduction is usually antegrade down through the AV node. This arrhythmia is benign although it may cause distressing symptoms.

The Lown–Ganong–Levine pre-excitation syndrome differs in that the accessory connection travels between the atrial muscle and the bundle of His. This

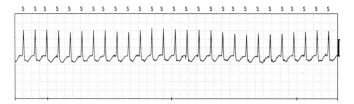

Fig. 2.48 ECG of a patient with recurrent palpitation who is known to have a Lown–Ganong–Levine (LGL) pre-excitation syndrome. The paper speed is 25 mm/s. The rhythm is regular and at a rate of 214/min. The QRS complexes are narrow. Atrial activity is difficult to identify. This is a reciprocating junctional tachycardia.

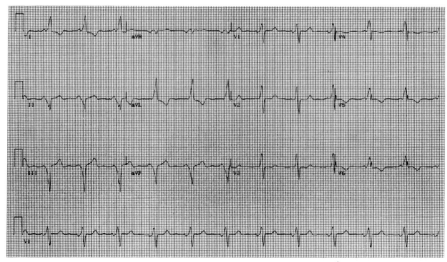

Fig. 2.49 ECG demonstrating the Wolff–Parkinson–White syndrome. The PR interval is very short (80 ms) and there is a delta wave which causes a slurred upstroke to the QRS complex.

manifests itself on the ECG as a very short PR interval without the delta wave (Fig. 2.50). Patients with this condition have re-entrant AV tachycardias.

Ventricular tachycardia

Ventricular tachycardia is defined as four or more ventricular extrasystoles in rapid succession. The rate is usually between 120 and 250/min. The ventricular complexes are abnormal in shape and duration (see Fig. 2.56). They are usually broader than 0.12 s, and they are usually slightly irregular. Atrial activity can continue to be initiated by the sinoatrial node and, because there is no retrograde conduction from the ventricles, continues to proceed independently. This can be seen in the ECG and may need to be specifically sought by examination of particular leads in order to make a diagnosis of the arrhythmia (Fig. 2.51). Alternatively, in some ventricular tachycardias there is retrograde atrial conduction so that each ventricular complex is followed by an inverted P wave which may be concealed in the T wave.

Torsade de pointes is an atypical ventricular arrhythmia that is characterized by repeated gradual changes in the QRS axis so that they appear to twist around the baseline like a twisted streamer (Fig. 2.52). It is important to recognize because its treatment is very different from that of the more common ventricular tachycardia. It can sometimes occur in conditions that produce a long QT interval; these can be hereditary in origin or can be caused by certain drugs such as the phenothiazines.

Ventricular fibrillation is the rapid, chaotic and incoordinate contraction of ventricular myocardial fibres (Fig. 2.53). It causes immediate circulatory arrest. When it occurs in a heart that was functioning satisfactorily in sinus rhythm, it is

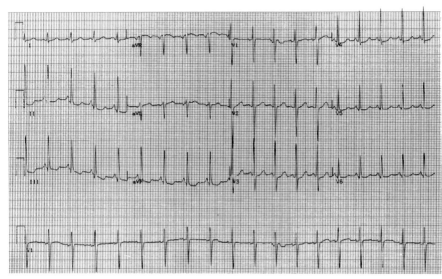

Fig. 2.50 ECG demonstrating the Lown–Ganong–Levine syndrome. The PR interval is very short but there are no delta waves. This patient had episodes of a re-entrant atrioventricular tachycardia, shown in Fig. 2.48.

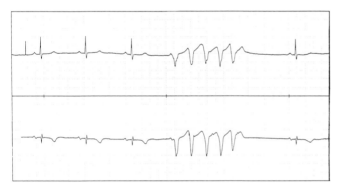

Fig. 2.51 An episode of ventricular tachycardia occurring during a 24-hour ambulatory recording. Two leads are recorded simultaneously: V_5 above and V_1 below. On the lower recording, P waves can be seen clearly within the ventricular tachycardia, and bear no relationship to the QRS complexes.

termed primary ventricular fibrillation; if it occurs in the context of heart failure or cardiogenic shock, it is called secondary. Successful treatment is very much less likely in the latter type.

Analysis of an arrhythmia

The analysis of an arrhythmia can be considered under two main headings. The analysis of the electrocardiographic recording is where most people will first

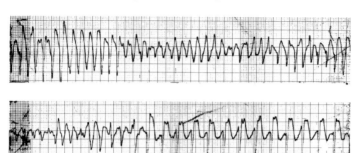

Fig. 2.52 Rhythm strip of a patient presenting with syncope. The rhythm is torsade de pointes – an atypical ventricular arrhythmia characterized by repeated gradual change in the QRS axis, which appears to twist round the baseline like a twisted streamer. To the left of the rhythm strip the point of the QRS complex appears downwards; by the middle of the strip it has rotated slowly round to point upwards and then to the right it is again pointing downwards.

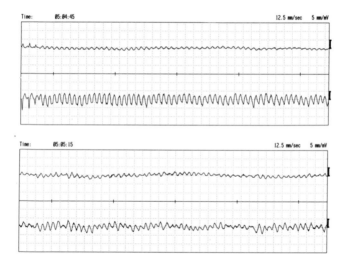

Fig. 2.53 Ventricular fibrillation occurring in a patient who collapsed during 24-hour ambulatory monitoring. Two leads are recorded simultaneously: V_5 above and V_1 below. The paper speed is 12.5 mm/s and the calibration (shown on the right) 5 mm/mV. The first two complexes in the top tracings are the patient's usual rhythm. He then develops a ventricular flutter/tachycardia which progresses to ventricular fibrillation.

turn. However, a lot of information can be gleaned from the clinical evaluation of the patient.

The clinical evaluation

Many arrhythmic episodes are asymptomatic. In the patient presenting with symptoms related to an arrhythmia, the mode of onset, the duration, the description of the sensation and the associated features are all useful information.

The knowledge of the situation in which the arrhythmia occurs is very helpful; the awareness of the heart action when under stress is very common. A patient may become aware of this sensation and present with the symptom of palpitation, an awareness of the heart action. In this instance palpitation may be physiological and related to a sinus tachycardia that is made obvious by the catecholamine release associated with the stress. The patient may well be able to describe the fact that the rhythm is regular and strong and the onset is gradual. In contrast, the patient with an AV re-entrant tachycardia of 180/min will describe the sudden onset of this rhythm and may illustrate this with non-verbal communication such as the flicking of the fingers. Extrasystoles can often be described accurately by patients; they are aware of extra beats that occur intermittently although they can be very frequent. They are sometimes aware of the powerful thump of the contraction that follows the compensatory pause. Alternatively, they may be aware of the gap that follows the extrasystole and become afraid lest the heart will stop. Patients with paroxysmal atrial fibrillation will often be aware of the extreme irregularity of the heart action.

At the bedside there is also information to be gleaned. If the patient is in atrial fibrillation the pulse will be irregularly irregular and remain so with exercise; there may be a pulse deficit when the apical rate is simultaneously counted; there will be a loss of the A wave in the venous pulse. In contrast, the patient with extrasystoles will have a pulse that is basically regular with an intermittent irregularity; this irregularity will disappear with mild exertion which speeds up the intrinsic normal rhythm. In the patient with a sustained tachycardia the features that suggest a supraventricular origin are: it is regular; the first heart sound is of the same intensity; and it may slow dramatically with carotid sinus massage which, by altering vagal tone, introduces a degree of block to AV conduction. If the rhythm is that of a junctional tachycardia there will be regular cannon waves at the same rate as the ventricular; these will be visible in the venous pulse in the neck. A ventricular tachycardia will usually be regular, the first heart sound will vary in intensity and there will be little change with carotid sinus massage; irregular cannon waves will be present in the venous pulse.

In the context of a patient with a bradycardia the following features will suggest complete, or third degree, AV block: a heart rate of less than 40/min that does not increase with exercise; and varying intensity of the first heart sound and intermittent cannon waves in the venous pulse. Cannon waves are caused by the atrium contracting at a time when the AV valve is closed or closing; the pressure wave is thus reflected up the neck as a characteristic flicking wave. A sinus bradycardia will have none of these features.

The electrocardiogram

Some arrhythmias are so simple to diagnose that only a few complexes are required to make the diagnosis. The more complex arrhythmia requires a long rhythm strip, ideally with several leads recorded simultaneously. The key to the analysis is the identification of the P wave; sometimes this is hard to find because it is buried in the T wave of the preceding complex. Once it has been identified, its relationship with the QRS complexes can be established and the mechanism of the arrhythmia determined. One of the more common and difficult problems is that of determining the mechanism of a rhythm such as that displayed in Fig. 2.54. The P waves cannot be found in any lead. The features that help distinguish a ventricular origin from a supraventricular one are shown in Table 2.6.

Table 2.6   Features that help distinguish a ventricular from a supraventricular arrhythmia

	Supraventricular	Ventricular
Duration of QRS complex	Narrow	Broad
Evidence of independent atrial activity	Absent	Present
Response to carotid sinus massage	Often responds dramatically	Little response
QRS complexes similar to ventricular extrasystoles	No	Yes
Shape in V_1	RSR	Rs or Qr
Similar QRS vector across chest leads	No	Yes

An important myth to dispel is that a ventricular tachycardia always causes severe haemodynamic upset. The rhythm can often be well tolerated. In contrast, a patient with a supraventricular arrhythmia who also has underlying heart disease or valve abnormality may be rendered extremely unwell.

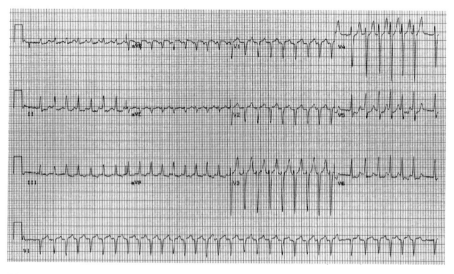

Fig. 2.54 ECG of patient who collapsed in the street. The ventricular rate is 196/min. There are no discernible P waves. The QRS duration is normal. The rhythm is atrial fibrillation with a fast ventricular response.

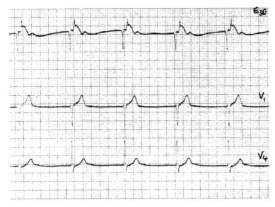

Fig. 2.55 Three leads of a patient with a bradycardia. Leads V₁ and V₄ show ventricular complexes without any P waves. The oesophageal lead placed 30 cm from the mouth (E30) shows the P wave hidden in each T wave. The rhythm can thus be confirmed to be a junctional bradycardia.

Other investigations can be employed to help diagnose the mechanism of an arrhythmia. An oesophageal recording electrode is easy to site and gives valuable information. The oesophagus lies just behind the left atrium. The atrial complex recorded from this site will be relatively large (Fig. 2.55). Not only will the atrial activity be more easily identified but the atrial vector, and therefore the site of the origin of the arrhythmia, also can be determined. This information may alternatively be obtained by introducing a pacing catheter into the atrium and recording from it. More sophisticated electrophysiological studies using numerous recording electrodes can be employed to map both normal and abnormal rhythms.

Adenosine given intravenously can help distinguish between a supraventricular and a ventricular tachycardia. It slows AV nodal conduction and can stop a supraventricular tachyarrhythmia but will have little effect on a ventricular tachycardia. It has a very short half-life.

Abnormalities of rhythm are often intermittent and difficult to document; 24-hour ambulatory monitoring is of considerable help because patients are able to carry on with their normal activities during the recording. Two leads are recorded simultaneously and the interpretation is aided by computer analysis (Fig. 2.56).

Treatment of arrhythmias

General measures

The treatment of an arrhythmia starts with a careful clinical assessment of the patient. It needs to be determined whether the rhythm abnormality is a manifestation of an underlying condition, such as heart failure, or whether it is occurring as an isolated abnormality. Conditions that influence the expression of an arrhythmia include the presence of underlying heart or valvular disease,

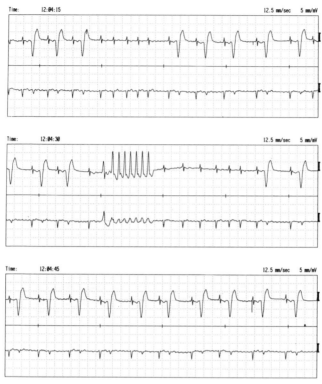

Fig. 2.56 Ambulatory monitoring analysis. Two leads are recorded simultaneously; this will aid analysis of the arrhythmias. The recording is at 12.5 mm/s and at 5 mm/mV calibration. In this patient the rhythm is atrial fibrillation with numerous ventricular premature beats, ventricular bigemini and ventricular tachycardia.

pulmonary disease, endocrine or autonomic imbalance, concurrent drug administration, electrolyte abnormalities, excess alcohol or caffeine or other drugs, excessive dieting and psychological disturbance.

Extrasystoles

Since extrasystoles are found in normal hearts, it is important that they are not treated unnecessarily. They may also occur in abnormal hearts and in association with some of the conditions mentioned above. The first step in their management is therefore to determine the context in which they are occurring. They very rarely require treatment in their own right; the management of the underlying condition is more important. The patient will need reassurance for the symptom of palpitation.

Bradycardias

The management of chronic conduction disturbances causing a persistent or intermittent bradycardia hinges on the question of the need for artificial electrical pacing. A sinus bradycardia does not usually require treatment. The sick sinus syndrome is a condition in which there is evidence of dysfunction of the sinus node and of AV conduction in association with atrial tachycardias and bradycardias. It is sometimes called the brady–tachy syndrome and can be very difficult to treat. Sometimes, if there are long pauses, pacemaker insertion is required and will improve the symptoms (Fig. 2.57). In patients with inter-mittent or permanent complete AV block causing Stokes–Adams attacks, permanent pacing is mandatory. Untreated syncopal attacks of this nature can be fatal. Even in the absence of these Stokes–Adams attacks the heart function may be improved by increasing the ventricular rate by pacing. Temporary pacing may be required in a patient who sustains an acute myocardial infarction and develops progressive AV block. This acute AV block will usually resolve over the ensuing 24 hours and the temporary pacemaker can be removed.

An artificial pacemaker is an electronic device that generates stimuli that are delivered to the endocardium or myocardium by a pacing electrode. The pacemaker may be used on a temporary basis when the problem is transient, or it may be implanted permanently. A permanent transvenous pacemaker can be implanted under local anaesthesia with minimal risk (see Fig. 1.32). Pacemaker technology has become very sophisticated, such that the pacemaker can both sense and stimulate the atria and the ventricles; it can also be programmed externally. A simple fixed rate pacemaker will deliver an impulse at a regular interval irrespective of any spontaneous ventricular activity. A demand pace-maker will stimulate the ventricle only if there is no spontaneous ventricular activity within a preset interval. An AV sequential pacemaker will sense atrial contraction and deliver the ventricular stimulus; in this way atrial transport is preserved and the pacemaker is responsive to the changing atrial rates that normally occur during the day and night.

Tachycardias

Some tachycardias cause little problem to the patient and will disappear spon-taneously if allowed to; more harm may come from treating them than by just giving firm reassurance! As a broad generalization, doctors tend to over-react to tachycardias and under-react to bradycardias.

Certain of the supraventricular tachycardias can be terminated by manoeuvres that increase vagal tone. These include carotid sinus massage, the Valsava manoeuvre, swallowing cold ice-cream and the induction of retching. These can

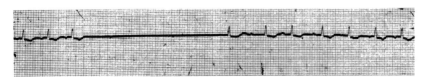

Fig. 2.57 Lead III rhythm strip of a patient presenting with dizzy spells. The first three sinus beats are followed by both sinus arrest and absence of any lower pacemaker for an interval of 3.84 s. There follows a junctional escape beat and three atrial beats with long PR intervals before sinus rhythm resumes.

all be taught to a patient who is troubled by recurrent tachycardias. The pressing on the eyeballs is not to be encouraged because it can cause a retinal detachment.

Drugs have a major role to play in the treatment of tachycardias but they all have limitations in their use. They can be classified in two ways: by their principal site of action (Fig. 2.58) or, alternatively, according to their effect on the transmembrane potential of the myocardial cell (Fig. 2.59).

Class I drugs (Fig. 2.60) impede the transport of sodium across the cell membrane and thereby reduce the rate of rise of the action potential (phase 0). This class has now been subdivided into:

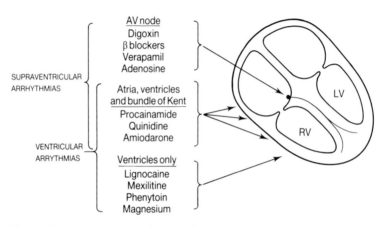

Fig. 2.58 The principal site of action of antiarrhythmic drugs on the heart.

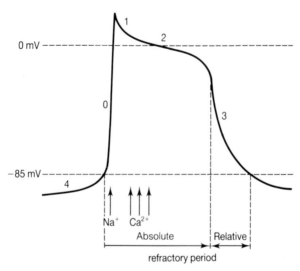

Fig. 2.59 Myocardial cell action potential, showing phases 0–4. The timing of the fast sodium channel is signified by '↑ Na' and the slow calcium channel by '↑ Ca²⁺'.

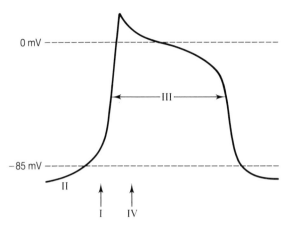

Fig. 2.60 Myocardial cell action potential showing site of action of classes of antiarrhythmic drugs.

IA. These drugs also prolong the action potential and therefore have a mild class III effect. Included in this group are quinidine and procainamide.

IB. These drugs also shorten the action potential. Included in this group are lignocaine and mexiletine and phenytoin

IC. These drugs also inhibit conduction down the His–Purkinje system. Included in this group are flecainide and propafenone.

Class II drugs are β-adrenergic blocking drugs.

Class III drugs act only on the repolarization phase of the action potential and prolong the action potential. They therefore prolong the QT interval. Included in this group are amiodarone, sotalol and bretylium. All these drugs have additional properties.

Class IV drugs inhibit the slow calcium channel. Included in this group are verapamil and diltiazem. The potassium channel openers are indirect calcium antagonists. They hyperpolarize the cell membrane, thereby moving the polarity away from that required to open the slow calcium channel. They are particularly useful in supraventricular tachycardia with a re-entrant circuit. Adenosine and adenosine triphosphate (ATP) are in this group.

If drugs are ineffective, or if the clinical circumstances necessitate an immediate return to sinus rhythm, DC cardioversion is the best approach. This technique is covered in Chapter 12. Artificial pacing can also be used to terminate an arrhythmia.

A number of drugs may be of prophylactic value in the treatment of intermittent supraventricular arrhythmias. Before embarking on prophylactic drug therapy it is important to recognize that, for a large part of the time, the patient will be in sinus rhythm; if the arrhythmia occurs spontaneously only once in every 3 months, is there much sense in treating the patient prophylactically? Sometimes the answer is yes, but often it may be wise to give the patient the appropriate drug to take whenever an episode occurs and does not respond to the usual measures. The drugs that can be used are shown in Fig. 2.58. Selection of the most effective and acceptable drug is usually one of trial and error. Some drugs have to be used with particular care because of their pro-arrhythmic effect; they can actually predispose to the generation of arrhythmias. This applies particularly to drugs in classes IA and III. If drugs are ineffective or cannot be tolerated, pacing techniques or ablation of part of the re-entrant circuit can be considered.

The main aim of treatment in chronic atrial fibrillation is to control the ventricular rate by slowing conduction through the AV node. The most useful and effective drug is digoxin. Restoration and maintenance of sinus rhythm is difficult unless the cause of the atrial fibrillation has been removed; an example of this is hyperthyroidism.

The principles of the treatment of intermittent ventricular tachycardia are similar to those of the supraventricular. The drugs that can be used are shown in Fig. 2.58.

The treatment of ventricular fibrillation is discussed in Chapter 12.

Further reading

Marriott, H. J. L. (1988) *Practical Electrocardiography*. Williams & Wilkins, Baltimore.

Rowlands, D. J. (1991) *Clinical Electrocardiography*. Gower Medical, Alder-shot.

3

CIRCULATORY FAILURE

The normal

In the normally functioning cardiovascular system, blood is transferred from the low pressure venous side to the high pressure arterial circulation. The heart provides an output of adequate volume tailored to the needs of the tissues. The venous and arterial circulations play their part by governing volume and peripheral resistance respectively. Changes in the factors controlling vascular tone and blood volume are important in the manifestations of circulatory failure.

Circulatory failure

Although cardiac output and venous return are inextricably linked in health and disease, it is helpful to consider circumstances in which one or the other is primarily at fault.

Circulatory failure is a general term that describes the inadequacy of the cardiovascular system to perform its basic function of providing nutrition to, and removing metabolic products from, the cells of the body. It may be caused by impaired function of the heart. In practice this must be distinguished from circulatory failure due to non-cardiac causes such as an inadequate blood volume typically due to bleeding, reduced venous return such as a vasovagal faint, peripheral vascular abnormalities as can occur in Gram-negative septicaemia, or an inadequate level of oxyhaemoglobin.

Circulatory overload or circulatory congestion are terms that refer to excess blood volume which may be caused by impaired function of the heart. It must be distinguished from the non-cardiac causes, which include conditions in which the primary defect is an increase in blood volume; this can be secondary to retention of salt and water caused by salt-retaining steroids or anti-inflammatory agents, to excess blood or fluid administration, or to other medical conditions such as an acute glomerulonephritis. An increased venous return can also result in a circulatory overload secondary to a high output heart failure; examples of this include arteriovenous fistulae or thiamine deficiency causing beriberi.

103

Table 3.1   A classification of circulatory failure and circulatory overload

Circulatory failure	Heart failure Non-cardiac circulatory failure: 1. Decreased return of blood to the heart because of inadequate blood volume 2. Increased capacity of vascular bed 3. Peripheral vascular abnormalities or disease 4. Inadequate oxyhaemoglobin
Circulatory overload	Heart failure Non-cardiac circulatory overload: 1. Increase in blood volume 2. Increase in venous return and/or decrease in peripheral vascular resistance

Symptoms of heart failure

Limitation of exercise tolerance

Limitation of exercise tolerance is a major manifestation of left or right ventricular disease. It is therefore important to establish whether such limitation is present, taking into account the patient's sex, age and background. Once the presence of a limited exercise tolerance has been established, its severity should be specified in terms of everyday activities which are readily defined. At its most severe patients may be breathless walking across a room or brushing their teeth; it can be further defined by the distance they can walk on the flat, on an incline or on flights of stairs. There are some more formal and objective measures of exercise tolerance.

Fatigue

Patients with heart disease are often very troubled by fatigue in addition to the exhaustion and breathlessness that are immediately related to exertion. This symptom is due to low cardiac output and poor peripheral blood flow; it can also occur as a result of excessive drug-induced diuresis.

Faintness on exertion

This is due to arterial hypotension and is an important symptom. It usually results from the combination of a fixed cardiac output and a normal reduction in peripheral resistance associated with exercise. It is seen in aortic stenosis, in pulmonary stenosis and can occur after exertion with hypertrophic cardiomyopathy. It may also occur in coronary artery disease, where it is an ominous sign of severe disease.

Breathlessness

Breathlessness on exertion is a very common symptom. The severity can be gauged on scales relating to activity.

Orthopnoea

This is the symptom of breathlessness that occurs when the patient lies down and is relieved by sitting up. The severity of the symptom may be judged by the number of pillows used. In severe cases the patient can sleep only when sitting in a chair. Although this symptom is very suggestive of a cardiac rather than a respiratory problem, some patients with bronchial asthma or with severe lung disease may be more comfortable sleeping while sitting up. Some patients may experience a dry cough when lying down which is also relieved by sitting up; this may have the same pathophysiological basis.

Paroxysmal nocturnal dyspnoea

The severity of this symptom may vary. In a mild form patients may wake with a sense of unease which is easily relieved by sitting at the side of the bed. In its most severe form patients typically describe suffocating breathlessness that wakes them up in the middle of the night and which is finally relieved by standing up or opening the window 'for some fresh air'. This condition can sometimes be termed cardiac asthma since there may be an associated wheeze due to broncho-spasm. It is important to distinguish it from bronchial asthma.

Acute pulmonary oedema

This is the most severe form of breathlessness and can sometimes result in death. The attack may begin with a dry cough and a feeling of intense breathlessness. The breathlessness increases, with profound anxiety and the production of pink frothy sputum representing intra-alveolar oedema.

Cheyne–Stokes respiration

This is observed in patients with either chronic pulmonary oedema or a low output state, and may also be a distressing symptom. It consists of alternating periods of hyperventilation and apnoea, which can be particularly frightening at night both to the patient and to the spouse. It may also contribute to the restlessness and insomnia that are associated with heart failure (Fig. 3.1).

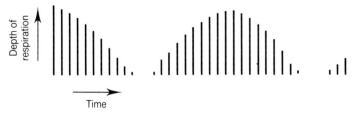

Fig. 3.1 Cheyne–Stokes respiration, demonstrating cyclical periods of hyperventilation and apnoea.

Pain

Chest pain or discomfort caused by myocardial ischaemia is described in Chapter 1. Patients with heart failure who have a high systemic venous pressure may experience pain due to distension of the liver capsule. This pain can be experienced over the lower part of the sternum or under the right costal margin. It can be mistaken for pain arising from a peptic ulcer or pain arising from myocardial ischaemia. Occasionally, because the liver is tender to touch, it can be incorrectly ascribed to pain arising from a ruptured abdominal viscus.

Sweating

Nocturnal sweating is a frequent symptom that is encountered in patients with heart failure. It may antedate the clinical evidence of heart failure; it is partly due to the release of catecholamines which occur as a compensatory mechanism in the failing heart and partly due to a need to lose body heat through sweating because it cannot be dissipated properly via the constricted skin circulation.

Weight loss

Cardiac cachexia may occur in the late stages of severe heart failure. Protein-losing enteropathy, hypermetabolism, poor appetite, mental depression and cellular hypoxia all contribute to this weight loss.

Signs of heart failure

A considerable amount of information about the presence or the nature and severity of heart disease can be obtained by careful clinical examination. In order to illustrate the importance of the examination and the information that can be gained from it, four thumbnail sketches are described. They will be referred to in the text.

Case 1

A 45-year-old insurance salesman presented with a history of increasing shortness of breath over 3 months. He had suffered three myocardial infarctions in the past 5 years. In the past week he had noted shortness of breath at rest and particularly when he lay down. He had noted swollen ankles for the past 5 days.

On examination he looked pale, clammy and unwell. He had mild central cyanosis. His blood pressure was 90/65/65 mmHg and he had a regular pulse of 124/min. His respiratory rate was 20/min. He had bilateral crackles at the bases. His venous pressure was elevated 10 cm above the sternal angle. He had some ankle oedema. His apex was displaced outside the mid-clavicular line and there was a gallop rhythm. There was reversed splitting of the second heart sound.

Case 2

A 35-year-old actress presented with a history of having fainted while at work. She had felt tired and easily fatigued over the previous 5 days. She was a heavy smoker and had a history of dyspepsia. On direct questioning it was clear that she had been having melaena for the past 2 days.

On examination she looked pale, clammy and unwell; this became more marked when she sat up, which caused her to become dizzy. Her peripheries were very cool to the touch. Her blood pressure was 90/65/65 mmHg and she had a regular pulse of 124/min. Her respiratory rate was 18/min. Her venous pressure was difficult to see but was thought to be low. Her lung fields were clear and the heart sounds normal.

Case 3

A 68-year-old female antique dealer was admitted through casualty after a fall on the ice. She was seen following her operation to repair her fractured femur because she was said to have heart failure. Her condition proved to be due to overenthusiastic intravenous transfusion with blood and colloids.

On examination she looked unwell. Her blood pressure was 110/75/70 mmHg. Her pulse was regular at a rate of 115/min. Her venous pressure was raised to 8 cm above the sternal angle. She had crackles at both her lung bases. Her heart apex beat was normal in character and site. Her heart sounds were normal and there was no gallop rhythm.

Case 4

A 65-year-old male lorry driver presented with a history of increasing shortness of breath. He had been a life-long smoker and was known by his general practitioner to have chronic bronchitis with obstructive airways disease. More recently his shortness of breath had become worse and he had noted ankle swelling.

On examination he looked unwell and was centrally cyanosed. He had a respiratory rate of 26/min. His pulse was irregular in rhythm and volume at a rate of between 110 and 120/min. His blood pressure was 110/75/70 mmHg. His venous pressure was elevated 9 cm above the sternal angle and rose with inspiration. His apex beat was normal in site and character. There was a parasternal heave. He had a gallop rhythm which was best heard at the left sternal edge. Pulmonary closure was accentuated. His lungs had widespread rhonchi or wheezes and some coarse crackles. There was both leg and sacral oedema together with ascites and hepatomegaly.

Physical examination

Observation of the patient

Careful observation of the patient can yield a lot of useful clinical information. The perfusion of the peripheries (i.e. the face, hands and feet) is affected in heart failure; the patient may be pale, clammy with cold hands and feet, together with a pinched appearance which can be associated with a tinge of central and peripheral cyanosis. These features are most marked in cases 1 and 2 where cardiac output is compromised: the first due to a cardiac cause and the second due to a circulatory problem.

The respiratory rate is a good index of the adequacy of gaseous exchange; this may be disturbed in heart failure. The work of both breathing and also giving a history may be difficult and be associated with a fast respiratory rate. The depth of respiration will tend to be shallow in heart failure, in contrast to the slower distressed breathing of a patient with asthma. In order to breathe most comfortably, the patient will want to sit upright in bed.

The arterial pulse

A sinus tachycardia is a common finding, in which case the pulse is regular in time and force (cases 1–3) and it may be poor in volume. Sinus arrhythmia does not occur. An excessive ventricular rate may be due to atrial fibrillation (case 4), in which case it will be irregular and of variable volume. In either case the ventricular rate may be well controlled at rest but rises rapidly at low levels of exercise.

Pulsus alternans

Pulsus alternans describes the situation in which alternate arterial pulses are weak and strong (Fig. 3.2). This occurs with regular sinus rhythm and must be distinguished from pulsus bigeminus which is due to alternate premature atrial or ventricular beats. Pulsus alternans is a reliable sign of ventricular disease.

Abnormality of the venous pulse

Careful examination of the jugular venous pulse enables a direct measurement to be made of the right atrial pressure (Fig. 3.3). This is clinically important in distinguishing patients whose poor circulatory state is due to inadequate blood volume (case 2) from those with venous congestion whether this is due to heart failure (cases 1 and 4) or some other cause (case 3). The commonest convention is to measure the vertical height in centimetres above the sternal angle which, apart from extremes of position, is about 5 cm above the centre of the right

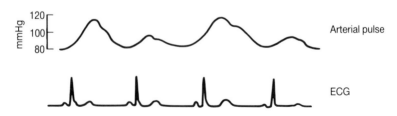

Fig. 3.2 Pulsus alternans, illustrating the alternating strength of the arterial pulse while the patient is in sinus rhythm.

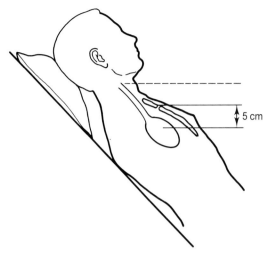

5 cm

Fig. 3.3 Examination of the jugular venous pulse, illustrating the ability to measure the right atrial pressure direct.

atrium. The unit of measurement is centimetres of blood. It is necessary to find the best position for the patient so that the top of the pulsating column is visualized; lying the patient at about 40 degrees is often the most satisfactory angle. If the venous pressure is low, the patient will need to be lying flatter in order for the venous pulsation to be seen above the clavicle; conversely, if the venous pressure is high then the patient may need to be sitting more upright. The change in position does not materially alter the vertical height of the venous pressure above the sternal angle or above the right atrium (Fig. 3.4). In health the height of the column above the sternal angle is no more than 3–4 cm; the normal right atrial pressure is therefore 8–9 cm of blood. To convert this to millimetres of mercury the pressure in centimetres of blood is divided by 1.36 (the specific gravity of mercury is 13.6).

The height of the venous pressure falls during inspiration as a result of the decreased intrathoracic pressure. A rise with inspiration suggests pericardial tamponade or right ventricular disease (case 4).

The waveform of the venous pulse will also give valuable information. The normal waveform consists of an a wave and a v wave together with the x and y descents (Fig. 3.5). The a wave reflects atrial contraction and is a brief, characteristically flicking, wave that precedes the onset of the upstroke of the carotid pulse. It becomes exaggerated when there is an increased resistance to right atrial emptying such as occurs in right ventricular hypertrophy. The x descent reflects atrial relaxation and the downward movement of the atrio-ventricular valve ring. In atrial fibrillation the a wave is absent. The v wave represents accumulating blood in the right atrium when the tricuspid valve is closed. The y descent signifies early diastolic filling of the right ventricle. An exaggerated v wave occurs in tricuspid regurgitation; with more severe tricuspid regurgitation the wave is more correctly referred to as a systolic wave or s wave, since it starts early in systole and then merges with the v wave.

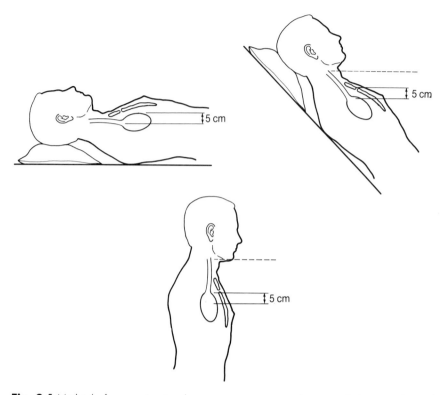

Fig. 3.4 Method of measuring jugular venous pressure as the vertical distance above the sternal angle, which is always 5 cm above the right atrial level regardless of the position of the patient.

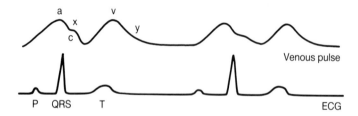

Fig. 3.5 Waveform of the normal venous pulse in relation to the ECG.

One of the main sources of confusion in trying to elicit the characteristics of the venous pulse is the need to use the internal jugular vein. The external jugular vein is not suitable because of its tortuous path through the clavipectoral fascia; it also has valves within it. The merit of the internal jugular vein is that it is a direct connection with the right atrium. The internal jugular vein lies deep to the sternomastoid muscle; it is in fact the movement of the muscle that is visualized. Therefore the patient's head must be relaxed and supported. Good light must fall from behind the patient onto the neck, thus creating a relative shadow at the front of the neck which facilitates visualization of the movement of the sterno-mastoid muscle.

Abnormality of the apex beat

Left ventricular disease may be accompanied by abnormalities of the apex beat. Hypertrophy of the left ventricle does not cause displacement but will cause a sustained or heaving apex beat. In normal subjects the apex beat moves outwards for the first third of systole only and thereafter retracts (Fig. 3.6). Failure of this retraction in late systole results in a sustained apex which is otherwise described as heaving or forceful. This type of apex beat is found in conditions in which there is an increase in the afterload on the ventricle such as in systemic hypertension or aortic stenosis.

Displacement of the apex beat occurs when the cavity of the ventricle is enlarged as in case 1. Abnormal pulsation may also be felt parasternally as in case 4. This parasternal heave arises from the right ventricle and reflects hypertrophy or volume overload.

In patients with coronary artery disease there may be a diffuse pulsation of the precordium internal to the apex beat. This reflects a left ventricular aneurysm or area of dyskinesia. This sign is commonly seen in a patient who has just sustained an anterior myocardial infarct. With recovery from the effects of the infarct the area of diffuse pulsation will disappear.

Added sounds

The third heart sound occurs 120–160 ms after the second heart sound (Fig. 3.7), at the end of the rapid filling of the ventricle. The sound is low pitched and is best heard with the bell of the stethoscope applied lightly to the skin. Although it is

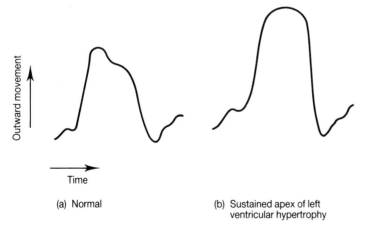

(a) Normal

(b) Sustained apex of left ventricular hypertrophy

Fig. 3.6 Movement of the apex: (**a**) in the normal person and (**b**) in a patient with left ventricular hypertrophy.

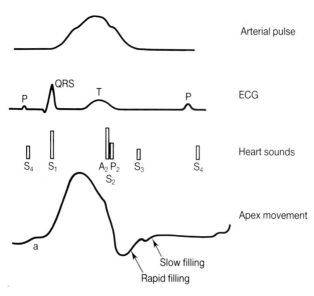

Fig. 3.7 The timing of the heart sounds in relation to the ECG, the arterial pulse and the movement of the apex. The third heart sound (S₃) occurs at the end of the rapid filling wave in the apex cardiogram. The fourth heart sound (S₄) occurs just after the P wave of the ECG and just before the a wave of the apex cardiogram which can sometimes be palpated.

normal in young people up to the age of about 20 years, the third heart sound occurs in situations in which there is rapid ventricular filling such as in mitral regurgitation or in high output states such as hyperthyroidism or pregnancy.

A fourth heart sound is due to increased atrial activity. A clearly audible fourth heart sound is significant and implies that there is some abnormality associated with the left or right atrium contracting against a non-compliant ventricle such as in cases 1 and 4. A fourth heart sound can sometimes be palpable at the apex.

The third and fourth heart sounds can become superimposed in the presence of a sinus tachycardia; a summation sound is then produced.

Under normal circumstances aortic closure is louder than pulmonary closure and occurs before it. With inspiration, as a result of the increased venous return to the right side of the heart, pulmonary closure occurs later and thus the second heart sound normally splits on inspiration. Reversed splitting whereby the sound is more widely split on expiration occurs with left ventricular disease (case 1). It may also be due directly to left bundle branch block. The loudness of pulmonary closure may be increased in the presence of pulmonary arterial hypertension (case 4).

Atrioventricular valve incompetence

The mitral and tricuspid valve cusps are supported by papillary muscles, chordae tendineae and the valve rings. Incompetence of these valves may occur as a component part of ventricular disease, particularly if cavity dilatation occurs.

The regurgitation produces a systolic murmur the characteristics of which may vary from day to day with the condition of the patient.

Basal crepitations

Crackles at the bases that do not clear on coughing may be present in patients with left ventricular disease as a manifestation of a raised left atrial pressure (case 1). They also occur in pulmonary disease (case 4).

Bilateral or right-sided pleural effusions occur. They consist of a transudate of a straw-coloured fluid of low protein content.

Peripheral oedema

Peripheral oedema is a late manifestation of fluid retention. In order for it to become apparent the extracellular fluid must have increased by 5–7 litres. Its distribution depends on the posture and activity of the patient. If the patient is active during the day it will collect around the ankles, whereas if the patient is in bed it will appear in the subcutaneous tissues over the sacrum. The fluid retention will be associated with weight gain.

Pericardial effusion

Pericardial effusions are common in patients with heart failure. They do not give rise to clinical consequences although they may contribute to the cardiac enlargement seen on the x-ray.

Ascites

Accumulation of ascites is a late manifestation of fluid retention. It is often associated with tricuspid regurgitation or pericardial disease. It is also often associated with hepatomegaly which, because of the stretching of the liver capsule, will cause discomfort and will be tender (as in case 4).

Cyanosis

Patients with severe chronic heart failure may have a dusky appearance of their face and extremities. Arterial oxygenation may be normal. The cyanosis occurs because of the extremely low venous oxygen content which reflects increased oxygen extraction by the tissues due to the low blood flow.

Pathophysiology of heart failure

In clinical medicine there is often a need for precise physiological definitions. Unfortunately there is still a considerable difference between the physiological and the clinical use of similar terms. This applies particularly to consideration of patients with heart failure.

The essence of heart failure is that, in spite of appropriate filling, the heart is unable adequately to supply the demands of the body. The logical extension of this argument is that the term heart failure could be applied whenever the demands for an increase in cardiac output are not met as a result of cardiac limitation. Any normal heart would therefore eventually fail if the demands were increased beyond its ability to generate output. This might occur in people with normal hearts during extreme exertion; the exertion is in fact stopped by fatigue or breathlessness.

Terminology

The term *congestive heart failure* is used clinically to describe a complicated and somewhat variable combination of symptoms and signs. These may include dyspnoea, tiredness, fatigue, peripheral oedema, tachypnoea and tachycardia, pulmonary crackles, cardiomegaly and a ventricular gallop. Congestive heart failure is that state in which abnormal circulatory congestion occurs as the result of both heart failure *and* the failure of the compensatory mechanisms. The term should not be used unless the congestion is of primary cardiac origin. When the cause of the pulmonary and/or peripheral congestion is not clear, it is wise to describe the symptoms or signs and avoid mistakenly diagnosing heart failure as illustrated in case 3.

Once the intravascular circulatory congestion has been present for some time, there is usually an increased transudation of fluid from the capillaries into the interstitial spaces. In the pulmonary circulation, if the rate of transudation exceeds the rate of lymphatic drainage, pulmonary oedema develops. In the systemic venous circulation the venous congestion may be visible and may result in the development of peripheral oedema (Fig. 3.8). The heart failure is usually

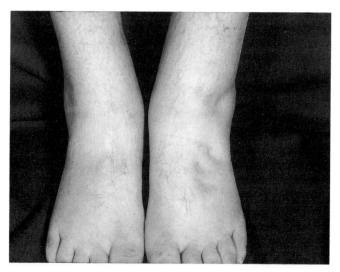

Fig. 3.8 Ankles of a patient with heart failure. The pitting nature of the oedema can be seen where firm pressure of the examiner's fingers has left indentations.

preceded by a period of myocardial dysfunction, during which the overall cardiac pump function and cardiac output may be maintained by compensatory mechanisms.

A hypothesis of backward failure was proposed by James Hope in 1832. It argues that the symptoms arise from the failure of the ventricles adequately to discharge their contents. The patient with *backward failure* has symptoms that result from elevation of the venous pressure behind the failing ventricle, which causes shortness of breath and oedema on the left and right sides respectively.

The forward failure hypothesis was proposed by James Mackenzie in the early part of this century. The classic features were thought to be a consequence of the inability of the ventricles to deliver blood under pressure to the arterial system. *Forward failure* implies that most of the patient's symptoms result from a low cardiac output; as a result the patient complains of tiredness, weakness, poor exercise tolerance, or may even be in a state of cardiogenic shock.

These terms, *forward* and *backward failure*, are still used but need not be regarded as contradictory.

Left heart failure and right heart failure are alternative terms used to refer to conditions in which the primary impairment is on one or other side of the heart. Because the two sides of the heart are in circuit, it is obvious that one side cannot pump significantly more blood to the other side in the absence of abnormal shunts or regurgitation. Experimentally produced pure failure of one ventricle will affect the output of the other; the biochemistry and haemodynamics of the other ventricle can be abnormal even in pure one-sided failure. The expression *left-sided heart failure* usually refers to symptoms and signs of elevated pulmonary venous pressure and congestion in the pulmonary veins and capillaries. The term *right-sided heart failure* refers to symptoms and signs of congestion of the systemic veins and capillaries. Nevertheless, significant amounts of sodium and water retention with subsequent formation of peripheral oedema may occur with pure left-sided heart failure without haemodynamic evidence of right-sided heart failure.

Systolic and diastolic function

Ventricular dysfunction usually involves both systolic and diastolic functions. In our attempts to understand the pathophysiology of heart failure, it is helpful to consider them separately. For instance, some patients can have a marked elevation of the left ventricular diastolic pressure, indicative of a diastolic problem, and will have consequent pulmonary congestion at a time when the systolic or pumping function of the ventricle is well maintained or perhaps even greater than normal; this may occur in hypertrophic cardiomyopathy or aortic stenosis.

The importance of diastolic function has been underestimated in the past. The ventricle must be able to fill as well as eject blood if it is to maintain its overall function. In the normal resting heart, the time available for filling may occupy the greater part of the cardiac cycle (Fig. 3.9). As the heart rate increases, the duration of diastole becomes relatively shorter than that of systole, reaching, at maximum rate, a time for filling that is half that of systole.

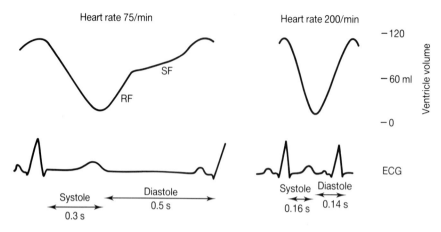

Fig. 3.9 Ventricular volumes in systole and diastole at two heart rates. RF, rapid filling; SF, slow filling.

The three phases of ventricular filling are complex and incompletely understood. Immediately after mitral valve opening there is a period of rapid filling, lasting up to 200 ms, when about 70 per cent of the ensuing stroke volume enters the ventricle. This is a very active process; blood is sucked into the ventricle and does not just passively move from atrium to ventricle. In mid-diastole the volume in the ventricle changes very little; the final 30 per cent enters during atrial systole. As the heart rate increases, so the initial rapid filling merges into atrial systole. The final proportion of ventricular filling may be increased in the presence of ventricular disease when the early filling is impaired. The atrial systole will increase the ventricular cavity size and fibre length and, thus, both stroke volume and the force of the succeeding contraction. Evidence of increased atrial activity is thus an important sign of ventricular disease.

Contractile function

The impaired contractile function of the heart results from the replacement of contractile cells by fibrous or scarred tissue. Fibrosis can occur as a consequence of a chronic imbalance between energy supply and excessive energy demand by the hypertrophied cell, leading to cell death. Alternatively, in the patient with coronary artery disease, coronary obstruction can cause cell death and scarring of the ischaemic region of the myocardium. There is a decrease in the myosin ATPase activity in the failing myocardium. The interaction between the contractile proteins actin and myosin is therefore decreased, leading to a reduction in both velocity and force of contraction. In most patients with heart failure there are phases of increased protein synthesis and of stable hyperfunction and hypertrophy of cells; these phases are probably initiated by a chronic increase in myocardial stress. The onset of myocardial failure is thought to be causally related to a decrease in the synthesis of normal protein.

Calcium plays an essential role in contractility and the initiation of systole. In the patient with heart failure impaired contractility is accompanied by impairment of both uptake and release of calcium from the sarcoplasmic reticulum; this results in impaired contraction and relaxation of the myocardium. Relaxation abnormalities are found particularly in the ischaemic myocardium, and are probably secondary to the fall in cellular ATP which provides the chemical energy for the movement of calcium out of the cell. A marked fall in cellular ATP in time leads to myocardial cell death. Fibrosis and scar tissue thus reduce the compliance of the heart, leading to relaxation abnormalities. Heart failure may also be associated with defects in the activity of the membrane transport enzyme Na^+/K^+ ATPase.

Depleted cardiac catecholamine stores can be demonstrated in patients with severe low output states and cardiac failure. They also have a reduction of β-adrenoceptor density in the myocardium which corresponds with the lack of response to isoprenaline stimulation. In some elderly individuals there may be involutional changes in the myocardium associated with decreased elasticity of the skeleton of the heart with mild fibrotic changes of the valves. The contractility and the adaptive reserve capacity of the heart are affected. Presbycardia, or the aged myocardium, has also been shown to have a diminished inotropic response to catecholamines and digitalis.

Breathlessness

The pathophysiology of shortness of breath caused by left ventricular dysfunction is complex. The lung circulation in normal humans has a low peripheral resistance and a low reflex vasomotor activity. As a result the pulsatile flow is maintained throughout the pulmonary arterial and capillary system. Pulmonary vascular resistance decreases as the blood flow through the lungs increases with exercise. The means by which these changes are effected are complex. There is a relationship between the intra-alveolar pressure, which tends to close lung capillaries, and the arterial and venous pressures, which tend to open them. Figure 3.10 displays the perfusion zones in the lung. In zone 1 no capillary blood

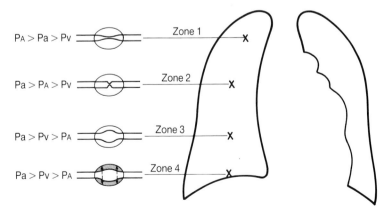

Fig. 3.10 Perfusion zones of lung in the erect position. PA, alveolar pressure; Pa, pulmonary arterial pressure; Pv, pulmonary venous pressure.

flow takes place because alveolar pressure exceeds both arterial and venous pulmonary pressures. In zone 2 blood flow begins at the level where pulmonary arterial pressure exceeds alveolar pressure. Zone 3 pulmonary venous pressure also exceeds pulmonary alveolar pressure and the capillary systems remain permanently open. In zone 4 regional blood flow falls because of a greater increase in transfer of interstitial fluid from the capillaries which occurs even in health. This contributes to the increase in intercapillary resistance to blood flow in this zone of the lung. If the left atrial or pulmonary venous pressure rises as a result of heart disease, there will be increased fluid transudation at the lung bases. This causes a reduction in blood flow through the capillaries in the lower zones and a redistribution of blood flow to the upper zones; this results in the radiological sign of upper lobe blood diversion.

These hydrostatic relationships indicate how vascular pressure adjustments as well as zonal distributions of blood flow can be achieved by physical means. At peak capillary flow rate such as might occur with exertion, the pulmonary arterial pressure will exceed the alveolar pressure in all areas of the lungs and all capillary systems will open to accommodate blood flow. During diastole the alveolar capillary systems will cease to conduct blood flow as the pulmonary arterial pressure falls in their zone. This will begin in the uppermost regions of the lung and extend downwards as arterial pressure continues to fall in diastole. Regional lung perfusion thus varies with time throughout the cardiac cycle in a tidal manner and is regulated by gravity. It also illustrates how areas of the lung are recruited when needed.

The pathophysiological basis of paroxysmal nocturnal dyspnoea and ortho-pnoea is not well understood. It is possible that it is related to the different function curves of the right and left ventricle in disease (Fig. 3.11). It can be seen, for instance, that at a filling pressure of 5 mmHg the normal right heart will pump 60 ml per beat into the pulmonary circulation. The left heart can pump 60 ml per beat only at the expense of a left atrial pressure of 15 mmHg. At this juncture the patient has a normal right-sided filling pressure and, therefore, a normal jugular venous pressure; the only abnormality is a high left atrial pressure which is difficult to detect clinically from the clinical signs. However, the patient will give a history of orthopnoea. This occurs because, as the patient slips down the bed and becomes flatter, the right atrial pressure rises slightly; it may only be by a trivial amount and is due to an alteration in the relative heights of the systemic venous reservoir and the right atrium. The increase in the right atrial pressure raises the stroke output of the right heart from 65 to 75 ml per beat. As seen in the Figure, the left heart can match this increase in stroke volume only with a rise in the left atrial pressure from 15 to 35 mmHg. This causes the rapid development of pulmonary oedema.

Compensatory mechanisms

Various compensatory mechanisms maintain the cardiac output of the failing heart, using the same mechanisms as the normal cardiovascular system (Table 3.2).

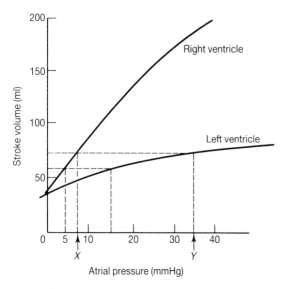

Fig. 3.11 The function curves of the two ventricles in someone with severe left ventricular disease. The right ventricular function curve is normal. At a right atrial pressure of 5 mmHg the right ventricular stroke volume is about 60 ml. The left ventricle can pump out this volume only at a pressure of 15 mmHg. If the patient lies flatter in the bed the right atrial pressure may rise a trivial amount (X); this produces an increase in stroke volume to 70–75 ml. The left ventricle can only cope with this volume at a pressure of 35 mmHg (Y), which causes the development of pulmonary oedema.

Table 3.2 Compensatory mechanisms

Frank–Starling mechanism
Neurohumoral mechanisms
Force interval relation
Hypertrophy
Peripheral oxygen delivery
Autonomic nervous system:
1. Heart:
   (a) Increased heart rate
   (b) Increased myocardial contractility
   (c) Increased rate of relaxation
2. Peripheral circulation:
   (a) Arterial vasoconstriction (increased afterload)
   (b) Venous vasoconstriction (increased preload)
Anaerobic metabolism

Frank–Starling mechanism

A landmark in the description and understanding of the ventricle's response to changing demand were the observations by Frank and Starling that increased tension of normal ventricular muscle in diastole prompted an increase in force of contraction in the heart–lung preparation. An extension of Starling's law to the intact heart describes a relationship between an increase in the wall tension in diastole and an increase in stroke volume. Similar, but not identical, relationships are obtained by plotting stroke volume against end-diastolic fibre length or end-diastolic volume. In the failing heart (Fig. 3.12) it can be seen that, despite an increase in the end-diastolic pressure, volume or muscle end-diastolic length, the stroke volume remains less than normal and may be inadequate to meet the needs of the situation. There is an upper limit to the advantageous increase in end-diastolic pressure before adverse effects occur; as it rises in the left ventricle so the left atrial and pulmonary venous pressures rise in concert, thus producing impairment of gaseous exchange in the lungs and the symptom of shortness of breath. The ventricle may dilate in response to a volume load, allowing an increase in ventricular work due to the Frank–Starling relationship. Dilatation may be excessive if the ventricle is damaged or the workload extreme. Unfortunately, as the dilatation progresses so the heart has to operate at an increasing disadvantage. This occurs because of the relationship between wall tension and intraventricular pressure described by Laplace. This means that a dilated heart must contract more forcibly than a normal heart in order to generate the same intraventricular pressure.

The primary defect in the patient with cardiac failure is the reduction in the intrinsic contractility of the myocardium, which leads to a decrease in cardiac output/volume at any given ventricular end-diastolic pressure (Fig. 3.12). It can be seen that in patients with an abnormality of the contractility of the myocardium there is a lower cardiac output for any given filling pressure. In addition to the systolic abnormalities there are associated diastolic abnormalities related to filling or relaxation. These contribute to the high ventricular filling pressures that are found in heart failure.

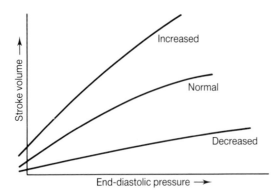

Fig. 3.12 The relation between end-diastolic pressure and stroke volume, showing displacement to the left with an increased contractility and to the right with a decreased contractility in a patient with left ventricular disease.

Neurohumoral mechanisms

Circulating catecholamine levels are elevated in patients with chronic cardiac failure (Fig. 3.13). These elevated levels contribute to the increase in systemic vascular resistance and also provide a chronotropic and inotropic stimulus to the myocardium. This continuous increase in circulating noradrenaline is thought to lead to a reduction of the β-adrenoceptor population and therefore to its lack of responsiveness.

The renin–angiotensin–aldosterone system is also activated, leading to an increase in plasma renin activity, angiotensin II and aldosterone. The secretion of renin is controlled by four main factors:

1. Changes in the wall tension in renal arterioles.
2. A macula densa receptor that detects changes in the rate of sodium and/or chloride reaching the distal tubule.

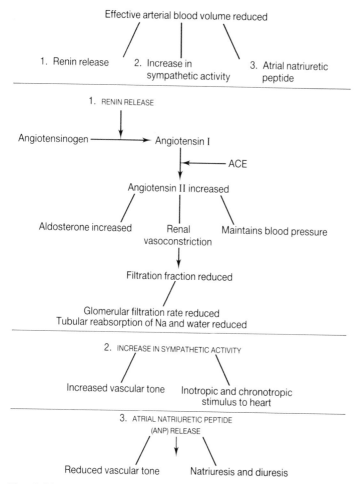

Fig. 3.13 Schema of the neurohumoral mechanisms in heart failure.

3. A negative feedback effect of circulating angiotensin.

4. The action of the central nervous system which influences renin secretion by the renal nerves, adrenal medulla and the posterior pituitary.

Angiotensin II has strong arterial vasoconstrictor properties and contributes to the increase in peripheral vascular resistance and the maintenance of blood pressure in heart failure when effective filling of the arterial circulation decreases. Angiotensin II is converted to angiotensin III which also has vasoconstrictive properties. Angiotensin II further constricts renal efferent arterioles, and in the brain it stimulates thirst. Angiotensin II also has some direct inotropic properties and may augment the release of noradrenaline from nerve endings. It stimulates secretion of aldosterone, which leads to salt and water retention and a further increase in blood volume. The sodium content of arteries and veins is increased, resulting in reduced compliance and increased impedance.

Antidiuretic hormone and arginine vasopressin levels are also increased in heart failure and may further contribute to salt and water retention and systemic vasoconstriction.

Atrial natriuretic peptide (ANP) is synthesized by atrial myocytes. The peptide release is influenced by a number of factors, of which the most important is the atrial pressure. ANP release produces a natriuresis and a diuresis. It also produces smooth muscle relaxation and a reduction in vascular resistance. It may also have some central effects. Thus a rise in atrial pressure will cause a release of ANP, which will produce rapid changes in vascular resistance and salt and water handling by the kidney. A number of these effects are opposite to those mediated by the renin–angiotensin–aldosterone system.

Force–interval relation

The development of tension and the shortening of cardiac muscle is controlled by the concentration of calcium ions released in the vicinity of the myofibrils. There is an intracellular store of calcium which is supplemented during each depolarization by an influx across the cell membrane. The intracellular store is replenished in part by the recycling of calcium from the previous beat and in part by the calcium entering the cell. The force generated by a particular heart beat is a function of several interacting factors, which include the duration of its action potential and the duration of the beat to beat interval that precedes it and follows it. These force–interval relationships are an intrinsic property of heart muscle and have been shown to have a regulatory role in normal cardiac function, and may be disturbed in disease. This relationship was first described by Bowditch in 1895 and predates the observations of Frank and Starling but has attracted little attention until recently.

Hypertrophy of the heart

Hypertrophy is one of the major adjustments of the heart to chronically increased stress. Hyperplasia, or an increase in the number of myocardial cells, does not occur in adults. Hypertrophy is associated with a significant increase in the number or size of sarcomeres within each myocardial cell. The hypertrophy is associated with a reduced compliance which will adversely affect ventricular filling.

Autonomic nervous system

One of the more important acute adjustments to heart failure is a reflex increase in autonomic sympathetic excitation to the heart and to most of the arteries and veins. This increase in sympathetic activity, in combination with an increased plasma concentration of noradrenaline and angiotensin II, produces a generalized arterial vasoconstriction and an increase in venous tone. There is an associated inhibition of cardiac parasympathetic activity. The increase in sympathetic impulses stimulates the local release of noradrenaline and thereby produces beta stimulation with an increase both in heart rate and in the force of myocardial contraction. Noradrenaline also increases the rate of ventricular relaxation, which further contributes to increased ventricular filling.

In patients with heart failure the actions of the autonomic nervous system and local autoregulatory mechanisms tend to preserve circulation to the brain and heart while decreasing the blood flow to the skin and skeletal muscles, splanchnic organs and kidneys. The arterial pressure is maintained, and the venous tone is increased resulting in a maintained venous return and ventricular filling. The arterial and arteriolar resistance is also increased by their increased sodium and water content.

Peripheral oxygen delivery

The redistribution of the diminished cardiac output is associated with a rightward shift of the oxygen dissociation curve, which facilitates the release of oxygen in the peripheral capillaries of underperfused tissues. Some tissues also utilize anaerobic metabolism; this mechanism is of very limited value to the myocardium or to the brain.

Investigation of ventricular disease

Chest x-ray

An increase in the transverse diameter of the heart is common in patients with chronic heart failure although severe failure may coexist with a normal heart shadow. Selective enlargement of the left atrium is well recognized in mitral valve disease but may also occur with conditions with an increased resistance to ventricular filling such as a hypertrophic cardiomyopathy.

Assessment of the pulmonary vasculature can give valuable information. An increase in the end-diastolic pressure in the left ventricle will cause an increase in the left atrial and pulmonary venous pressures. The effect of this on the pulmonary venous drainage is to facilitate drainage from the upper zones of the lung and impede it from the lower. This causes upper lobe blood diversion which is recognized by the vessels in the upper zones appearing larger than those to the lower. Septal lines also occur; these horizontal lines are seen in the lower lung fields and represent oedema in the interlobular fissures. There may also be peribronchial cuffing due to the oedema. In acute heart failure there will be alveolar pulmonary oedema which is often distributed in a bat's wing distribution (Fig. 3.14).

Abnormalities are often seen in the pulmonary vasculature of patients with right ventricular problems due to acute pulmonary embolism, cor pulmonale or primary pulmonary hypertension.

Electrocardiogram

There are no specific electrocardiographic abnormalities that indicate the presence of heart failure. Indirect information can be extracted from this investigation. Left ventricular hypertrophy may manifest itself as an increase in the QRS

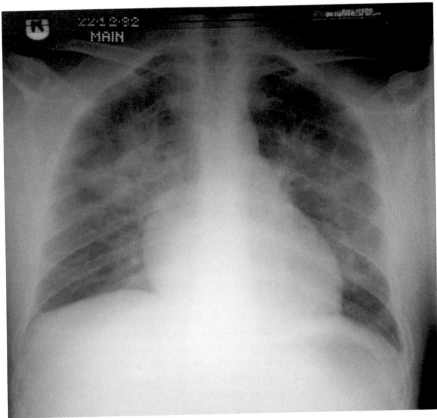

Fig. 3.14 Portable anteroposterior view of the chest, demonstrating a bat's wing distribution of alveolar pulmonary oedema due to acute heart failure.

voltage and/or by T wave changes. The most commonly used criteria are those of the sum of the R wave in V_6 with the S wave in V_1 amounting to more than 35 mm (Fig. 3.15). These ECG changes have a sensitivity and a specificity in the order of 70 per cent. It is thus possible for severe left ventricular hypertrophy to coexist with a normal ECG and for the criteria of left ventricular hypertrophy to exist with a normal ventricle.

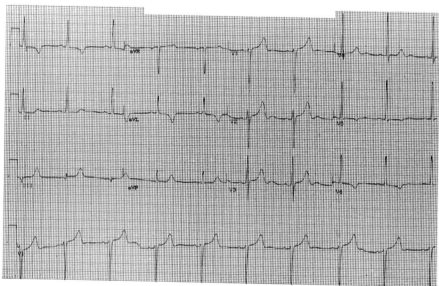

Fig. 3.15 ECG showing the QRS voltage changes of left ventricular hypertrophy. The sum of the R wave in V_6 and the S wave in V_1 is greater than 35 mm. See Chapter 2 for discussion of criteria for the diagnosis of left ventricular hypertrophy.

The presence of left bundle branch block is usually associated with left ventricular abnormalities. A right bundle branch block can be a normal finding but may be a feature of right ventricular dysfunction. Other manifestations of right ventricular problems include the presence of right ventricular hypertrophy or right axis deviation.

Pathological Q waves are characteristic of an acute or a previous myocardial infarction (see Chapter 1). They can also occur as a result of septal hypertrophy in hypertrophic cardiomyopathy.

Evidence of left atrial hypertrophy may be present in patients with left ventricular disease as well as in those with mitral valve disease. This shows itself as a broad and bifid P wave in the standard leads with a predominantly negative P wave deflection in V_1 (Fig. 3.16). Right atrial hypertrophy may be present in patients with right ventricular disease. This shows itself as abnormally peaked P waves (Fig. 3.17).

Rhythm abnormalities are commonly seen in patients with heart failure. These may be detected on the ECG or during 24-hour ambulatory monitoring.

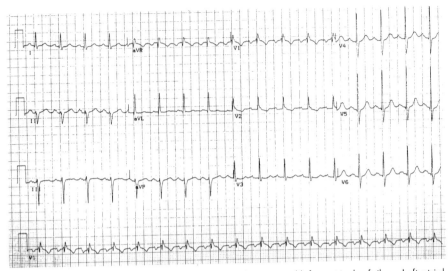

Fig. 3.16 ECG of a patient with coronary artery disease and left ventricular failure. Left atrial hypertension is present, as manifest by a broad and bifid P wave in lead II and a predominantly negative deflection in V_1.

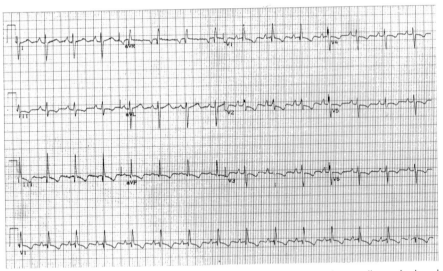

Fig. 3.17 ECG showing right atrial hypertrophy. The P waves are abnormally peaked and enlarged. This is seen best in leads I and V_{2-4}. A right bundle branch block pattern is also present.

Exercise testing

Exercise testing provides an objective measure of functional impairment in chronic heart failure. Maximal or submaximal tests on a treadmill or bicycle ergometer, with the measurement of exercise time or oxygen consumption, can be useful in the follow-up of symptomatic patients.

Systolic time interval

Systolic time intervals can be used to assess ventricular function. Well defined landmarks in the cardiac cycle are measured from simultaneously recorded indirect carotid pulse, phonocardiogram and ECG. The most useful measurement is the pre-ejection period, which represents the time necessary for ventricular activation. Left ventricular disease is associated with a prolongation of isovolumic contraction and thus with delay in aortic valve opening and a long pre-ejection period (Fig. 3.18).

Echocardiography

This technique is covered in Chapter 6. It can give useful structural information about the heart. The size of the chambers can be demonstrated, their wall thickness measured and movements documented. The presence and amount of pericardial fluid can also be shown. The echocardiographic features will reflect the underlying ventricular abnormality. In patients with coronary artery disease two-dimensional echocardiography may show a segmental reduction in wall movement or a localized left ventricular aneurysm. In the patient with a dilated cardiomyopathy the left ventricular dimensions may be increased and the amplitude of wall motions reduced globally. In a hypertrophic cardiomyopathy there may be eccentric hypertrophy of the interventricular septum; the cavity is small and may become obliterated in systole. Myocardial infiltrations such as amyloid, may produce characteristic reflection patterns from the myocardium.

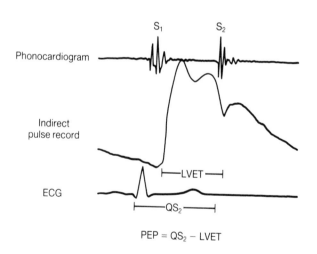

$$PEP = QS_2 - LVET$$

Fig. 3.18 The use of the phonocardiogram, ECG and indirect carotid pulse record for the measurement of systolic time intervals. Left ventricular ejection time (LVET) is measured from the beginning of the upstroke of the pulse record to the dichrotic notch of the pulse. QS_2 is measured from the Q wave of the ECG to the aortic component of the second sound. The pre-ejection period (PEP) is calculated by subtracting LVET from QS_2. S_1, first heart sound; S_2, second heart sound.

In patients with right heart failure there may be abnormalities of septal movement, right ventricular hypertrophy or cavity dilatation.

Nuclear cardiology

This technique is considered in Chapter 1. Ventricular function can be assessed using first-pass angiocardiography in which the radiolabelled isotope is rapidly injected intravenously and its passage through the heart recorded. Direct assessment can be made of transit times, ventricular ejection fractions, ventricular volumes and regional wall motion. Alternatively, the equilibrium gated blood pool technique can be employed, in which the ECG is used as a means of sampling data from various phases of the cardiac cycle over multiple heart beats until sufficient data have been accumulated to allow analysis. Assessment can be made of the size of each chamber, the size and relationship of the great vessels and the thickness of the interventricular septum. Ventricular volumes can be calculated and the changes in spatial information during the cardiac cycle can be used to generate colour-coded images representing the amplitude and phase of regional wall motion.

Cardiac catheterization and angiography

Bedside monitoring of the right-sided pressures can be useful in the management of patients with acute heart failure. A balloon-tipped catheter positioned with its tip in the pulmonary artery (Fig. 3.19) allows accurate measurement of

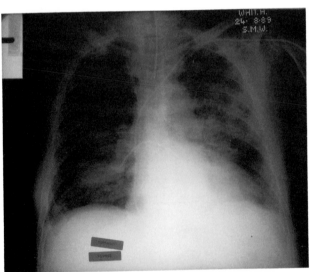

Fig. 3.19 X-ray of a patient in whom a Swan–Ganz catheter has been positioned in the pulmonary artery. With the balloon deflated, the pressure in the pulmonary artery can be measured from the tip of the catheter. With the balloon inflated, the tip will record the pulmonary artery wedge or indirect left atrial pressure. (The patient also has an endotracheal tube in place and is on a ventilator.)

the pulmonary artery, the pulmonary artery wedge or indirect left atrial, and also right atrial pressures. In this way the filling pressures of both ventricles can be measured and modified by treatment as necessary.

Because of the increasing sophistication of non-invasive imaging techniques, formal catheter studies are rarely necessary for the investigation of the patient with chronic heart failure other than to exclude the presence of coronary artery disease or to determine the suitability for transplantation.

Endomyocardial muscle biopsy

The biopsy is performed with a biotome passed through a long sheath introduced into a vein or artery. The muscle biopsy is taken from either the right or the left ventricle. It is useful for diagnosing or confirming the presence of specific heart muscle disease such as amyloid or sarcoid. It can be helpful in distinguishing between a chronic myocarditis or a dilated cardiomyopathy. It is also a useful technique in determining whether rejection is taking place in a transplanted heart. It has not proved to be as helpful as hoped in relating histological, ultrastructural or biochemical changes to the aetiology of the heart disease nor in determining the prognosis.

Treatment of ventricular disease

The main components of treatment of heart failure are:

1. To identify and manage the specific aetiology wherever possible
2. To discover and manage the precipitating causes so as to decrease the workload on the heart
3. To control the heart rate and rhythm
4. To increase myocardial contractility
5. To decrease the congestion by increasing the excretion of salt and water
6. To decrease the preload or afterload
7. To manage surgically where appropriate

Aetiology

The approach to the possible aetiology can be divided into the following:

1. Direct myocardial damage; e.g. myocardial infarction, viral myocarditis
2. Ventricular overload:
   (a) volume overload; e.g. valvular incompetence or a shunt
   (b) pressure overload; e.g. systemic hypertension, aortic or pulmonary stenosis
3. Restriction of diastolic filling; e.g. mitral stenosis or constrictive pericarditis

Precipitating causes

These include occult infection, severe anaemia and hyperthyroidism. The toxic effects of alcohol and other drugs must not be forgotten; they might alternatively be considered under the aetiology.

Heart rate and rhythm

Controlling the heart rate is important. It is necessary to distinguish the abnormalities of heart rate or rhythm from the compensatory sinus tachycardia mediated by sympathetic activity. Prophylactic antiarrhythmic drug therapy is contraindicated in heart failure, especially in view of the high incidence of bradyarrhythmic deaths. The treatment of symptomatic arrhythmias is first to identify any cause, such as hypokalaemia. Most effective antiarrhythmic drugs reduce left ventricular function and are therefore best avoided if possible.

Myocardial contractility

Increasing myocardial contractility can be achieved by the use of certain drugs.

Cardiac glycosides
The mechanism of the action of digitalis is related to the inhibition of the Na^+/K^+ ATPase enzyme system in the cell membrane. This leads to an increase in intracellular sodium concentration. Ca^{2+} is subsequently exchanged for the Na^+, thus increasing the intracellular calcium concentration and the force of contraction. Slowing of the heart rate secondary to vagal stimulation and decreased conduction velocity through the AV node is also beneficial in the patient with atrial fibrillation and heart failure. In the patient with sinus rhythm the drug is undoubtedly useful in the short term and probably useful in the long term.

Phosphodiesterase inhibitors
Drugs that inhibit phosphodiesterase III activity (such as milrinone) cause increased levels of cyclic AMP in cardiac tissues. They may also produce an increased sensitivity of the contractile proteins to Ca^{2+}. They acutely improve the haemodynamic state and may have more long-lasting benefit. Their vasodilatory effects have been described more recently and the drug can be conveniently described as an inodilator.

Adenyl cyclase activators
Drugs are currently being developed which induce stimulation of this enzyme. The changes in contractility parallel an increase in cyclic AMP concentration and calcium transport into the myocardium.

Receptor-mediated inotropic drugs
An increase in myocardial contractility can be obtained by the stimulation of various types of receptors in the heart. These include the adrenergic (α and β), dopaminergic, histaminergic and serotoninergic.

The postsynaptic adrenoceptors are the most important mediators although the presynaptic α_2- or β_2-adrenoceptors may play a modulatory role. Catecholamines increase contractility by stimulating β_1-adrenoceptors on the myocardial surface. The clinical usefulness of adrenaline, noradrenaline and isoprenaline is limited by their relative chronotropic and peripheral receptor effects (Table 3.3). Noradrenaline is the endogenous catecholamine that is synthesized and stored in granules in the adrenergic nerve endings in the myocardium. It is released from its stores and stimulates specific β_1-adrenoceptor sites on the myocardial cell surface. Most of the released noradrenaline is subsequently taken up by the same adrenergic nerve endings and stored for further release. A subpopulation of β_2-adrenoceptors is also found in the heart with effects similar to those of the β_1-receptors; in severe heart failure the β_2-receptors dominate. Noradrenaline has marked α-agonist properties which may be beneficial in hypotension but the benefit is offset by the increase in afterload. The increased myocardial oxygen consumption compromises left ventricular function and reduces peripheral organ perfusion. Isoprenaline, a β_1-adrenoceptor agonist, is a potent inotrope but its beneficial effect is compromised by its powerful chronotropic effect, resulting in tachycardia and provocation of arrhythmias. In addition, the β_2-mediated systemic vasodilatation may be disadvantageous by diverting the increased cardiac output to the large vascular splanchnic and skeletal muscle beds and away from vital organs. Xamoterol is a relatively new orally active compound which is a partial agonist at the β_1-receptor. It can be used only in mild heart failure and has been shown to be dangerous in patients with more severe heart failure.

Table 3.3   Receptor activity of catecholamines

	Receptors				
	α_1	α_2	β_1	β_2	Dopaminergic
Noradrenaline	+ +	+ +	+ +	0	0
Adrenaline	+ +	+ +	+ +	+ +	0
Isoprenaline	0	0	+ +	+ +	0
Dopamine	+ +	+	+	0	+ +
Dobutamine	+	0	+ +	+	0
Prenalterol	0	0	+ +	0	0
Salbutamol	0	0	0	+ +	0
Xamoterol	0	0	+	0	0

Dopamine and dobutamine are more selective in their effect and are useful agents (Table 3.3). Dopamine is an endogenous precursor of noradrenaline and has both a direct sympathomimetic action and, by releasing noradrenaline from its stores, an indirect effect. At low doses it has a specific vasodilator effect on the renal vasculature; this effect results from stimulation of the structurally specific dopaminergic receptor. At high doses, dopamine behaves like noradrenaline, having a predominantly vasoconstrictor effect on peripheral vascular beds mediated by α-receptor stimulation. Dobutamine, which is a derived analogue of dopamine, has an effect that is similar to isoprenaline although the β_2-peripheral effect is less. Newer inotropic agents are being developed.

Increased excretion of salt and water

Diuretics increase the excretion of the excess salt and water that occur in heart failure. Thiazide diuretics are often quite satisfactory. The loop diuretics are now more commonly used; they inhibit the reabsorption of sodium in the ascending loop of Henle. They can cause hypokalaemia and hypomagnesaemia, which may predispose the patient to arrhythmias particularly if digoxin therapy is used concurrently. The diuretics also have acute haemodynamic effects which are often not noticed because of the overall benefit to the patient. They can depress heart function due to an increase in the afterload. Venodilatation may also occur which will contribute to the fall in the pulmonary artery pressure; this, in conjunction with the ensuing diuresis, may cause an abrupt fall in the left ventricular filling pressure and a deterioration in cardiac output.

Decreased preload or afterload

The compensatory mechanisms of arterial and venous vasoconstriction impede left ventricular ejection and shift blood centrally from the venous capacitance vessels. This increases both preload and afterload which adversely affect ventricular performance. Vasodilators may produce venodilatation, arteriolar dilatation, or both. There may also be other benefits in the form of relief of myocardial ischaemia or altered diastolic function of the ventricle. The vasodilators may be classified according to their effects (Table 3.4).

Table 3.4 A classification of the vasodilators

Venodilators	Nitrates
Mixed dilators	Prazocin
	Sodium nitroprusside
	ACE inhibitors
Arteriolar dilators	Nifedipine
	Hydralazine
	Phentolamine

The angiotensin-converting enzyme (ACE) inhibitors inhibit the conversion of angiotensin I to angiotensin II. Elevated levels of angiotensin contribute to the increased systemic vascular resistance in heart failure (Fig. 3.20). The introduction of an ACE inhibitor reduces a number of the adverse effects of angiotensin II.

Several ACE inhibitors are available. They produce considerable symptomatic benefit to the patient with heart failure and may also improve the duration of life. They are not without side effects; the drug needs to be introduced carefully because of the hypotensive effects that will occur, particularly if the filling pressure in the ventricles is less than adequate. Other problems include rashes, angioneurotic oedema and hyperkalaemia, particularly in the presence of renal impairment. Cough is a particular side effect that occurs in a small proportion of

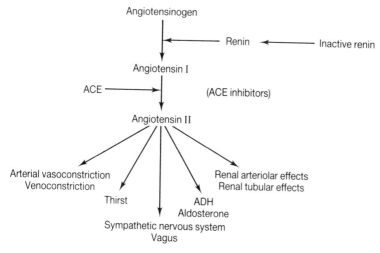

Fig. 3.20 The effects of angiotensin II.

patients. It is thought to be related to the effects that the drug has on the metabolism of other substances such as bradykinin.

Surgery

Surgery has an important role in the management of heart failure in certain circumstances. If the patient has developed heart failure due to severe aortic regurgitation caused by infective endocarditis, an aortic valve replacement may cure the heart failure. Other instances include mitral regurgitation due to ruptured chordae, resection of a left ventricular aneurysm due to myocardial infarction or a traumatic ventricular septal effect due to a knife wound. Surgery of course has an important role in the prevention of heart failure; for instance, the patient with aortic valve stenosis is followed carefully in outpatients over some years in order to choose the correct time to replace the aortic valve before left ventricular function has been compromised.

Summary

The aims of therapy are different in acute and in chronic heart failure. In acute heart failure the reduction of the pulmonary capillary or wedge pressure and the right atrial pressure are sought, together with an improvement in the cardiac output if this is also compromised. In chronic heart failure the aim of therapy is to translate the haemodynamic benefits of vasodilator and inotropic therapy, or inodilator therapy, into improving the functional capacity of the patient without compromising the duration of life or its quality.

In mild to moderate chronic heart failure the search for an ideal orally active and effective drug with both inotropic and vasodilatory properties is still underway. In more severe heart failure the peripheral component of therapy will need to become more dominant because the myocardial problem will increasingly limit the response to inotropic therapy.

Conditions causing ventricular disease

The conditions that cause ventricular disease are:

1. Valvular abnormalities
2. Coronary artery disease
3. Congenital heart disease
4. Cardiomyopathy
5. Specific heart muscle disease
6. Respiratory diseases
7. Altered cardiac rhythm
8. Systemic hypertension

These conditions may progress to heart failure; some can be identified early in their natural history and treated, thus preventing the development of failure. A number of these conditions are fully covered in other chapters of this book.

Cardiomyopathies and specific heart muscle disorders

Cardiomyopathies are, by definition, heart muscle disease of unknown cause. The specific heart muscle diseases are either of known cause or associated with a general disorder. These terms replace the former subdivision into primary and secondary cardiomyopathies. Three categories can be identified by their distinctive pathological and haemodynamic characteristics:

1. Dilated cardiomyopathy
2. Hypertrophic cardiomyopathy
3. Restrictive cardiomyopathy

Dilated cardiomyopathy

Dilated cardiomyopathy was previously known as a congestive cardiomyopathy. The condition is common world wide. The main characteristic is the dilatation of the left or right, or both, ventricular cavities. The dilatation is associated with an impairment of systolic and diastolic function which varies in severity. Disturbances of ventricular or atrial rhythm are common and death may occur suddenly.

Dilated cardiomyopathy has been attributed to a previous myocarditis, heavy alcohol intake or hypertension. The condition is probably the outcome of a number of different factors operating in a susceptible subject. On inspection of the heart the muscle is pale and flabby. Hypertrophy may accompany and probably follows the dilatation. The coronary arteries are normal. The interior of the left ventricle shows flattening of the trabeculae, and thrombi may be seen protruding from the trabecular crevices. Microscopy shows hypertrophy of the myocardial fibres which vary in size. Interstitial fibrosis varies in amount but there is no cellular infiltration in contrast to an active myocarditis.

The presentation is usually with heart failure, arrhythmias or embolism. The initial presentation with shortness of breath is often associated with a cough and may be mistaken for a chest infection. Asymptomatic patients may be picked up during an incidental medical examination or a routine ECG or chest x-ray.

The clinical features depend on the severity. They vary from no detectable abnormality to those of heart failure.

The ECG abnormalities found most commonly are non-specific; they include widening of the QRS complex, repolarization abnormalities, multiple ectopic beats or incomplete left bundle branch block pattern. The x-ray (Fig. 3.21) may show the heart to be slightly or markedly enlarged. The echocardiogram (Fig. 3.22) shows that the left ventricular cavity is dilated and poorly contract-

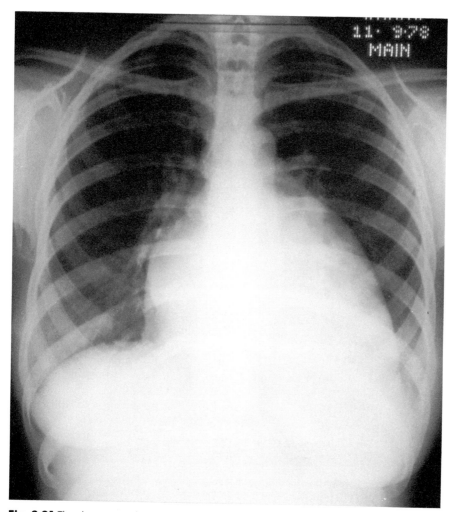

Fig. 3.21 The chest x-ray of a patient with a dilated cardiomyopathy, showing a large cardiac sillhouette and clear lung fields.

ing. The left atrium and right ventricular cavities may also be large. The thickness of the left ventricular walls is usually normal although, in contrast to the very large cavity, the walls look thinned.

Hypertrophic cardiomyopathy

Hypertrophic cardiomyopathy is characterized by unexplained hypertrophy of the left ventricle and, occasionally, of the right ventricle; this typically involves the septum more than the free wall. The left ventricular volume is normal or reduced. The diastolic pressure is usually raised.

The condition may be inherited as an autosomal dominant.

The heart is overweight due to a marked increase in myocardial mass. Histology shows a bizarre form of myocardial fibre hypertrophy and disarray. The myocardial cells are thicker, shorter and more bizarre in shape than in any other condition, and the nuclei may appear abnormal. The coronary arteries are usually abnormally large. The basic cellular defect is unknown.

Hypertrophic cardiomyopathy may be seen at any age from the neonate to the octogenarian. Many patients are asymptomatic. The commonest symptom is shortness of breath resulting from a raised left atrial pressure caused by the stiff left ventricle with its high diastolic pressure. The patient may have angina; the

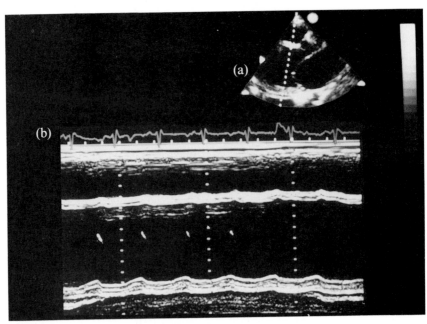

Fig. 3.22 Two-dimensional echocardiogram frame (top right) and M-mode of a patient with a dilated cardiomyopathy. The two-dimensional frame shows a dilated left ventricle. The function of the left ventricle can be assessed from the wall movements on the video film recording. The M-mode shows that the interventricular septum and posterior left ventricular wall are moving very little, reflecting grossly impaired left ventricular systolic function.

large muscle mass requires a large coronary blood flow. Arrhythmias are common.

The clinical features are variable. The heart beat is regular and the arterial pulses are increased in volume and jerky in character. The left ventricular impulse is prominent and preceded by a palpable atrial beat; this gives a double impulse. There may be a mid-systolic murmur heard internal to the apex which does not radiate widely.

The ECG is nearly always abnormal. It usually shows left ventricular hyper-trophy with ST segment and T wave abnormalities. Sometimes steep T wave inversion simulates a previous infarction. A deep Q wave in the precordial leads may simulate a previous infarction but in fact represents depolarization of the very thick septum. Echocardiography is very valuable and will often demon-strate the increase in the left ventricular wall thickness, particularly of the septum. The left ventricular cavity is normal or reduced in size (Fig. 3.23). The impaired diastolic function is demonstrated by a reduced diastolic closure rate of the mitral valve (Fig. 3.24). The heart may be normal in size on x-ray. In severe cases the lungs will show evidence of a raised left atrial pressure.

Restrictive cardiomyopathy

Restrictive cardiomyopathy is the least common of the cardiomyopathies. It includes endomyocardial fibrosis (EMF), previously called tropical endomyo-cardial fibrosis, and eosinophilic endomyocardial disease, also called Löffler's endomyocardial disease. The cause of EMF is unknown but appears to be related to the humid zone in the equatorial belt throughout the world. The episodes of fever and irregular exacerbation are suggestive of an infective aetiology. There is not such a dramatic eosinophilia in this form as in eosinophilic endomyocardial disease. In the latter the marked eosinophilia may be caused by a variety of different conditions. The similarity in the pathology suggests that the sinister role of the eosinophil may be common to both conditions. There is increasing evidence that prolonged release of the protein from the eosinophil cell causes the endocardial, subendocardial or myocardial fibrosis. Endomyocardial biopsies have documented an acute necrotic phase, a thrombotic phase and a late fibrotic phase. The fibrosis is maximal at the apex of the heart and also involves the papillary muscles, producing valvular regurgitation. Systolic emptying of the ventricles is initially preserved but the endomyocardial scarring restricts filling.

The acute illness of EMF is characterized by oedema, breathlessness and fever. Following the initial illness there may be intermittent further episodes with intervening good health; alternatively, a state of chronic ill health super-venes during which evidence of cardiac damage emerges with the onset of symptoms and signs. Once developed, the condition must be differentiated from constrictive pericarditis which it can mimic. In the latter, appropriate treatment is very effective; in the former, treatment is unrewarding.

The chest radiograph may show slight cardiomegaly; if there is a pericardial effusion the heart may appear very large. The ECG will show non-specific changes. The echocardiogram may demonstrate concentric ventricular hyper-trophy, normal or decreased ventricular size and decreased ventricular systolic

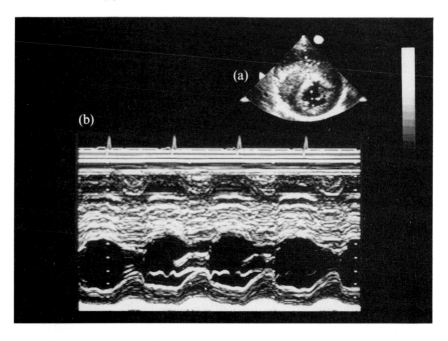

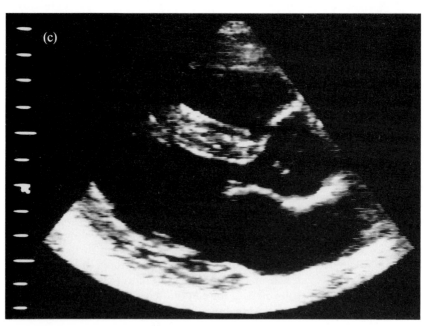

Fig. 3.23 (a) Two-dimensional echocardiogram frame at the level of the mitral valve in the short axis. (**b**) M-mode. (**c**) Long axis view of a patient with hypertrophic cardiomyopathy. The M-mode shows the very thick interventricular septum; the posterior wall is also thickened but not as markedly as the septum. The long axis view taken in diastole shows the very thick septum (scale in cm shown at the left of the recording).

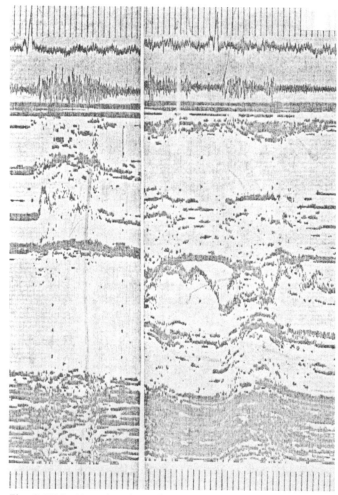

Fig. 3.24 An M-mode echocardiogram of a patient with a hypertrophic cardiomyopathy. The view on the left is through the aortic valve and left atrium; the view on the right is through the left ventricle at the level of the mitral valve. The very thick interventricular septum is well shown. The movement of both the mitral valve and the aortic valve is abnormal, reflecting the reduced rate of filling of the ventricle (reduced E–F slope) and the obstruction to outflow that can sometimes occur (early closure of the aortic valve and systolic movement of the mitral valve in systole (SAM)).

and diastolic function. Two-dimensional echocardiography may show the presence of thrombus or obliteration of the apices by the fibrotic process.

Specific heart muscle disease

In most of the specific heart muscle diseases the myocardium shows a generalized reduction in contractile force together with dilatation of the cavity of the ventricle. Some of these conditions will predominantly affect systolic function rather than diastolic and some, such as amyloid, will adversely affect both.

The specific heart muscle diseases can be classified as follows:

1. *Infective*. Viruses have been incriminated. Other agents include rickettsiae, protozoa such as trypanosomiasis causing Chagas' disease.
2. *Metabolic*. Endocrine causes include diabetes, thyrotoxicosis and acromegaly.
   Storage diseases include the glycogen storage disease and the mucopolysaccharidoses.
3. *Infiltration and granulomas*. These include haemochromatosis, amyloid and sarcoid.
4. *Systemic disease*. These include scleroderma, systemic lupus erythematosis, rheumatoid arthritis and polyarteritis nodosa.
5. *Muscular dystrophies* and *neuromuscular dystrophies*. These include Friedreich's ataxia and dystrophia myotonica.
6. *Sensitivity* and *toxic reactions*. Drugs include antimonials, emetine and some chemotherapeutic drugs. Alcohol, barbiturates and cobalt have all been incriminated.
7. *Deficiency states*. These include magnesium deficiency and nutritional deprivation as in kwashiorkor or thiamine deficiency causing beriberi.

Conditions primarily affecting right ventricular function

Cor pulmonale

The term cor pulmonale was introduced to denote right ventricular hypertrophy and eventual heart failure, associated with a wide variety of diseases of the lung parenchyma, airways, respiratory control mechanisms and thoracic cage. Right ventricular hypertrophy is a consequence of the high afterload produced by the pulmonary arterial hypertension; this is itself caused by the consequences of the pulmonary disease. The diseases associated with cor pulmonale are listed in Table 3.5

Table 3.5   Some conditions associated with the development of cor pulmonale

Diseases of lung parenchyma	Chronic obstructive airways disease
	Fibrosing alveolitis
	Bronchiectasis
	Severe asthma
	Pneumoconioses
Disorders of the thoracic cage	Kyphosis
	Scoliosis
Neuromuscular causes	Skeletal myopathies
	Myasthenia gravis
Obstruction of extrathoracic airways	Large tonsils or adenoids
Disturbances of respiratory control	Extreme obesity
	Cerebrovascular disease
Chronic thromboembolic disease	

Pathogenesis

Until recently it was thought that the destruction of the lung parenchyma led to obstruction of pulmonary blood flow and the development of secondary changes in the heart. However, this theory does not explain the development of the condition where the primary problem lies outside the lungs themselves. A distinct type of pulmonary vascular abnormality is present whether the primary process is pulmonary disease or not. The changes in the pulmonary arteries are now thought to be related to hypoxia although other factors may play a contributory role. This hypoxia causes pulmonary vasoconstriction, which causes the pulmonary hypertension and the increased afterload. Figure 3.25 outlines the probable steps involved.

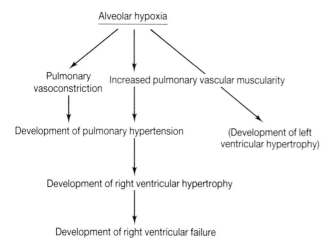

Fig. 3.25 Steps involved in the development of cor pulmonale.

The left ventricle may become hypertrophied in cor pulmonale in the absence of any left-sided problem. It is likely that this occurs because of the hypoxia.

The clinical features of the condition will be largely dominated by the primary disease process. Other signs may be present that reflect the stage of the disease and will include signs of pulmonary hypertension, right ventricular hypertrophy and heart failure (case 4).

Blood gas analysis will show the arterial hypoxia; the carbon dioxide tensions will vary with the underlying condition. The ECG will reflect the changes in the right ventricle; there may be evidence of right ventricular and right atrial hypertrophy (Fig. 3.26). Some of these changes will be masked by the underlying pulmonary disease. There may also be abnormalities of rhythm such as atrial tachycardia, atrial fibrillation or nodal rhythm. A right bundle branch block may also be present.

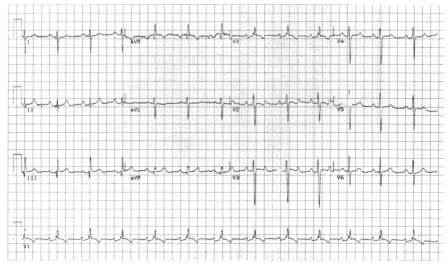

Fig. 3.26 ECG of a patient with cor pulmonale. There is right axis deviation and evidence of both right ventricular and right atrial hypertrophy.

Treatment

The ideal aim of treatment is to reduce the workload on the right ventricle by lowering pulmonary vascular resistance and pulmonary artery pressure. Its success depends on the ability to:

1. Treat the primary disease and relieve respiratory failure
2. Use supplemental oxygen to reduce hypoxia and reduce pulmonary vascular resistance
3. Reduce the oedema with the use of diuretics
4. Reduce the pulmonary artery pressure with the use of vasodilators
5. Reduce the viscosity by venesection
6. Increase ventricular contractility; there is some evidence that digoxin is useful in this condition

Pulmonary embolic disease

Most pulmonary emboli are caused by the dislodgement of venous thrombi and their impaction in the pulmonary circulation. Another fairly common and often unrecognized cause is fat embolus resulting from soft tissue trauma or fractures of bones. Rarer causes of pulmonary emboli include amniotic fluid emboli and tumour emboli.

The causes of venous thrombosis can be conveniently subdivided under three headings which comprise Virchow's triad: stasis, damage to the vessel wall and alteration in the coagulability of the blood. This condition is considered further in Chapter 10.

The true incidence of pulmonary embolic disease is unknown. Estimates of its frequency will depend on the characteristics of the population studied and the basis on which the diagnosis is made and, in particular, whether it was a clinical or a postmortem study. It has been estimated to cause about 21 000 deaths per year in the UK. There is some scope for prevention: early mobilization after an illness such as a myocardial infarction or a pneumonia will reduce the likelihood of venous thrombosis and pulmonary emboli. A high risk group of patients are those undergoing abdominal or pelvic surgery, those over the age of 50 years and those with a previous history of deep venous thrombosis or pulmonary emboli. Measures such as heparin prophylaxis, slight elevation of the bottom end of the operating table and firm special stockings will reduce the likelihood of the problem.

Pulmonary embolism due to venous thrombi can present in three distinct ways, which depend on the volume of the embolic material and the duration of the disease (Table 3.6).

Table 3.6 Clinical syndromes of pulmonary embolic disease

Clinical syndrome	Symptoms	Signs
Acute minor embolism	Pleurisy Haemoptysis	Pleural rub Crackles
Acute massive embolism	Collapse Chest pain Sudden shortness of breath	Acute right heart failure Shock Ventilation/perfusion mismatch
Chronic thrombo-embolic disease	Gradual onset of shortness of breath Effort syncope	Pulmonary hypertension

Acute minor embolism

This occurs when a small amount of venous thrombosis impacts in a small distal pulmonary artery. It is often a 'silent' event and recognized only subsequently with a chest x-ray. Symptoms and signs occur when it involves the pleural surface; pleuritic pain, haemoptysis, pleural rub or fine crackles may then become manifest. The term pulmonary infarction is sometimes used in this setting. In fact, actual infarction with necrosis does not occur in previously normal lungs because of the dual blood supply. It can occasionally occur in diseased lungs with problems in one or other blood supply. This 'pulmonary infarct' is caused by exudation of fluid and cells into the alveolar spaces of the afflicted area of the lung. These radiological shadows appear suddenly and usually resolve completely over a few days although they may leave a linear scar. There are no specific ECG changes, as there are no significant haemodynamic alterations.

Specific treatment of the embolus that has already occurred is not required. Appropriate treatment to prevent further emboli is required as described in Chapter 10.

In the differential diagnosis other causes of pleuritic chest pain, such as a pneumonia, will need to be considered.

Acute massive embolism

This occurs when a large amount of embolic material obstructs the pulmonary arterial tree and causes significant haemodynamic disturbance. In excess of 50 per cent of the pulmonary artery tree is obstructed and the haemodynamic disturbance dominates the presenting clinical picture. Most of the embolic material blocks the central pulmonary arteries; pleural involvement is present in less than a third of patients and will often represent a previous minor premonitory embolus.

The presentation can be considered under three main headings:

1. Acute reduction of cardiac output
2. Acute right heart failure
3. Acute disturbance of ventilation and perfusion

As a result of the obstruction to the pulmonary blood flow, the left ventricular filling pressure drops and cardiac output falls abruptly. This is the cause for one of the classic presentations with collapse. It may be a short episode or may result in sudden death. If the patient survives, there may be a low or unrecordable blood pressure, a sinus tachycardia with a small volume sharp upstroke pulse, peripheral vasoconstriction and evidence of impaired cerebration.

The acute right heart failure is caused by the sudden dilatation of the ventricle as a result of the acute obstruction to the right ventricular outflow. The right ventricle cannot suddenly develop sufficient pressure to overcome the resistance to flow; therefore the signs of pulmonary hypertension and right ventricular hypertrophy are absent. The dilatation of the ventricle may be the cause of the chest pain that can accompany this syndrome; it may be indistinguishable from the discomfort of a myocardial infarction. In the latter the patient will want to sit up because the main insult is to the left ventricle, causing left ventricular failure, whereas in the former the patient will prefer to lie flat and may lose consciousness or become dizzy if upright.

The signs of acute right heart failure include an elevated venous pressure, a gallop rhythm, a tachycardia and delayed closure of the pulmonary valve.

The disturbance in the ventilation and perfusion relationships causes the acute onset of shortness of breath and tachypnoea. A degree of arterial desaturation is usually present and, as a result of the consequent hyperventilation, there is usually a low arterial P_{CO_2}. The mechanism responsible for the desaturation is not well understood; it may be a consequence of right to left shunting across a patent foramen ovale or the perfusion of some atelectatic zones of the lung.

The diagnosis of acute massive embolism is made when a patient presents with the signs of right heart failure, shock and acute shortness of breath, particularly when they prefer to lie flat rather than sit up!

The ECG may show evidence of acute right heart strain (Fig. 3.27). The plain chest radiograph may help in confirming the diagnosis. Impaired perfusion to the affected areas of the lung causes a reduction in the radiologically visible

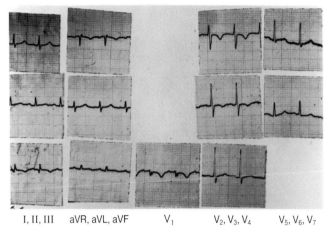

I, II, III   aVR, aVL, aVF V_1 V_2, V_3, V_4 V_5, V_6, V_7

Fig. 3.27 ECG of a patient with an acute massive embolism. The characteristic features are: (1) an S wave in lead I, Q wave and T wave inversion in lead III ($S_1 Q_3 T_3$ pattern); (2) T wave inversion in the right precordial leads; and (3) a partial right bundle branch block.

pulmonary vascular markings; this oligaemia may be the only abnormality present. Sometimes the affected pulmonary artery has an abrupt cut-off rather than the normal tapering. There may also be more peripheral shadows as described under 'Acute minor embolism', above; these will usually represent prior emboli. The diaphragm on the affected side may be elevated due to the resulting loss of lung volume.

The investigation of choice to clinch the diagnosis is pulmonary angiography. The advantage of this test is that it confirms the diagnosis immediately and the catheter inserted into the pulmonary artery can then be used to treat the patient. The disadvantage is that it requires skilled personnel to perform the test. Digital subtraction angiography is an alternative investigation that requires less skilled personnel but does not give quite such accurate information and cannot be used therapeutically. Emboli are seen as filling defects within the pulmonary arteries. At the time of the test the angiographic catheter can sometimes be usefully employed to break up the emboli into smaller fragments, thus aiding their passage more peripherally and often reducing the acute load on the right ventricle. The catheter can also be left in place for the infusion of heparin or a thrombolytic agent such as streptokinase or tissue plasminogen activator (t-PA).

An alternative investigation is that of perfusion scanning using a peripheral vein to inject a radioisotope. This may be combined with the inhalation of an isotopically labelled gas to perform ventilation/perfusion scanning. A normal perfusion scan can exclude the possibility of a major pulmonary embolus; unfortunately, false positives can occur. The ventilation/perfusion scan is more specific (Fig. 3.28).

The treatment of massive pulmonary embolism can be considered under two headings: the immediate resuscitation and the definitive treatment. The immediate resuscitation centres upon helping the right ventricle and reducing the hypoxia. The right ventricular function is critically dependent on the filling

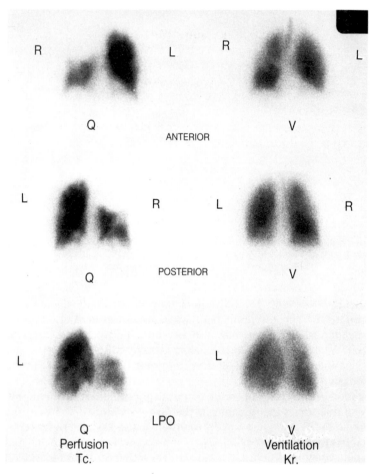

Fig. 3.28 Ventilation/perfusion (V/Q) of a patient with a large pulmonary embolism. The ventilation scan is normal; the perfusion scan shows a large defect in the upper zone of the right lung and smaller defects in the left lung.

pressure; any measure that causes this to fall will potentially kill the patient. Thus any venodilating drug such as the opiates is specifically contraindicated. Many patients will actually benefit from intravenous fluids to raise their right ventricular filling pressure even though the venous pressure is 'normal' or raised; the optimal filling pressure for the acutely stressed ventricle may be very high. The use of inotropes can also be useful. To treat the hypoxia, 100% oxygen should be given by facemask.

Definitive treatment consists of heparin or a thrombolytic agent given intravenously or into the pulmonary artery. Emergency pulmonary embolectomy is occasionally required if the patient does not respond to the above measures.

Differential diagnosis includes other cause of collapse or shock such as myocardial infarction or septicaemic shock.

Chronic thromboembolic disease

This condition is rare and somewhat speculative. Patients typically present with increasing breathlessness which may also be episodic in nature. They may also develop syncope associated with exertion. The physical signs are those of pulmonary hypertension and include a large A wave in the venous pulse, a parasternal heave, delayed and loud closure of the pulmonary valve and, in some patients, the immediate diastolic murmur of pulmonary regurgitation.

The diagnosis is confirmed by catheter studies in which the pulmonary arterial hypertension is determined and angiography demonstrates the occlusions of the pulmonary arteries.

Shock

Definition

The word 'shock' is readily understood in lay terms. In the Shorter Oxford English Dictionary it is defined as 'a sudden debilitating effect produced by over-stimulation of nerves, intense pain, violent emotion, or the like; the condition of nervous exhaustion resulting from this.' The response to injury, pain, fear or sudden bad news will induce a recognizable state in which the victim may be pale, clammy and with a racing pulse. What these conditions have in common is the body's response, that is an increase in adrenergic tone and circulating catecholamines. A similar situation may be seen in clinically definable states that include blood loss, loss of circulating blood volume due to internal fluid movements, and poor output due to a cardiac cause; the appearance of 'shock' is associated with severity and the risk of a poor outcome. Once the measurement of blood pressure became possible, it was noted that a feature in common was hypotension – a lesson that then had to be unlearned when it became evident that the arterial blood pressure might be well maintained in spite of a cardiac output so low that the kidneys and other organs were seriously compromised by poor flow. Perhaps a low cardiac output is the central feature? Not necessarily, because the output may be increased in overwhelming infection, a condition that has become known as septicaemic shock. In pain or distress there may be pallor, sweating and tachycardia but the cardiac output is normal and the arterial pressure may be increased. In attempts to unravel this problem and desperate to find a unifying concept, clinical teachers started defining shock as 'any condition in which there is a failure of tissue perfusion'. Unfortunately, not only is this rather hypothetical and untestable but it can also be used to lump together clinical states, irrespective of whether the blood pressure is high or low, the cardiac output is up or down, or the patient is pale or plethoric. Care should therefore be taken in the use of the word 'shock'.

Individual states such as septicaemia, anaphylaxis, dehydration, blood loss, hypovolaemia, cardiogenic shock and acute anxiety may be specifically recognized and defined. While the failure of the circulatory system to deliver the necessary substrates to, and remove metabolites from, the tissues is a recurring theme, in clinical practice it can be less than helpful. In working practice the features of a poor cardiac output are pallor, peripheral cooling, tachycardia and oliguria. These must first be recognized and then the underlying cause identified.

Approach to the patient presenting in shock of unknown cause

The problem can be approached from a practical point of view. The human circulation can deteriorate to the point close to death in a number of different ways. If the process of deterioration is to be reversed, we need to make a diagnosis and then introduce measures that are appropriate for that condition. Unfortunately, with such a sick patient we are often presented with a dilemma: the diagnosis should come before the treatment is started. However, the physical signs on which we base our diagnosis will tend to disappear as the haemodynamic state deteriorates and the patient approaches death. For instance, the patient with an intestinal catastrophe who presents with severe hypotension may have no abnormal abdominal physical signs. Once fluid has been given and the circulation slightly improved, these signs become more obvious. We have to accept that, in this serious state, we will have to arrive at the diagnosis in stages and will need to give some supportive treatment that will not obscure the underlying condition.

A systematic approach to the patient with a major acute circulatory disturbance (shock) of unknown cause is displayed in Figs. 3.29 and 3.30. The initial measures to be instituted are basic resuscitation. Some of these measures are fully covered in Chapter 12. The early exclusion of a tension pneumothorax is important; it should present no difficulty in diagnosis provided the condition is considered in the first place!

Measurement of the venous pressure is a key step in the diagnostic and

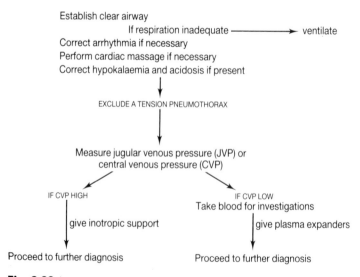

Fig. 3.29 A systematic approach to the patient with shock.

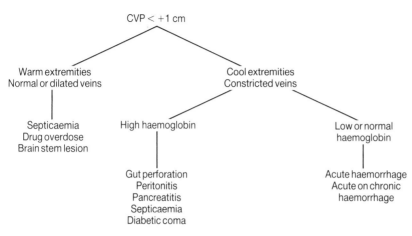

Fig. 3.30 The patient with a low central venous pressure and shock.

treatment pathway. If the jugular venous pressure can be measured accurately, the scheme shown in Fig. 3.29 can be followed immediately. However, in sick patients the venous pressure may be extremely difficult to visualize and the insertion of a central venous catheter is required. The catheter is introduced into the vena cava via either the subclavian or the internal jugular vein. The pressures must then be measured from a predetermined fixed point; the sternal angle or the mid-axillary line are the two main choices but it is very important that the normal range of pressures for each is known and the units of measurement are clearly defined.

If we first consider the low venous pressure group, we can try to discriminate between two main groups; one group will be characterized by having a cool periphery with constricted veins and the other by being warm peripherally with no venous constriction (Fig. 3.30).

If the cause of the low venous pressure is a fall in venous tone, the limb veins will appear to be of normal calibre or may sometimes be dilated. This may occur in opiate or barbiturate overdoses, septicaemia or some brainstem lesions. These patients may retain a reasonable output, as manifest by continuing urine flow, even though the arterial pressure is as low as 50–60 mmHg. The initial management of these patients involves raising the central venous pressure towards the normal range. Because there is a low systemic vascular resistance the arterial pressure will not be restored to the normal range by these measures. Perfectly adequate flow can be obtained in these patients by achieving an arterial systolic pressure in the range of 85–95 mmHg. To strive further to raise the arterial pressure by giving more fluids is unnecessary and is a common iatrogenic cause of pulmonary oedema.

If a low circulating blood volume is the cause of the low venous pressure, the normal intact compensatory mechanisms will produce venoconstriction and cold extremities. If the haemoglobin level is high, evidence of gastrointestinal or renal losses of fluids should be sought. The gastrointestinal losses may be into the lumen of the gut, into the peritoneal cavity or into both. Causes will include perforation, pancreatitis, pyloric stenosis, dysentery and toxic megacolon. Renal losses may occur in diabetic ketoacidosis or the polyuric phase of renal tubular acidosis. If the haemoglobin level is low or normal the likeliest cause is acute haemorrhage. This may not yet be clinically apparent if the bleed occurred into the gut. The treatment of this group of patients involves replacement of the fluid that has been lost and, when appropriate, definitive treatment of the underlying condition. The rate of replacement of fluid is crucial; although it would seem wise to replace a similar volume as has been lost and as quickly as possible, this can lead to serious problems. This is best illustrated in Fig. 3.31. During the initial loss of fluid the venous pressure is maintained by the increasing venous tone. The venous pressure can only be maintained by this compensatory means up to a limit; with the ensuing fall in venous pressure the cardiac output and arterial pressure fall. These changes are described by the curve ABCDE in Fig. 3.31. If ideal circumstances prevail, the replacing volume will allow the curve ABCDE to be reversed. However, if there are circumstances that will keep the venous tone high, the venous pressure may follow a different path, EFGH. Conditions that will cause the veins to remain constricted include anxiety, stress, acidosis or hypoxaemia. By following the path EFGHA the patient may develop pulmonary oedema.

In the group of patients who have a major circulatory disturbance in the presence of a raised venous pressure, the diagnosis can often be made on the basis of the clinical examination, the ECG and the chest x-ray. The conditions

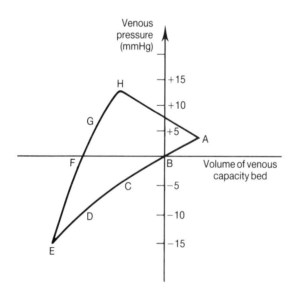

Fig. 3.31 Diagram of venous pressure against venous volume. As venous volume falls along the curve ABCDE, so the venous pressure falls. If ideal circumstances prevail, replacement volume will allow the curve to be reversed. If the haemodynamic and metabolic consequences of being at point DE on the curve are sufficiently severe, the patient will return via curve EFGH; this may produce pulmonary oedema.

that present in this way include myocardial infarction, acute massive pulmonary embolism, acute cardiac tamponade and septicaemia.

Cardiac tamponade may present with a high venous pressure that rises with inspiration, a paradoxical arterial pulse, a tachycardia and a low blood pressure. It is discussed in Chapter 8.

Acute massive pulmonary embolism is discussed above.

Septicaemia has a number of different effects on the cardiovascular system; these effects can vary between patients and can also vary in the same patient at different times. This has implications for both making the diagnosis and the treatment, which may need to be radically changed if the haemodynamic effects of the septicaemia alter. The principles of management of the patient with septicaemic shock depend on defining the particular haemodynamic and other disturbances present at the time. The circulation can then be supported appropriately until such time that the sepsis is successfully treated by antibiotics and any other required measure. The fluid losses are replaced with plasma expanders. The left and right heart filling pressure may need to be modified in order to produce the optimal output without risking pulmonary oedema. Inotropes may be required to maintain an adequate cardiac output. The associated ventilation/perfusion mismatch or intrapulmonary shunts of blood may need to be treated by an increased inspiratory oxygen concentration (FiO_2) together with intermittent positive pressure ventilation (IPPV). The IPPV has to be introduced with care since the positive inspiratory pressure will impede venous return and may cause a pronounced drop in blood pressure. It will improve the hypoxaemia due to ventilation/perfusion mismatch and, if the haemodynamic state will allow the introduction of positive end-expiratory pressure (PEEP), will reduce the tissue exudation into the lungs.

Disseminated intravascular coagulation (DIC) is a frequent complication of septicaemia. In the acute form there is the onset of generalized bleeding associated with a reduction in the circulating blood volume. The laying down of fibrin has been incriminated as one of the causes of the resulting organ damage. The most serious manifestation is renal involvement producing either renal tubular necrosis or irreversible renal cortical necrosis. The skin is also affected and areas of gangrene may form. The fibrin may also play a role in the development of the adult respiratory distress syndrome (shock lung). The DIC can be cured only by effective treatment of the septicaemia; however, the haemostatic state can be maintained with the use of clotting factor and platelet transfusions.

The term cardiogenic shock is used to described the clinical syndrome of hypotension (<90 mmHg), oliguria (<20 ml/h for a few hours) and peripheral vasoconstriction occurring as a result of myocardial disease in patients whose left ventricular filling pressure is adequate. It may occur in such conditions as myocardial infarction or the end-stage of an aortic stenosis. It is associated with mental confusion. The term cardiogenic shock should be reserved for patients in whom the clinical picture occurs in the absence of an arrhythmia or unrelieved chest pain. Occasionally a patient presents with the clinical picture of cardiogenic shock but whose left ventricular filling pressure is low as a result of diuretic therapy. Unfortunately, and potentially misleading, the right-sided filling pressure, as manifest by the venous pressure, may be normal or even high. The patient's condition can be transformed by the infusion of fluids.

The results of treatment of cardiogenic shock due to myocardial infarction are uniformly depressing, mortality rates remaining in excess of 80 per cent. Treatment of cardiogenic shock can be considered under the following headings.

Optimal filling pressure

The measurement of the pulmonary artery wedge pressure reflects the filling pressure of the left ventricle. The damaged left ventricle will require a higher filling pressure for an equivalent output. It may be possible to produce the optimal filling pressure without producing pulmonary oedema. However, inspection of the flat function curve of the damaged ventricle (Fig. 3.11) shows that a substantial increase in the filling pressure may produce a negligible change in the stroke volume. Moreover, as the filling pressure rises, so the likelihood of pulmonary oedema increases.

Inotropes

Inotropic agents have been used for many years without improving the prognosis. The newer agents may have some benefits.

Balloon counter-pulsation

A balloon is introduced into the upper part of the descending aorta; the inflation and collapse of the balloon is ECG triggered. The balloon is deflated in systole and inflates during diastole, thus aiding both coronary flow and forward flow down the aorta. Although the shorter term prognosis may be improved slightly, this technique has not improved the longer term outlook. It does have a role in the patient with a ruptured septum following an infarct since it enables the individual to be supported until the time of surgical repair.

Vasodilatation

Forward flow may be helped by reducing the afterload. However, when the arterial pressure is already low this treatment is potentially dangerous. It must be remembered that, to increase forward flow, the filling pressure must be kept constant. Most vasodilator drugs will produce both venodilatation and arteriolar dilatation; it may therefore be necessary to give fluids to raise the filling pressure in advance of giving the vasodilator.

Further reading

Hurst, J. W. (Ed.) (1990) *The Heart*. McGraw-Hill, London and New York.
Opie, L. H. (Ed.) (1991) *Drugs for the Heart*. W. B. Saunders, Philadelphia.

4

VALVULAR HEART DISEASE

A clear understanding of the normal cyclical pressure changes in the ventricles, atria and great vessels (Figs. 4.1 and 4.2) is essential to an understanding of the symptoms, signs and pathological consequences of valvular heart disease. In each cardiac cycle the ventricles fill through the respective atrioventricular valves which present no resistance to the flow of blood. The final priming of the ventricles is achieved by atrial systole and then, early in systole, the valves close with a soft first heart sound. Once the ventricular pressures exceed those of the

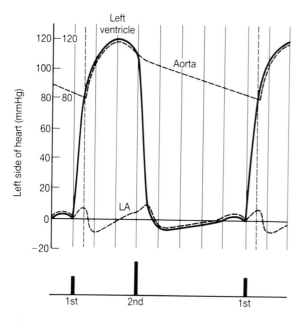

Fig. 4.1 Pressure changes on the left side of the heart. Vertical marks are at 0.2 s intervals. LA, left atrium.

153

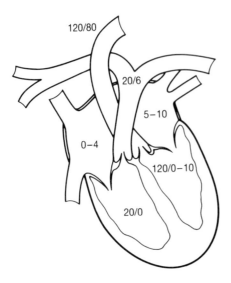

120/80

20/6

5–10

0–4

120/0–10

20/0

Fig. 4.2 Typical pressures in the cardiac chambers of the great vessels at rest.

aorta and pulmonary artery respectively, their valves open and again blood flows silently, without resistance. At the end of systole the valves close with a more abrupt second sound. On inspiration, the pulmonary component of the second heart sound is slightly after the aortic valve sound. The timing of systole and diastole from palpation of the pulse, and recognition of the relationship of the heart sounds to the cardiac events, is fundamental in interpreting the physical signs in valvular heart disease.

The mitral valve

Normal anatomy

The mitral valve annulus is part of the fibrous skeleton of the heart which normally completely separates atrial from ventricular muscle and is traversed only by the bundle of His (a point of importance in maintaining normal sinus rhythm). Its orifice is rather oval, flattened on one side and measures about 2 × 3 cm to give an orifice area of 4–6 cm². It has two cusps and, although they bear little resemblance to the halves of a bishop's hat, it is always called the mitral valve (never the bicuspid valve) by clinicians. The anterior cusp is larger in surface area, and is sometimes known as the septal cusp, or, confusingly, as the aortic cusp because of its anatomical contiguity. The posterior (or mural) cusp is narrower, with a larger circumferential attachment. The two papillary muscles, from which chordae run to the undersurface and the margins of the nearest parts of the two cusps, protrude into the ventricular cavity, approximately beneath the anterolateral and posteromedial commissures.

Normal physiology

The valve opens widely and silently as the left ventricular pressure falls below left atrial pressure (5–10 mmHg) at the rapid filling phase of diastole. The pressures across the valve are identical while the valve is open, both pressures tending to fall as the relaxing left ventricle sucks blood in. The cusps tend to waft together, to open again briefly with atrial systole (see M-mode echocardiograms, Fig. 6.9). At the onset of ventricular systole the valve closes and the cusps and chordae take·the strain, creating the normal soft first sound, as the ventricular pressure rapidly rises. While the mitral valve is closed the pressures in the atrium and ventricle become very different, with an increasing pressure difference across the valve.

Mitral stenosis

Cardiac pathology

There are some very rare examples of isolated congenital abnormalities of the mitral valve which are to some degree obstructive, but virtually all cases of mitral stenosis seen in adults are believed to be a consequence of rheumatic fever (see later). The changes in the valve are the results of the inflammatory process. Particularly characteristic is the development of commissural fusion such that the orifice becomes a buttonhole of about 1 × 0.5 cm (Fig. 4.3). Later changes are fibrous thickening of the cusps, and thickening and matting of the subvalvar apparatus. Finally, what was a delicate structure ends up a thickened and calcified mass.

The atrium hypertrophies and becomes enlarged, partly due to back-pressure, but the muscle itself may also be damaged by the rheumatic process. Atrial fibrillation is likely and the atrium may become massively dilated. Back-pressure causes elevated pulmonary vascular resistance and, in due course, dilatation of the pulmonary artery and the right heart chambers. In long-standing severe mitral stenosis, only the left ventricle and aorta, the structures downstream of the obstruction, are spared. Stasis in the enlarged, fibrillating atrium provides an environment in which thrombus may form, resulting in stroke or peripheral arterial embolism.

Clinical presentation and symptoms

Mitral stenosis is twice as common in women as in men. It is more common in those from the Third World, Mediterranean countries or a poor environment.

Usual symptoms are breathlessness on exertion, orthopnoea and sometimes paroxysmal nocturnal dyspnoea. Palpitation, systemic embolization or haemoptysis may be the presenting symptom in some cases or occur at some time in the course of the disease.

Dyspnoea

As a direct consequence of the stenotic valve the atrial pressure is above the normal resting pressure of 5–10 mmHg and rises further on exertion with the

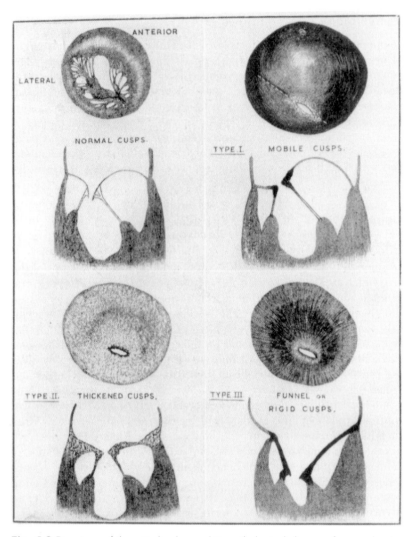

Fig. 4.3 Drawings of the mitral valve and its pathological changes from a classic paper by Thomas Holmes Sellors in 1953, when mitral valvotomy was a common and well-established operation. He described the mobile valve with commissural fusion which was amenable to commissurotomy, and more severe examples with thickened cusps and chordae, and the end stage is an immobile funnel. (Reproduced, with permission, from Holmes Sellors, 1953, *British Medical Journal*, **2**, 1060.)

sudden increase in venous return. Also with exercise there is an increase in heart rate, with shortening diastole limiting the time for ventricular filling through the stenotic valve. As hydrostatic pressure approaches and exceeds the oncotic pressure, water accumulates in the lungs, making them stiff, reducing oxygen transport and causing breathlessness.

Orthopnoea and paroxysmal nocturnal dyspnoea

Dyspnoea on exertion is a non-specific symptom but the characteristic history of orthopnoea (breathlessness on lying down) is of more diagnostic value in identifying cardiac breathlessness due to a raised left atrial pressure (the pathophysiology is described in Chapter 3). A history of paroxysmal nocturnal dyspnoea (PND) is of particular diagnostic help. In its most florid form, patients wake an hour or so after going to bed, gasping for breath and coughing frothy fluid. They characteristically throw open a window and usually gain relief over a few minutes, due to the effect of gravity on the venous return rather than any soothing qualities of the night air. This symptom is partly due to mobilized peripheral fluid increasing venous return, further elevating the left atrial pressure after lying down. These patients tend to sleep propped up once these symptoms develop and thus avoid orthopnoea. PND does not tend to happen after the first few episodes even if the patient does wake breathless having slipped down in bed. This is because of changes in the lung capillary membranes which protect the alveoli from becoming waterlogged even at high left atrial pressures.

Palpitation

The onset of atrial fibrillation, which at first may be intermittent, may be the first symptom appreciated by the patient. Direct questioning about palpitation is important in taking the history because it may be the event that causes a previously tolerated degree of mitral stenosis to become symptomatic. Alternatively, this period of varying atrial rhythms may cause systemic embolization, with thrombus forming during a period of fibrillation and escaping when sinus rhythm returns.

Systemic embolism

Mitral stenosis may present for the first time tragically with a stroke. This can occur in 10 per cent of cases with unrelieved mitral stenosis. Embolism to the leg or mesenteric circulation also occur.

Physical signs

The appearance of the patient varies greatly, depending upon the severity of the stenosis and the length of history. Early in the natural history the patient may appear to be entirely healthy and the discovery of significant mitral stenosis, for example during pregnancy, may come as a complete surprise. Long-standing cases fit the more classic description of a little woman with a malar flush. The mitral facies, a dusky reddening high on the cheeks over the zygoma (or malar bone), is now relatively uncommon in mitral valve disease and is, in any case, non-specific.

The pulse tends to be small volume and may be in atrial fibrillation. Blood pressure is unhelpful in making the diagnosis and the jugular venous pressure reflects the degree of right-sided abnormality that has resulted.

The heart is usually normal in size in cases presenting for the first time. In long-standing cases the heart may be very large but displacement of the apex beat is more likely to be due to the enlarged left atrium rather than a large left

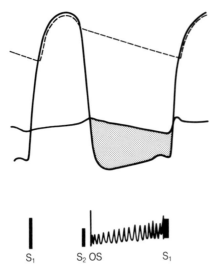

S_1 S_2 OS S_1

Fig. 4.4 Pressures in the left heart in mitral stenosis. S_1 and S_2 are the first and second heart sounds; OS, 'opening snap'. The shaded area represents the pressure difference across the valve.

ventricle. The apex beat is characteristically 'tapping' in quality, due to a palpably increased first sound. There may be a right ventricular heave. Sometimes, in a severe case with a thin chest, a diastolic thrill can be felt as the jet of blood strikes the apex.

On auscultation, the most striking finding is the loud first sound. This and the tapping apex are most evident if the valve cusps are still pliable. The stenotic valve which has been bulging into the left ventricle throughout diastole tenses abruptly in the opposite direction. This occurs at the onset of diastole when, instead of wafting open gently as the ventricular pressure falls, it bulges abruptly into the ventricle, creating the opening snap. There is a rumbling diastolic murmur which may be the most difficult sign to elicit. Some gentle exercise in the form of leg raising may increase the murmur due to increasing the flow, and rolling the patient towards the left makes it easier to hear. The tighter the stenosis, the higher is the left atrial pressure, the longer the murmur and the closer the opening snap is to the second heart sound (Fig. 4.4). Often the murmur becomes more accentuated at the very end of diastole.

Other signs that should be sought are a systolic murmur as evidence of mitral or tricuspid regurgitation and a loud pulmonary second sound which may provide evidence of pulmonary hypertension. Aortic valve disease may coexist.

Investigations

Chest x-ray
The chest radiograph should be examined carefully. There are three signs of left atrial enlargement (Fig. 4.5):

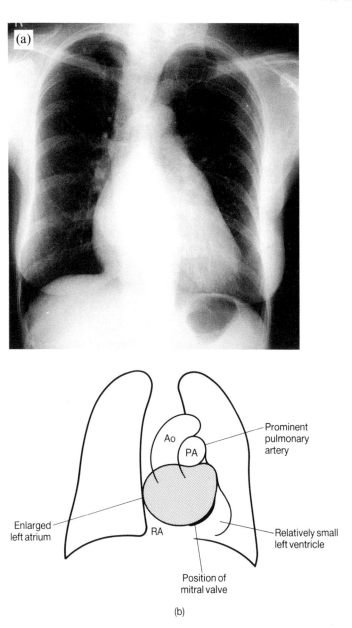

(a)

(b)

Ao
PA
Prominent
pulmonary
artery
Enlarged
left atrium
RA
Relatively small
left ventricle
Position of
mitral valve

Fig. 4.5 X-ray of the heart in mitral stenosis, with a line drawing to help identify the pathological changes. Ao, aorta; LA, enlarged left atrium; PA, pulmonary artery.

1. A double shadow at the right border of the heart where the two atria bulge in the front of and behind the atrial septum.

2. The angle beneath the tracheal bifurcation is normally less than 90 degrees. If the left atrium, which lies immediately beneath, is enlarged, the left main

bronchus runs more horizontally and the bifurcation is splayed to over 100 degrees.

3. The left atrial appendage is normally indiscernible on the chest x-ray but if it is enlarged it bulges out to fill in the concavity below the left hilum.

The aorta is relatively small and the pulmonary artery enlarged; this, with the left atrial enlargement, produces a straight left border to the heart. In addition, enlargement of the upper lobe vessels and the presence of Kerley* B lines, or interlobular oedema as the appearance is now known, are evidence of raised left atrial pressure.

Electrocardiography

Electrocardiography will confirm atrial fibrillation if present, but if the heart is still in sinus rhythm the notched, slightly widened, M-shaped pattern of p mitrale may be seen. In severe cases, right axis deviation and prominent R waves in V_{1-3} are in keeping with right ventricular hypertrophy, secondary to pulmonary hypertension (Fig. 4.6).

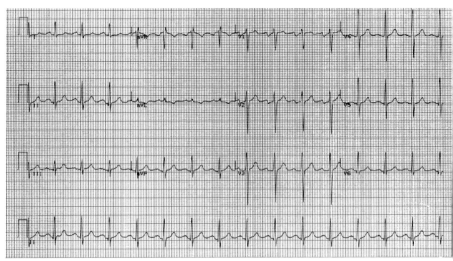

Fig. 4.6 ECG of a patient with mitral stenosis. Note that sinus rhythm is still present and there is 'P mitrale'; the duration of the P wave in lead II exceeds 120 ms and there is a larger negative deflection than positive in the P wave in V_1.

Echocardiography

M-mode echocardiography is particularly valuable in the diagnosis of mitral valve disease. The normal anterior leaflet describes a characteristic 'M' against the time base as it opens in diastole and reopens in atrial systole. This is lost and the leaflets are thickened (Fig. 4.7).

Doppler

The use of echo-guided pulsed Doppler provides information about flow while the echo techniques only show structure.

* Peter James Kerley, British radiologist

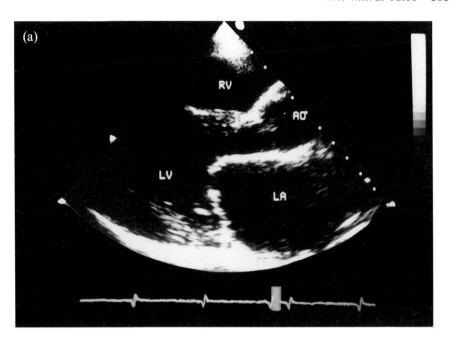

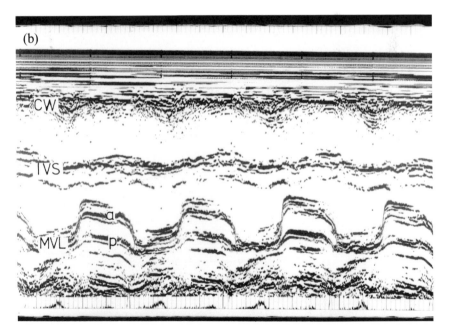

Fig. 4.7 (**a**) Two-dimensional and (**b**) M-mode echocardiogram from a patient with mitral valve stenosis. On the echocardiogram the mitral valve is thickened and its movements are restricted. On the M-mode the characteristic features are the large number of echoes coming from the leaflets and the slow EF slope. a and p = anterior and posterior mitral valve leaflet.

Cardiac catheterization

Invasive investigation is not necessary for the diagnosis of mitral stenosis itself. Its value is in measuring the pulmonary artery pressure, assessing the severity of coexisting abnormalities such as clinically detected aortic regurgitation, which is common in rheumatic heart disease, and in examining the state of the coronary arteries.

Natural history

Rheumatic mitral valve disease can run a very long course. One or more episodes of rheumatic fever may occur in childhood or adolescence (see 'Rheumatic fever' later). First symptoms may occur during the 20s or 30s with the onset of breathlessness or may be brought to light by pregnancy. The course may be punctuated by events such as the onset of atrial fibrillation or, in 30 per cent of cases, a systemic embolus. Exercise tolerance deteriorates through the 40s and 50s, and eventually right heart failure develops with a new set of symptoms and the development of peripheral oedema and ascites.

   Although the course may be long in some cases, it should not be forgotten that this is potentially a lethal disease. In large numbers of patients whose progress was documented in the days before surgery, the median survival was about 15 years in asymptomatic cases, only 7 years in those with mild symptoms and less than 2 years in those who were judged to have moderate to severe symptoms (Fig. 4.8). We should not be lulled into thinking this is a benign disease because

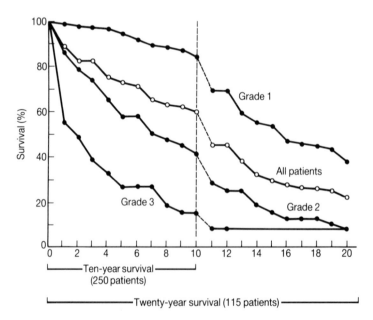

Fig. 4.8 Twenty-year survival in mitral stenosis by grade of severity. (Reproduced, with permission, from J. C. Rowe, E. F. Bland, H. B. Sprague and P. D. White, 1960, *Annals of Internal Medicine*, **52**, 741, © American College of Physicians.)

of the few long-term survivors returning year after year to be seen in our outpatient clinics.

The course of rheumatic heart disease is now punctuated by surgical interventions. In many of the cases seen in the developed world, a mitral valvotomy performed 10–30 years previously dramatically relieved symptoms and increased the average survival of this group by at least 10 years. Nowadays the mitral valvotomy can be performed with a balloon introduced via the femoral vein and approaching the valve via the right atrium and puncture of the interatrial septum. Mitral valve replacement has also been successful in relieving symptoms and improving prognosis, but has added its own pattern of 'prosthetic valve disease', discussed later in this chapter.

Management

The first line of treatment in haemodynamically significant stenosis is to relieve the stenosis by balloon valvotomy or by surgical commissurotomy. If there are significant symptoms, mitral valvotomy is justified on those grounds alone. Even if there are no symptoms, there will be a steady deterioration in the state of the heart and lungs, the onset of atrial fibrillation and the ever present risk of systemic embolism and stroke. It is probably a fair principle that we should aim to relieve any significant degree of mitral stenosis.

In atrial fibrillation, the ventricular rate should be controlled, usually with digoxin. Patients with unrelieved mitral stenosis in atrial fibrillation should be given anticoagulants. Patients still in sinus rhythm are at risk of atrial fibrillation, and it can be argued that we should give anticoagulants in all cases.

If there is pure mitral stenosis, mitral commissurotomy has a very good chance of success. The history of mitral valve surgery is of interest. The concept of valvotomy was suggested by Lauder Brunton, a physician at St Bartholomew's Hospital, in a communication to the *Lancet* in 1902 but was summarily dismissed in an editorial a few weeks later. The first commissurotomy was performed by Souttar at The London Hospital in 1925 but again it was not appreciated. For some reason that is hard to understand the eminent physicians were reluctant to accept that the obvious gross abnormality of the valve contributed much to the patient's state, in spite of Souttar's argument that the problem was 'to a large extent mechanical'. However, it remains true that the degree of involvement of the left ventricular muscle influences the long-term benefits of valve surgery.

Soon after World War II, surgeons who had gained considerable confidence in handling thoracic and cardiovascular injuries, learned to open the adherent commissures with a finger inserted into the beating heart via the left atrial appendage. Closed mitral valvotomy, where the skill has not been lost, remains an excellent low risk operation with a mortality of less than 1 per cent. Many operations are now performed with the heart open and the patient on cardiopulmonary bypass. If there is severe calcification or coexistent regurgitation, the valve must be replaced and then the risk is higher, at about 5 per cent.

Mitral regurgitation

Cardiac pathology

Unlike mitral stenosis, which is due, in virtually all cases, to rheumatic heart disease, mitral regurgitation may be due to one of a number of causes. A variety of congenital abnormalities involve the mitral valve, including those in the spectrum of atrioventricular septal defects. Parachute valve and a variety of uncommon malformations result in mitral regurgitation which usually presents in infancy and childhood.

Various abnormalities of connective tissue may involve the mitral valve and cause it to become regurgitant. These include Marfan's syndrome (see Chapter 7), pseudoxanthoma elasticum and Ehlers–Danlos syndrome, but most frequent among these is floppy mitral valve. In this condition the valve is thicker than normal and increased in area, and redundant. It has a yellowish appearance and in its most florid form has the appearance of omelette. The chordae are elongated and may rupture, and the annulus is enlarged. The valve may prolapse or a leaflet become flail causing regurgitation.

Acute rheumatic carditis may cause mitral regurgitation or there may be predominant regurgitation in a chronic case. After surgical valvotomy, there may be significant regurgitation. Infective endocarditis may occur on any mitral valve abnormality and cause or exacerbate regurgitation.

Ischaemia may cause mitral regurgitation through various mechanisms. The failing ventricle may dilate and 'functional' regurgitation may occur purely due to annular dilatation. Left ventricular aneurysm may distort the subvalvar apparatus such that there is malalignment. Ischaemic papillary muscles do not function satisfactorily. After infarction there may be complete rupture of a papillary muscle, causing sudden severe regurgitation.

An uncommon but well described cause of mitral regurgitation is chordal rupture due to a bursting effect of blunt chest trauma, such as against a steering wheel in a deceleration injury.

Apart from the valve itself, the pathological appearances depend upon whether regurgitation has developed acutely or if it is a chronic state. In acute regurgitation due to some acute process such as papillary muscle necrosis, the chambers are of normal size. In chronic disease the left atrium and ventricle are both very much enlarged as a result of a chronic volume load. In due course the right-sided chambers become enlarged due to a pressure load. Note that in their pure forms dilatation and hypertrophy of cardiac chambers can be distinguished and may occur under different circumstances. In mitral regurgitation the enlargement is due to a varying combination of the two.

Clinical presentation and symptoms

The clinical picture of mitral regurgitation similarly depends on whether it is acute or chronic. Acute mitral regurgitation, as occurs with a sudden rupture of a chorda or a papillary muscle, results in a large proportion of the left ventricular stroke volume refluxing into a small atrium and creating back-pressure on the pulmonary veins. Reflex tachycardia and peripheral vasoconstriction due to poor cardiac output make the situation worse. The major symptom is breathlessness, perhaps with paroxysmal nocturnal dyspnoea, orthopnoea and frothy sputum typical of acute pulmonary oedema. Other symptoms are those of the underlying condition, which might be myocardial infarction or infective endocarditis.

Chronic cases may be free of symptoms in spite of severe regurgitation. If the condition develops gradually the atrium dilates and the addition of the regurgitant volume creates little change. The ventricle dilates gradually and generates the additional stroke volume required at little increase in end-diastolic pressure. In the absence of myocardial ischaemia or other major complicating factor, these patients may have very few symptoms.

There are also cases of trivial regurgitation that come to light because of the discovery of a mid-systolic murmur or a click. Because they do not have mitral regurgitation to any extent, they are discussed later under the heading 'Floppy mitral valve'.

Physical signs

The state of the periphery and the pulse depend upon the cardiac output, and may be normal or impaired. They are of value in assessing the patient's state but not of the presence or severity of regurgitation. Similarly, the jugular venous pressure tells us something of the right-sided consequences.

The apex beat is displaced laterally because of overall enlargement of the heart in these cases. The heart sounds are dominated by a pansystolic murmur, which overruns the second sound, heard best to the left of the sternum, radiating well over towards the axilla. The regurgitant volume has to re-enter the ventricle with the pulmonary venous return and there may be a delayed diastolic murmur due to the much increased flow across the valve. There is also a third sound of ventricular filling (Fig. 4.9).

Investigations

Chest x-ray
Left atrial and ventricular enlargement are seen in proportion to the severity and chronicity of the leak. The whole heart may be very large in the absence of major symptoms.

ECG
The ECG may be normal. There may be evidence of left ventricular hypertrophy or evidence of underlying disease such as myocardial infarction.

Echo-Doppler
The M-mode echocardiographic features of mitral regurgitation are difficult for the non-expert to appreciate, but two-dimensional echocardiography has made it easy to see valve prolapse, ruptured papillary muscles or chordae. Doppler studies show retrograde flow into the left atrium during systole and can be quantified.

(a)

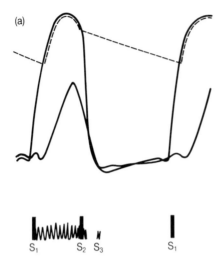

S_1 S_2 S_3 S_1

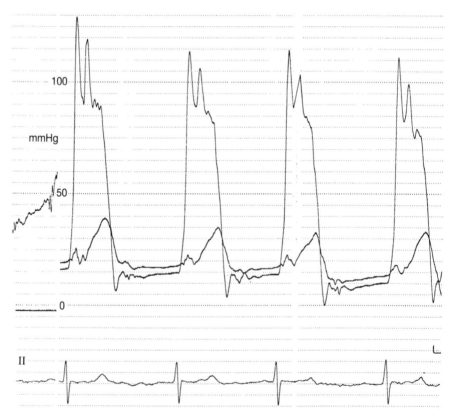

Fig. 4.9 (a) The diagram shows a left atrial pressure wave in mitral regurgitation. **(b)** An actual example of left ventricular and left atrial pressures recorded simultaneously.

Cardiac catheterization
Left ventricular angiography shows the state of the left ventricle and the degree and direction of the regurgitant jet. The coronary arteries can be visualized.

Natural history

Acute severe mitral regurgitation, complicating myocardial infarction or infective endocarditis, may be rapidly fatal unless the patient can be saved by valve replacement.

The natural history of mild regurgitation is benign. Patients who have progressed slowly over many years have a good outlook despite a large heart and dramatic chest x-rays.

Regurgitant mitral valves are particularly prone to endocarditis.

Management

The options for treatment include valve replacement, valve conservation and repair, and medical management.

In asymptomatic cases, in a condition with a relatively benign prognosis, there may be little to gain by replacing the valve. On the other hand, if the condition progresses, valve replacement later is more dangerous and will not reverse the deterioration. The decision can be a very difficult one. If the heart is getting larger over a period of months or years, it is usual to recommend valve surgery to halt the deterioration. Symptomatic cases are usually much improved by operation, sometimes very dramatically. After elective mitral valve replacement, the likelihood of leaving hospital alive is about 95 per cent.

Surgery is undoubtedly life saving in severe acute cases but carries a commensurately higher risk. Urgent valve replacement in the week following myocardial infarction has a mortality of about 35 per cent with or without coronary grafting. Elective surgery where valve replacement is combined with coronary artery grafting for ischaemic heart disease has an in-hospital mortality of up to 10 per cent.

Floppy mitral valve

A group of clinical syndromes and echocardiographic and pathological appearances will be discussed under this heading. They seem to be manifestations of a common underlying abnormality but this is not entirely clear. The terms myxomatous mitral valve degeneration, mitral leaflet prolapse, billowing mitral valve syndrome and Barlow's syndrome are used, more or less as synonyms.

Pathology

Valves removed surgically are not representative of the syndrome as a whole because they are from a selected minority who have a haemodynamic problem. Those seen have a range of appearances but in its most florid form the cusp tissue is soft, thickened, redundant and ballooning. The valve seems to be too large even for a dilated annulus and there seems to be extra tissue at the commissures, giving the appearance of a quadricuspid valve. The chordae are yellow, thin and elongated. Chordal rupture is one of the reasons they come to operation. Histologically there is acid mucopolysaccharide in the valve, hence the name myxomatous degeneration.

The strong association between mitral valve prolapse and well recognized abnormalities of connective tissue in Marfan's disease and Ehlers–Danlos syndrome suggests that there is a primary abnormality of collagen in its aetiology. However, the description of myxoid change is not uncommon in pathology and is by no means specific.

The tricuspid valve may be involved but surgical removal of the tricuspid valve for this condition must be very rare.

Symptoms and clinical presentation

Patients who present with severe acute regurgitation due either to ruptured chordae or to endocarditis have the symptoms and signs of those conditions and are managed as already described, irrespective of the underlying cause. The management of chronic severe mitral regurgitation has also been dealt with. In this section we are primarily concerned with those without significant mitral regurgitation.

The symptoms include palpitation and atypical chest pain. Much has been made of the observation that some of these patients are very anxious and even psychiatrically disturbed. It has been suggested that the neurotic symptoms are caused or perpetuated by the discovery of something wrong with the heart. Alternatively, with such a common echocardiographic abnormality, patients with coincidental abnormalities will be included. Nevertheless, there are many examples of patients whose symptoms have been discounted as neurotic because doctors did not understand the disease.

Clinical signs

The signs of interest are a mid-systolic click and a late systolic murmur. The murmur is due to the redundant, billowing posterior cusp spilling blood back into the atrium during late ventricular systole. The murmur is typically preceded by a click caused by abrupt tensing of the mitral valve and its subvalve apparatus as it is pushed backwards into the left atrium in mid-systole. Sometimes several clicks are heard due to prolapse of individual scallops of the mitral valve. If there is prolapse without regurgitation there is a click but no murmur.

Investigations

Chest x-ray
The heart is normal in appearance. Straight thoracic spine and pectus excavatum have been described. They may be associated with the condition, if it is a true tissue abnormality, or alternatively influence the echocardiographic visualization of the mitral valve.

ECG

Non-specific ST and T wave changes in the inferior leads are sometimes seen and have led to the suggestion that papillary muscle ischaemia might be part of the problem, either as a cause, permitting prolapse, or as a consequence of abnormal tensions. Arrhythmias can be documented.

Echocardiography

The diagnosis is dependent on echocardiography revealing cusp prolapse. If echo criteria alone are used, 5 per cent of the population has the syndrome. A small minority of these have the full syndrome, including the murmur and click. For the majority, there are serious doubts about the relationship between the echocardiographic diagnosis and the symptoms (Fig. 4.10).

Natural history

Floppy valve disease is particularly prone to endocarditis and is a common underlying cause. Unquestionably, a small proportion of patients suffer ruptured chordae and develop severe mitral regurgitation. Sudden death from arrhythmia occurs very rarely. For most people the condition is quite benign and associated with a normal life span.

The aortic valve

Normal anatomy

The aortic valve has three semilunar cusps, each opposite a shallow bulge in the aortic root, the sinuses of Valsalva. The coronary arteries give their names to the cusps and to the sinuses from which they arise. The left coronary ostium is in fact more or less posterior; so, therefore, is the left coronary cusp, and the right coronary artery arises directly anterior which is therefore the position of the right coronary cusp. The non-coronary cusp lies to the right (Fig. 4.11). The nomenclature is potentially confusing.

The aortic valve sits in the middle of the heart. It is related to the right atrium and right ventricle which lie in front and the left atrium behind. It is in continuity with the anterior leaflet of the mitral valve and is closely related to the bundle of His. Disease of the aortic valve and sinuses can involve all these structures.

Normal physiology

At the end of isovolumic contraction the valve opens widely and silently, with each cusp accommodated in its respective sinus so that the stream of blood is presented with a channel of even width and is ejected without turbulence. At the end of systole, eddy currents in the sinuses, behind the valve, encourage the cusps to begin closing; closure is completed, producing the aortic component of the second sound. The pressure in the aorta then falls gently, governed by the peripheral run-off. The pressure in the ventricle falls rapidly and the valve holds a pressure difference, with a maximum of 80 mmHg during diastole (see Fig. 4.1).

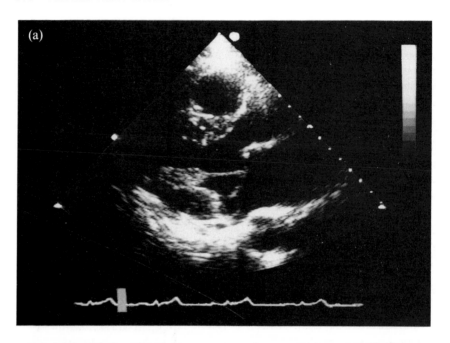

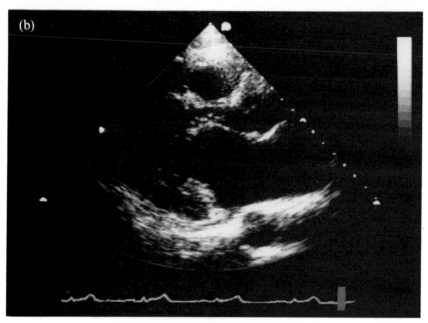

Fig. 4.10 A systolic (**a**) and diastolic (**b**) frame of a two-dimensional echocardiogram of a patient with mitral valve prolapse. The systolic frame shows the closed mitral valve which is bowing, or prolapsing, back into the left atrium. The diastolic frame shows the mitral valve in the open position.

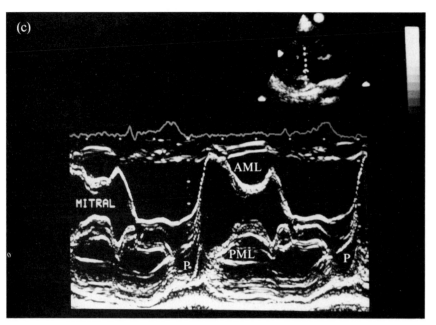

Fig. 4.10 (c) The M-mode reveals the characteristic pattern of movement of the mitral valve in systole, which is shown by the posterior displacement (P) occurring at the end of ventricular systole. AML, anterior mitral valve leaflet; PML, posterior mitral valve leaflet.

Aortic stenosis

Cardiac pathology

Severe degrees of congenital abnormality of the aortic valve present in infancy and childhood. These are described in Chapter 5. Milder degrees of abnormality are compatible with normal health but are subject to stiffening and calcification with time, and are one of the three common causes of stenosis of the aortic valve presenting in adult life. The other two are rheumatic and senile calcific aortic stenosis.

In milder congenital abnormalities of the aortic valve there is usually deficient development of one of the commissures, resulting in a bicuspid valve. In its most frequent form there is a common cusp to the left, representing fusion of left and right coronary cusps. A common anterior cusp due to fusion of the right and non-coronary cusps is also seen. Sometimes both these commissures are absent and there is a single cusp with an eccentric orifice. Rarely, there are no commissures identifiable (Fig. 4.12). In general, the more abnormal the anatomy, the earlier the presentation.

In rheumatic aortic stenosis there is thickening of the valve tissue and more or less symmetrical fusion of the commissures. In senile calcification the anatomy appears to be normal but the cusps have become rigid with calcification. By the time any of these valves presents as aortic stenosis there is extensive calcification, but the underlying cause can usually be readily determined.

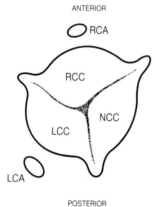

Fig. 4.11 Diagram of the aortic valve to illustrate the nomenclature. LCA, left coronary artery; LCC, left coronary cusp; NCC, non-coronary cusp; RCA, right coronary artery; RCC, right coronary cusp.

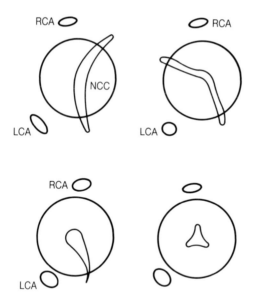

Fig. 4.12 Typical patterns of aortic valve abnormality described in the text, in order of frequency seen.

The left ventricle is massively hypertrophied with a small cavity, although in advanced cases there is dilatation and the external dimensions of the heart become enlarged. There may be poststenotic dilatation of the aortic root, although this is a very variable feature. In the more severe forms of congenital abnormality the aortic root may be distorted and there is sometimes further narrowing at the level of the commissures. Other parts of the heart are normal, other than in advanced cases.

Clinical presentation and symptoms

The three cardinal symptoms of aortic stenosis are effort syncope, angina and breathlessness on exertion.

The typical history of syncope is sudden loss of consciousness after unaccustomed exercise such as carrying a heavy suitcase upstairs or running for a train. The patient may recover from one or more such episodes before presenting, or die at the first attack. It is likely that effort syncope is a result of sudden severe arterial hypotension which occurs because the limited flow through the stenotic valve cannot keep pace with exercise-induced peripheral vasodilatation. Arrhythmia may follow, in an ischaemic hypertrophied ventricle, but is unlikely to be the primary cause of effort syncope.

Angina due to aortic stenosis has all the characteristics of that associated with coronary stenoses. The simple explanation is that, on effort, the hypertrophied left ventricle requires more blood than can be supplied. An additional explanation is that the jet of blood actually robs the coronaries by drawing blood retrogradely from their orifices by a Venturi effect. Of course, in these patients, who are often elderly, coronary artery disease may coexist.

Breathlessness on exertion develops insidiously and is discounted as being due to age. It is not usually associated with orthopnoea but may well be a result of an increase in left ventricular end-diastolic pressure (LVEDP) and, therefore, left atrial pressure.

Occasionally, aortic stenosis presents with transient ischaemic attacks or amaurosis fugax due to cerebral or retinal platelet emboli from the irregular valve.

Advanced cases may present stuporose and oliguric with an extremely poor cardiac output. (Under these circumstances there may be no murmur.)

Infective endocarditis may be the first manifestation, although this is more commonly associated with regurgitant aortic valves.

Some are detected without symptoms because a murmur is heard or an abnormality detected on chest x-ray or ECG. Interestingly, many of these 'asymptomatic' patients feel better after relief of their aortic stenosis by valve replacement, illustrating how insidious the symptoms may be.

Clinical signs

The general appearance of the patient is normal. The pulse is regular but there is a reduction in the rate of rise of the pressure wave, which is best appreciated by palpation of the carotid artery where a 'judder' may also be felt, particularly on the left. In expert hands, this is the best way of deciding clinically if a patient with a systolic murmur has significant stenosis. The blood pressure is of no diagnostic help. The pressure-controlling mechanisms are downstream of the diseased valve and, provided they are intact, endeavour to maintain normal pressure. Hypertension may occur. Hypotension is a near terminal event. The relationships between pressures and heart sounds are illustrated in Fig. 4.13.

The jugular venous pressure is not usually elevated although a prominent a wave may be detected due to the hypertrophic septum reducing the normal compliance of the right ventricle.

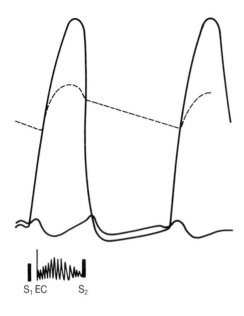

S₁ EC   S₂

Fig. 4.13 A pressure diagram showing changes in aortic stenosis (cf. Fig. 4.1). 'EC' indicates ejection click in a young patient with a bicuspid valve (above). Below is the situation in the more typical calcified valve, demonstrating the reduced intensity of aortic closure.

The cardiac impulse may be abnormally forceful but is not displaced unless the heart is enlarged. A thrill may be palpable over the aorta.

On auscultation the most striking sound is a loud, harsh, ejection systolic murmur. This may be audible at the apex but the diagnostic feature is that it radiates into the neck. An early diastolic murmur is audible when aortic regurgitation coexists. This is best heard with the patient leaning forwards in complete expiration. There is always some regurgitation in rheumatic aortic stenosis.

Cases presenting in terminal state may have no murmur and be virtually pulseless.

Investigations

Chest x-ray

The heart size is not usually enlarged, on the basis of a cardiothoracic ratio (0.5), but there may be a prominence of the left border. The ascending aorta also may be prominent and these two together give a characteristic shape to the heart. Aortic valve calcification may be seen on the lateral film, above the oblique fissure (Fig. 4.14).

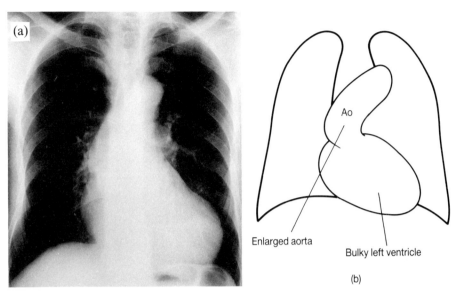

Fig. 4.14 (a) An x-ray of the heart in aortic stenosis, with (**b**) a drawing showing the changes in the aorta and left ventricle.

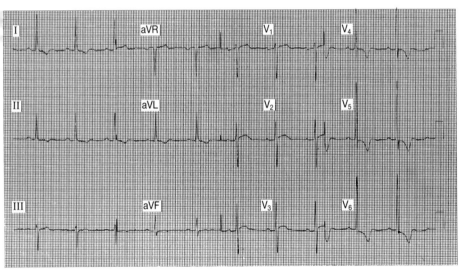

Fig. 4.15 ECG showing sinus rhythm with a normal QRS axis. There is left ventricular hypertrophy and strain pattern.

ECG

Usually there is sinus rhythm. The features of left ventricular hypertrophy should be present. The voltage of the QRS complex in the chest leads are increased, with flattening and, later, inversion of the T waves in V_5 and V_6. The usual criteria are that the S wave in lead V_1 or V_2 plus the R wave in lead V_5 or V_6 should total 35 mm (7 large squares) (Fig. 4.15).

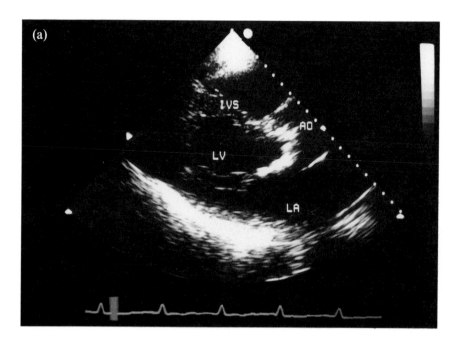

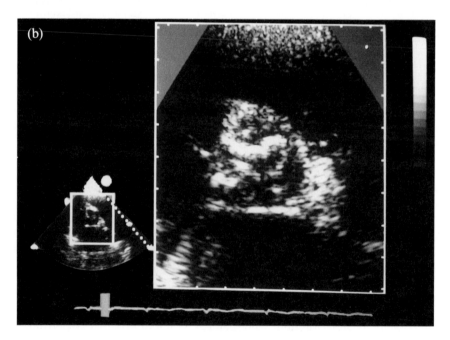

Fig. 4.16 The long axis (**a**) and short axis (**b**) views of the level of the aortic valve in a patient with calcific aortic valve stenosis. There are dense echoes arising from the aortic valve; with the moving image it can be recognized that the opening of the aortic valve is severely restricted.

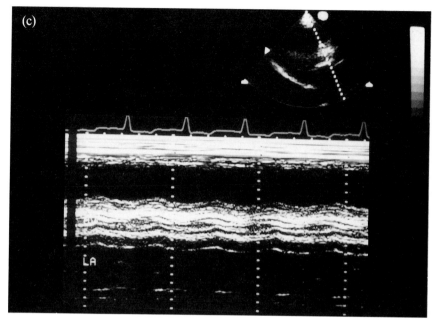

Fig. 4.16 (**c**) The M-mode of the same distorted aortic valve shows a lot of echoes arising from it. These pictures should be compared with the views of a patient with a normal aortic valve. (See also Fig. 6.8.)

Echocardiography

The heavily calcified valve gives off bright echoes. Left ventricular hypertrophy and left ventricular function can be assessed. The abnormal anatomy may be seen with two-dimensional echocardiography (Fig. 4.16).

Cardiac catheterization

The gradient is usually measured by passing an arterial catheter retrogradely across the aortic valve and then withdrawing it back into the aorta. The smaller the orifice and the greater the flow, the bigger the pressure drop across the valve. At presentation it is typically between 60 and 100 mmHg (Fig. 4.17). Coronary artery disease, aortic regurgitation and associated lesions can be diagnosed at the same time.

Natural history

Aortic stenosis leads to sudden death in an important minority of cases. From the onset of symptoms the median survival is under 2 years and the development of heart failure is particularly ominous. Patients who have had syncopal attacks should be warned to avoid exertion because they are at risk at any time.

The gradient across the valve increases as it stiffens but then falls as the cardiac

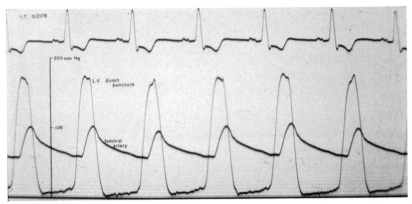

Fig. 4.17 A recording of the ECG, a direct left ventricular pressure and a femoral artery pressure recording. The patient had aortic valve stenosis. The pressure difference across the valve is about 75 mmHg.

output falls. In the presence of good left ventricular function, a gradient of 60 mmHg should be regarded as carrying a bad prognosis. If the cardiac output is reduced for any reason, a lower gradient may be significant. Cardiac function deteriorates quite rapidly.

Management

Clinically or haemodynamically significant aortic stenosis should be relieved. There are few exceptions. Fit patients with symptoms or a significant gradient should be offered elective surgery. Age itself is no barrier. Patients with terminal low cardiac output have no prospect of survival unless the obstruction is relieved.

Elective valve replacement can be performed, with a mortality of under 3 per cent; associated coronary artery disease can be bypassed at the same time, with little difference in the risk. The risk is higher if there is severe impairment of left ventricular function. Relief by balloon valvuloplasty may buy time in the worst cases.

Aortic regurgitation

Cardiac pathology

There are many causes of aortic regurgitation. Congenital abnormalities of the valve may present as regurgitation in adult life. Bicuspid aortic valve, a very common malformation (which is described in this chapter, under 'Aortic stenosis', and in Chapter 5) is particularly likely to lead to regurgitation, and then presents at a much younger age than with stenosis. Bicuspid valves are particularly prone to infective endocarditis and may present either acutely with infection or be seen with healed endocarditis but a damaged valve. Congenital abnormalities that may be associated with aortic regurgitation are high ventricular septal defect, when the right coronary cusp may prolapse, and subvalvar stenosis, when the poststenotic turbulence may damage the valve cusps.

Rheumatic heart disease is the commonest cause of abnormality of the valve itself. This rarely presents as pure aortic regurgitation but is seen as a mixed lesion with aortic stenosis or rheumatic mitral stenosis, or both. The list of rare causes of acquired disease of the aortic valve includes systemic lupus erythematosus.

The aortic valve may be regurgitant due to annular disease as is seen in Marfan's syndrome (see Chapter 7), syphilis, yaws, Reiter's syndrome, ankylosing spondylitis, osteogenesis imperfecta and hypertension. In these conditions the valve cusps are fairly normal but the annulus is so dilated that they no longer master the orifice. Quite rarely, aortic dissection is survived and remains undiagnosed to present with aortic regurgitation.

The left ventricle is enlarged, both hypertrophied and dilated, and there may be dilatation of the aorta in response to the volume load.

Clinical presentation and symptoms

Aortic regurgitation may be well tolerated (see 'Mitral regurgitation' earlier in this chapter) because the heart accommodates the volume load well. Breathlessness is a feature once symptoms start and some patients may have angina, particularly on lying down.

The condition may be detected by discovery of an abnormal x-ray or ECG or some other chance finding.

Clinical signs

The signs of aortic regurgitation may be very dramatic even though the symptoms are few. With severe long-standing regurgitation the whole neck pulses in a dramatic way and the head may bob in time with the pulse.

The pulse pressure is very wide, with a high systolic pressure collapsing almost completely in diastole. This collapsing pulse gives rise to several signs of interest. The brachial artery can be made to tap the examiner's fingers which, in the past, reminded physicians of the sensation of the Victorian physics teachers' 'water hammer' as water falls through a vacuum. Auscultation over the femoral arteries may produce a pistol shot sound or a to-and-fro murmur. The diastolic pressure is low and the sounds may be heard even when the cuff pressure has fallen to zero.

The murmur of aortic regurgitation may be difficult for the learner to detect because it is usually soft in quality and quite localized, but once heard it is diagnostic. It is a blowing murmur heard at the left sternal edge, which may be made more easily audible if the patient leans forwards and breathes out completely. It can also be brought out by squatting. In addition, at the apex, there may be a lower-pitched diastolic murmur due to the anterior leaflet of the mitral valve fluttering in the regurgitant jet, the Austin Flint murmur (see 'Echocardiography', below).

Investigations

Chest x-ray
The heart is usually enlarged but this may remain modest for many years. Progressive increase in heart size is an important and ominous observation that indicates deterioration. Enlargement or calcification of the aorta may help in diagnosis.

ECG
Sinus rhythm with evidence of left ventricular hypertrophy and strain are the usual features.

Echocardiography
M-mode echocardiography shows the fluttering of the anterior mitral leaflet, which both excludes mitral stenosis (because the valve is mobile and opens widely) and confirms aortic regurgitation.

Cardiac catheterization
Aortography permits quantification of the aortic regurgitation and diagnosis of other abnormalities such as aortic stenosis, mitral valve disease or coronary artery disease.

Natural history

There may be a stable state for many years with the extra volume load on the left ventricle tolerated well. Eventually, but rather unpredictably, the ventricle dilates and the deterioration in left ventricular function is only partly retrievable. Average survival is only 2–3 years after cardiac enlargement or ECG changes begin to progress.

Management

If symptoms are severe or the left ventricle is enlarging, and, in particular, if the left ventricular end-systolic dimension is greater than 55 mm, aortic valve replacement is indicated. If the clinical state deteriorates abruptly, due to endocarditis for example, valve replacement is needed urgently. Inpatients with mild symptoms and no more than moderate regurgitation the decision is very difficult. Early operation subjects a patient with few symptoms and a good prognosis to major surgery. If the decision is delayed too long, a sick patient is subjected to a more hazardous operation with less prospect of benefit.

The tricuspid valve

Normal anatomy

The cross-section of the right ventricle is approximately triangular. The septum is functionally part of the left ventricle and from the right ventricular side is gently convex, forming one side of the triangle. The anterior and diaphragmatic surfaces meet at an acute angle, marked externally by the acute marginal artery. The annulus is much less clearly defined than the mitral annulus, as are the commissures. The cusps fit this triangular configuration and are named septal, anterior and posterior (actually inferior). The cusp tissue and the chordae are thinner and more delicate than those of the mitral valve.

Pathology

The tricuspid valve may be congenitally abnormal in association with the mitral valve in atrioventricular septal defects, and in its own right in Ebstein's anomaly (see Chapter 5).

Acquired organic disease of the tricuspid valve is relatively rare. It can be involved with the rheumatic process but tricuspid stenosis is rare. It is more commonly regurgitant, secondary to pulmonary hypertension and right ventricular dilatation, most commonly associated with left heart disease, but can occur with primary pulmonary vascular disease.

Carcinoid tumours that have metastasized to the liver produce serotonin (5-hydroxytryptamine) which damages the right-sided valves. Tricuspid endocarditis is seen in drug addicts; they are prone to endocarditis on other valves also but the repeated injection of dirty, particulate-laden drugs damages and infects the tricuspid valve.

Tricuspid regurgitation

Clinical presentation and symptoms

The symptoms of tricuspid regurgitation are the consequence of chronically elevated right atrial pressure. Dependent oedema, ascites, and abdominal pain and tenderness due to liver engorgement are typical.

Clinical signs

Oedema, ascites and hepatomegaly should be assessed.

The jugular venous pulse should be carefully examined. In tricuspid regurgitation it may be so high that no pressure wave can be determined but if the patient is sat up vertically, and the top of the venous column can be seen, the wave is in time with systole (s wave).

The murmur of tricuspid regurgitation has to be distinguished from mitral regurgitation. It is a pansystolic murmur, which is increased on inspiration, heard best to the left of the lower end of the sternum.

Natural history

The course of tricuspid valve disease is dominated in most cases by the natural history of the associated condition. Most frequently, tricuspid regurgitation forms part of multiple valve disease. In one particular circumstance tricuspid regurgitation is seen as an isolated lesion – after tricuspid resection in drug addicts. We know that it is poorly tolerated and although these patients have survived without a tricuspid valve, they are very symptomatic and long-term survivors have needed tricuspid valve replacement.

Management

The condition of patients with tricuspid regurgitation is improved by bedrest and diuretics but it returns as they become active again.

If a patient with tricuspid regurgitation is being operated upon for other valve disease, it is possible to improve the situation by valve replacement or annuloplasty, although in some cases, if the left-sided disease is controlled, the tricuspid regurgitation improves secondarily. This is a difficult judgement to make.

Valve surgery

History

Mitral valvotomy was the first valve operation. It is performed within the beating heart without the need for cardiopulmonary bypass and remains a highly successful operation for relieving pure mitral stenosis. A little of its history was given earlier. It came into routine use in the late 1940s and the operation was performed in large numbers in the 1950s when many patients with what was a common disease obtained excellent benefit at low risk. The operation is hazardous in the presence of atrial thrombus or valve calcification, much less effective in severely thickened valves, and inapplicable in mitral regurgitation. Early attempts at closed operations to help cope with mitral regurgitation were hopeless. The operation remains highly successful in the relief of pure mitral stenosis, but is limited to this application.

The principles of closed valvotomy were extended to the pulmonary valve by Holmes Sellors in 1947 and Brock in 1948, and were particularly useful in the palliation of Fallot's tetralogy. Attempts at closed aortic valvotomy in the early 1950s did not come to much. The only valve replacement possible before cardiopulmonary bypass was a ball valve prosthesis (the Hufnagel valve) inserted in the descending aorta in an attempt to limit aortic regurgitation.

Cardiac surgery was limited to extracardiac operations (e.g. closure of patent ductus, coarctation), the various forms of valvotomy, and operations that could be performed in the few minutes of circulatory arrest permissible at 30°C (see the section on atrial septal defect in Chapter 5). Cardiopulmonary bypass was first used by Gibbon in 1953 in the Mayo Clinic to close an atrial septal defect, and from then it became possible to operate within the heart and direct surgery on valves became feasible (Fig. 4.18).

The development of replacement valves has followed two separate but parallel lines: mechanical and tissue valves (Fig. 4.19). There have been many but the ones described here not only were landmarks in historical development but also are all in current use. The first consistently successful prosthesis was of ball and cage design, called the Starr–Edwards valve after its developers, a cardiac sur-

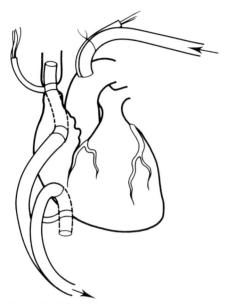

Fig. 4.18 The heart prepared for full bypass.

Valve protheses

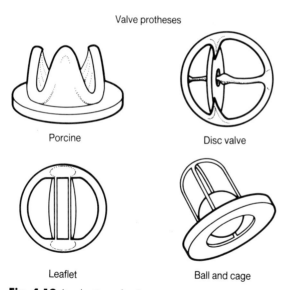

Porcine

Disc valve

Leaflet

Ball and cage

Fig. 4.19 A selection of valve types.

geon and an engineer. It was first used in the early 1960s and remains the most durable mechanical valve. There have been a number of prostheses on the caged ball principle but few others are still used. Their disadvantages are that the occluder sits in the middle of the flow, creating turbulence and resistance to flow, and the cage is bulky. Tilting disc valves overcome these two disadvantages; the best known is the Björk–Shiley valve, again after a surgeon and an engineer. From time to time there have been problems with disc valves jamming shut, the disc embolizing or the whole device clotting, with predictably disastrous results. The next step in the evolution of mechanical valves was a bileaflet valve, which avoids the finality of these catastrophes in that half the valve can still function and give some time in which the situation can be salvaged. The St Jude valve is the archetype of this pattern. As a group, mechanical valves are durable but all need life-long anticoagulation.

Human cadaveric grafts, reported separately by Ross and Barratt Boyes in 1962, were the first tissue valves used to replace the aortic valve. These are generally called homograft valves although, by modern convention, they are allografts. A variety of preservation and sterilization methods have been tried over the years but the methods that have been most successful are fresh storage in antibiotic solutions and freeze drying. Homografts were adapted for use in the mitral position without great success. Carpentier produced the first serviceable, glutaraldehyde-preserved, stent-mounted porcine valves in 1968 and, with various modifications, these have become the standard tissue valve. They are known as xenografts. They can be used to replace the aortic, mitral or tricuspid valve. Man-made valves of preserved calf pericardium are an alternative type of tissue valve. As a group, tissue valves are much less prone to thromboembolic problems but are much less durable. A few fail unpredictably in the first few years, but, from about 7 years after implantation, some failures can be expected from wear and calcification. At 10 years, 80 per cent are still functioning, and median valve survival is about 12–13 years.

Outline of the surgical techniques

Valve replacement is performed on cardiopulmonary bypass, which supports the patient while the heart is non-working and open. The whole body's venous return is drained to the bypass machine either by a single large cannula in the right atrium or, if the heart itself has to be opened or displaced, separate cannulae are placed in the superior and inferior venae cavae. After oxygenation the blood is returned under pressure to a cannula placed in the ascending aorta.

During the cardiac part of the operation, the commonest procedure is to arrest the heart by a technique called cardioplegia. Cold (4°C) potassium-rich (20 mmol/l) blood or electrolyte solution is infused into the aortic root or into the coronaries directly.

The native valve is excised and all annular calcification is removed so that the valve can be seated well. Great care must be taken not to damage surrounding structures and to avoid entering adjacent chambers of the heart. The replacement valve has a sewing ring with a cuff of material through which continuous or multiple interrupted sutures are placed. Once the valve is in place, the heart is closed, air is excluded, it is reperfused with blood and begins to beat again.

It is usually possible to complete the intracardiac part of the operation within an hour and the whole procedure, for a routine single valve replacement, takes about 3 hours.

Risks of operation

All cardiac operations performed in the UK are subjected to an annual audit. The hospital (or 30-day) mortality for about 5000 valve replacements in total averages 5 per cent, being slightly more for mitral valve replacement and less for aortic valve replacement. Individuals may have predictably higher or lower risks, these identifiable features being called 'risk factors'. Some factors that increase the risk of perioperative death are, in approximate order of their influence: attempts to retrieve patients from a moribund state; the presence of endocarditis; recent myocardial infarction; chronic right-sided failure and hepatic dysfunction; pulmonary hypertension; multiple valve operation; reoperation; combined valve and coronary operation; and increasing age. It is important to recognize them because they go into the estimate of risk and benefit that helps to decide if surgery is the best management of an individual case. If none of the risk factors applies in, for example, an otherwise fit patient having an elective single valve operation, the chances of survival are close to 100 per cent. In an elderly moribund patient in renal failure caused by severe mitral regurgitation due to uncontrolled infection on a calcified xenograft (this problem does occur!), the chances of success approach zero.

Immediate risk

Death in the operating theatre is now very uncommon but results if the state of the heart is so poor that it will not take over after cardiopulmonary bypass or if haemorrhage cannot be controlled. The causes of death in the first few hours after surgery are poor cardiac output, haemorrhage, tamponade and cardiac arrhythmia. The postoperative care of these patients therefore includes careful monitoring of the ECG, arterial pressure, central venous pressure, central and peripheral temperature, urine output and blood loss.

Early complications

Arrhythmias of every type occur after cardiac surgery – frequently supraventricular tachycardia, rarely ventricular tachycardia and sometimes complete heart block. Cardiac output may be poor due to left and/or right ventricular disease. Renal failure and hepatic failure are now uncommon but, if they occur, the chances of a successful outcome become remote. The chest requires special attention after surgery and anaesthesia, and more so after chest operations and artificial ventilation. Infection has become uncommon but sternotomy wound infection is a very major problem and prosthetic valve infection is a disaster. Neurological complications occur in 1–2 per cent of cases, and range from the (now rare) catastrophes of failure to wake after surgery or major hemiplegia to minor visual field defects. Most are due to perioperative embolism of air, clot or particles of calcium. Many patients have a more subtle alteration in their cerebral state which may impair memory and concentration.

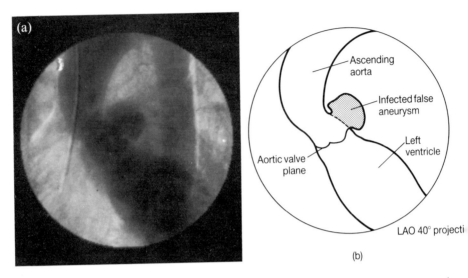

Fig. 4.20 Intravenous digital subtraction angiogram of a patient, showing aortic root and infected false aneurysm in the 40 degree left anterior oblique projection. (Reproduced, with permission, from G. Hunter, H. Thomas, T. Treasure, M. F. Sturridge and H. S. Swanton, 1988, *British Heart Journal*, **60**, 252.)

Late complications and their avoidance

All patients with cardiac abnormality are at risk from endocarditis (Fig. 4.20) (see later), particularly those with an artificial valve. All dental work and other possible sources of bacteraemia should be covered by prophylactic antibiotics. A simple and probably effective regimen for dental work is amoxycillin 3 g an hour before treatment, and a further dose 6 hours later. Most cardiac surgical units provide patients with a card (either their own or from the British Heart Foundation) detailing the indications for and nature of antibiotic prophylaxis.

All patients with artificial valves are at risk from embolism. Stroke is a particularly tragic complication. All mechanical valves must be anticoagulated for life to reduce this risk but anticoagulation itself carries a risk of haemorrhage of about 2 per cent per year.

The outlook for a patient with an artificial valve is thus far from perfect. If we add the risks of endocarditis, embolism and haemorrhage, the likelihood of eventual tissue valve failure, the progression of some aspects of heart disease and the persistence of others, the chances of being free from heart-related disease are not great.

Rheumatic fever

Rheumatic fever is due to a hyperimmune response to a bacterial antigen resulting from a *Streptococcus pyogenes* infection. In its typical form the disease is an acute febrile illness characterized by inflammation of the joints, heart, skin and nervous system and often preceded by a pharyngitis caused by this streptococcus in the Lancefield group A. Chronic disease of the heart valves may ensue.

The streptococcal components that cross-react with human tissue are known to damage the myocardium, the sarcolemma and the glycoproteins of the heart valves. Large amounts of immunoglobulin G (IgG) and complement are often found in the heart muscle of children dying from acute rheumatic fever.

Epidemiology

The incidence of rheumatic fever and rheumatic heart disease is declining in developed countries. In contrast, it is still a scourge in countries where over-crowding, malnutrition and other poor environmental conditions prevail. About 90 per cent of the initial attacks of rheumatic fever occur in the 4- to 14-year-old age group. In some tropical countries juvenile rheumatic heart disease is a common and aggressive disease. Many of these young people have severe pulmonary hypertension; mitral valve commissurotomy is not uncommon under the age of 20 years!

Pathology

The pathology of rheumatic fever is characterized by diffuse proliferative and exudative inflammatory lesions in the connective tissues, particularly around small blood vessels. The disease is unusual because of its unique lesions of the heart and its tendency to spare other organs from serious damage.

The hallmark of rheumatic fever is the Aschoff granuloma (Fig. 4.21). It consists of a central area of fibrinoid degeneration which is surrounded by lymphocytes, monocytes and polymorphonuclear leucocytes. Aschoff nodules may persist for years after the attack of acute rheumatic fever.

Acute rheumatic endocarditis is characterized by a verrucous valvulitis which causes swelling, oedema and deformity of the valves; it leads to permanent valvular deformities over the ensuing years (Fig. 4.22). Healing of the valvulitis may occur with fibrous thickening and adhesions of the valve commissures and chordae tendineae, leading to varying degrees of stenosis or regurgitation.

Microscopically, an important feature of the affected valves is the presence of blood vessels in the cusps which are normally avascular. Capillaries grow into the cusps from their base early in the first attack of rheumatic fever. Some of these subsequently enlarge and grow into arterioles and venules. Capillarization is followed by acute inflammatory oedema (Fig. 4.23).

Superficial ulceration occurs at and around the parts of the valve cusps that are in contact during closure. This is due to the loss of endothelium resulting from the impact of valve closure on the inflamed oedematous cusps. Platelets and fibrin are deposited and build up to form vegetations. The acute changes are followed by organization of the vegetations and more diffuse fibrous thickening of the cusps.

The residual effects with permanent distortion are usually confined to the mitral and aortic valves. Pulmonary valve lesions are uncommon, and tricuspid valve involvement is seen in only about 10 per cent of cases.

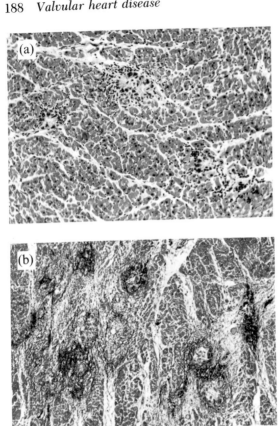

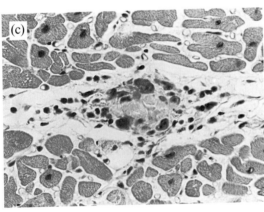

Fig. 4.21 Rheumatic myocarditis. (**a**) The acute stage, showing several Aschoff bodies. ×80. (**b**) Later stage, showing fibrosis around the Aschoff bodies (Masson's trichrome stain: collagen appears dark). ×48. (**c**) Early Aschoff body in the myocardium of a child who died of heart failure during an attack of acute rheumatic fever. Central hyaline material is surrounded by macrophages, some with large or multiple nuclei, and by lymphocytes etc. ×310. (Reproduced, with permission, from J. R. Anderson (Ed.), 1985, *Muir's Textbook of Pathology*, 12th edn, Edward Arnold, London.)

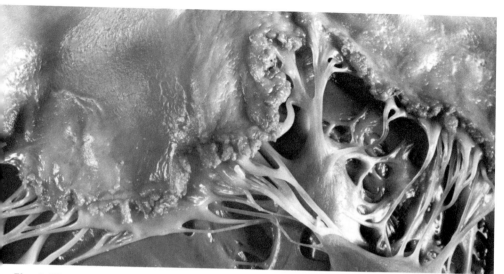

Fig. 4.22 Mitral valve in acute rheumatic endocarditis, showing the small vegetations which form along the line of apposition of the cusp. ×2. (Reproduced, with permission, from R. N. M. MacSween and K. Whaley (Eds.), 1992, *Muir's Textbook of Pathology*, 13th edn, Edward Arnold, London.)

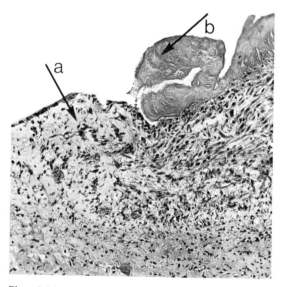

Fig. 4.23 Section of the mitral valve in acute rheumatic endocarditis. The cusp shows inflammatory oedema (**a**) and cellular infiltration, and appears to be vascularized. Where the cusps meet, the oedematous tissue has ulcerated and platelets have been deposited on the ulcerated surface to form the early vegetations (**b**) ×80. (Reproduced, with permission, from R. N. M. MacSween and K. Whaley (Eds.), 1992, *Muir's Textbook of Pathology*, 13th edn, Edward Arnold, London.)

The pericarditis is exudative with effusion of serous fluid and deposition of fibrin on both pericardial surfaces (Fig. 4.24).

The diagnosis of acute rheumatic fever

The symptoms and signs of acute rheumatic fever vary greatly. Some major and minor criteria have been developed which are helpful in making the diagnosis (Table 4.1). A high probability of rheumatic fever is present when two major criteria, or one major plus two minor criteria, exist in the context of proven recent streptococcal infection. It must be emphasized that the prevalence of the disease in a community will have a marked effect on the specificity and sensitivity of these criteria.

Table 4.1 Major and minor criteria used for diagnosis of rheumatic fever

Major criteria	Minor criteria
Carditis	Fever
Polyarthritis	Arthralgia
Erythema marginatum	Previous rheumatic fever or rheumatic heart disease
Chorea	Elevated ESR
Subcutaneous nodules	Prolonged PR interval

Major criteria

The carditis that occurs is a pancarditis involving the myocardium, pericardium and endocardium. Pericarditis occurs in about 10 per cent of cases and is always associated with rheumatic valvular involvement. A friction rub, and sometimes a pericardial effusion, is present. Unexpected heart failure is indicative of myocardial involvement. The involvement of the atrium in the rheumatic process may largely determine the individual susceptibility to the future development of atrial fibrillation. Endocarditis is manifest by the presence of a heart murmur. Murmurs vary in character and intensity during the course of the disease; a short rumbling mid-diastolic mitral murmur (Carey Coombs murmur) may be present due to blood flow over acutely inflamed valves. Systolic murmurs may be present; these may reflect flow across an inflamed aortic valve or the increased flow associated with fever and anaemia.

The polyarthritis involves the large joints. Two or more joints should be involved and will be red, swollen and tender; there will be some limitation of joint movement. The pain and joint involvement are fleeting or migratory.

Rheumatic chorea has become less common and occurs in only 2–3 per cent of cases.

Subcutaneous nodules occur in about 5 per cent of patients. They are found over the extensor surface of the body, particularly at tendon insertions or joints. They are also noted over the occipital region, the vertebral spine and the extensor surfaces of the elbows, knees and wrists.

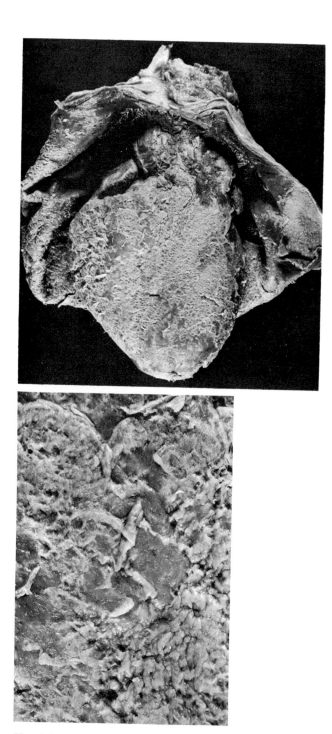

Fig. 4.24 Acute pericarditis: showing a thick, irregular deposit of fibrin on the pericardial surface. The appearance has been likened to that when a butter sandwich is pulled apart ('bread and butter' pericarditis). (**a**) ×0.7; (**b**) ×3. (Reproduced, with permission, from R. N. M. MacSween and K. Whaley (Eds.), *Muir's Textbook of Pathology*, 13th edn, Edward Arnold, London.)

Erythema marginatum is a fleeting ringed erythematous eruption. It is seen predominantly on the trunk and proximal parts of the body.

Minor criteria

The prolongation of the PR interval is considered by some to be a major criterion; it has become less common a manifestation. Other minor criteria include a raised ESR, fever, anaemia, leucocytosis, arthralgia, pleurisy and a previous history of rheumatic fever. Occasionally, abdominal pain reflects rheumatic peritonitis.

Differential diagnosis

Acute rheumatic fever may be mistaken for juvenile rheumatoid arthritis, congenital heart disease, osteomyelitis, systemic lupus erythematosus, gonococcal arthritis or a viral carditis. Occasionally an atrial myxoma may mimic acute rheumatic fever.

Treatment

Rest should be advised while there is evidence of active disease. If there is definite evidence of carditis, bedrest should be continued for at least 6 weeks.

Drug therapy

The symptoms of acute rheumatic fever may be helped by salicylates or corticosteroids. However, neither of these drugs reduces the likelihood of subsequent chronic valvular disease.

Heart failure may need to be treated with digoxin, diuretics or vasodilators.

Prophylaxis

Penicillin will reduce the likelihood of further attacks from 70 per cent to less than 4 per cent in populations at risk. It is the drug of choice and can be given by intramuscular injection every 3 weeks or, alternatively, as oral phenoxymethyl-penicillin twice daily. An alternative to penicillin, but not quite so effective, is a sulphonamide drug. The drug therapy needs to be continued until early adult life; if there is a recrudescence in spite of treatment, the treatment must be continued for life.

Prognosis

The mortality from acute rheumatic fever is approximately 7 per cent. Ten years after the onset of acute rheumatic fever about 50 per cent of the patients have chronic rheumatic heart disease.

Infective endocarditis

Pathology

Endocarditis requires a combination of a vulnerable intracardiac site and exposure to a suitable organism. The cases we see most commonly now are of infection on abnormal cardiac valves, either the patient's own valve, which is in some way abnormal, or an artificial heart valve. Bicuspid, previously asymptomatic, aortic valves and regurgitant, typically floppy, mitral valves are now the most common but rheumatic, stenotic valves are also vulnerable. It affects congenitally abnormal hearts, ventricular septal defect particularly, and congenital abnormalities outside the heart itself (patent ductus arteriosus, coarctation) where the term 'endarteritis' is more specific but the same principles apply. It affects previously healthy valves under unusual circumstances, such as the endocarditis that is seen in intravenous drug users.

The transient occurrence of organisms in the blood stream is not a rare event and bacteraemia can be demonstrated under a variety of circumstances, in particular after dental work. The gingival margin has a close relationship with blood vessels, and the resident flora of the mouth can be demonstrated in the circulation on a fairly regular basis after dental treatment. Scaling and polishing, which appear to be minor, comprise an assault on the gingival margin on a broad front and should not be underestimated. Instrumentation of the urogenital and gastrointestinal tracts may also be responsible for some cases. It is difficult to be confident about the cause and effect relationship between any particular event and the occurrence of endocarditis. Endocarditis has an insidious course and there is a time lapse between the presumed bacteraemia and clinical presentation. Bacteraemia is common and dental treatment, cystoscopy etc. are carried out commonly without apparent harm. A causative organism is not always identified.

Virtually any organism can cause endocarditis, which is a reason for avoiding the old term 'subacute bacterial endocarditis', which has become so firmly entrenched as the abbreviation 'SBE'. The viridans streptococci group of organisms (*Streptococcus mutans*, *milleri* and *mitis*) are still responsible for about half the total cases, and for the majority of cases that follow the more classic pattern. Staphylococcal infection is more commonly responsible for a newer pattern of disease which affects prosthetic valves. A proportion of these are due to the skin commensals, coagulase negative staphylococci (*Staphylococcus aureus* species) probably introduced at the time of surgery but taking months to present. Enterococci (*Strep. faecalis*) are also seen, sometimes with a recognized colonic source.

Flow through the normal heart is smooth and non-turbulent, and it is where the endothelium might be damaged by turbulence that endocarditis seems to occur. It is usually seen on the downstream side of a stenotic lesion (on the right side of a ventricular septal defect, in the pulmonary artery with a patent ductus arteriosus) or where a jet lesion impinges. Deposits of platelets and fibrin, with organisms within them, form vegetations at these sites. The infection tends to invade tissue, destroying the valves. In the aortic valve in particular, it burrows into the annulus, forming abscesses around the aortic root and into the septum.

Vegetations may break off, producing a variety of consequences including stroke, visual field defects and abscess formation elsewhere.

Symptoms and presentation

The initial symptom is nearly always with an influenza-like episode with fever, generalized aches and malaise. If an antibiotic is given at this time, the patient usually feels better, perhaps for a couple of weeks, but the symptoms recur. It is quite possible that an unknown proportion of very early cases of endocarditis, with sensitive organisms, are in fact cured by antibiotics at this stage. This is no excuse for what is at the very least an illogical practice, that is treating what you believe to be a viral illness (a cold or 'flu') with a drug that acts against bacteria. In the cases that are subsequently seen, this practice has served only to delay the diagnosis and permit the endocarditis to do more damage.

Patients with artificial valves or any other cardiac lesion are warned about the risk of infection on the valve and many are given a card or booklet. The existence of a vulnerable cardiac lesion is a vital part of the history.

Clinical signs

A patient with endocarditis may be moribund with florid signs or appear remarkably well. A high index of suspicion is required in some cases but a febrile patient with a cardiac lesion should be considered to be a case of endocarditis until a better explanation is found.

Clubbing and anaemia occur in long-standing cases. Splinter haemorrhages in the nails should be sought and noted, to distinguish between the consequences of minor trauma and the appearance of new ones. Osler's nodes are tender nodules in the pulp of the fingers. The explanation for them is not clear but they are thought to be caused by a vasculitis due to immune complexes rather than recurrent systemic particulate microemboli from valve vegetations.

In the cardiovascular system, any abnormality of the heart is important in confirming that the patient is a candidate for endocarditis. Any new murmur, or a change in one heard in the past, is suggestive. In particular, with prosthetic valve endocarditis the detection of a new regurgitant murmur is virtually diagnostic. These murmurs should be carefully listened for. Even when the diagnosis is made, one should listen for changes because then they are critically important in deciding on management.

Splenomegaly may occur. A neurological examination and a record of the peripheral pulses should be entered in the notes, and retinal emboli should be looked for.

Daily clinical examination is important to assess the progress of treatment of the infection and to monitor cardiac failure, which is now the commonest mode of death in this condition. If there is a haemodynamic lesion, usually valvar regurgitation, or a ventricular septal defect, urgent surgery may be the only way of reversing a downward trend.

Investigations

The critical investigation is blood culture. A series of cultures should be taken. Antibiotic should be delayed until these have been secured, which can be done in the first few hours after admission. Taking blood as the temperature rises may increase the chance of detection, and using multiple venous sites reduces the chance of a false result due to contamination. About 20 per cent of cases are culture negative.

Haemoglobin may be low; the white cell count and erythrocyte sedimentation rate may be raised. The chest x-ray shows evidence of the underlying abnormality but change in heart size is most critical in monitoring progress of a regurgitant lesion. The lung fields should be searched for evidence of lung abscess, which is common with right-sided lesions.

ECG may show, in particular, a lengthening PR interval which is indicative of the formation of a septal abscess.

Echocardiography (Fig. 4.25) is very valuable. If vegetations are seen, the diagnosis is confirmed. It also permits progress of the disease to be followed, both evidence of valve destruction and cardiac function. Cardiac catheterization is usually avoided because of the risk of embolization of dislodged vegetation.

Natural history

Before antibiotics were available, endocarditis was uniformly fatal. Even now, the mortality is 25–30 per cent. If the infection is due to a sensitive organism and treated early enough, cure should be possible in most cases. Delayed diagnosis, prosthetic endocarditis and resistant organisms all reduce the chance of cure.

The infection invades tissue and destroys the valves. Development or worsening of regurgitation is usual and may require urgent valve replacement. Severe and worsening left ventricular failure is the usual terminal event under these circumstances.

The valve annulus may be attacked; infection burrows down into the septum from the aortic valve annulus and results in heart block. Vegetations may embolize and all the usual consequences of systemic emboli may occur, plus the consequences of infection.

Management

In view of the high mortality of this condition and the possibility of cure if the best decisions are made at the best time, there is an argument for some of these cases being looked after in a surgical centre unless there is prompt response to treatment. A team of microbiologist, cardiologist and surgeon, working together, offers the best chance of cure. Surgery is of value in a minority of cases but will not succeed if it is not considered until the patient is in extremis.

As soon as blood cultures are taken, intravenous antibiotics should be given in adequate doses for a period usually not less than 6 weeks, although the later part of the treatment may not have to be intravenous. There is debate about whether to use central or peripheral lines, the central line being a potential source of

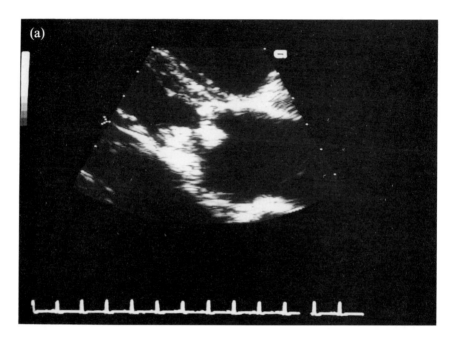

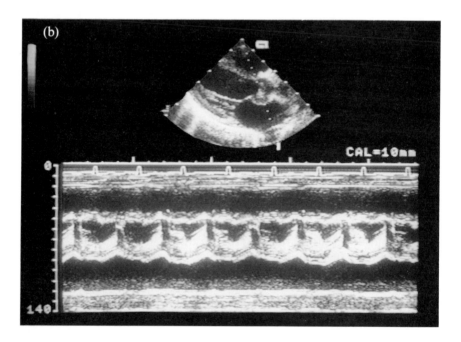

Fig. 4.25 (**a**) Two-dimensional echocardiogram and (**b**) M-mode of a patient with infective endocarditis. A mass of echoes are seen on the aortic valve.

further bacteraemia in spite of its convenience for long-term therapy. Some also favour continuous rather than intermittent therapy. It is usual to start with a broad spectrum combination that tackles streptococci and staphylococci. Gentamicin, penicillin and flucloxacillin are most used but obsessional care in checking drug levels of gentamicin is important. The treatment is then modified according to the results of culture and the advice of a microbiologist, preferably one with an interest and experience in endocarditis.

Surgery should be used very selectively and only when the prospects of saving the patient on medical treatment are beginning to look unlikely (not when all hope has gone!). Usual indications are:

1. An important haemodynamic lesion amenable to correction (e.g. valve regurgitation or a shunt)
2. The development of heart block, indicating abscess formation (see Fig. 4.20) and infection beyond the reach of antibiotics alone
3. Failure to bring infection under control with medical treatment
4. Embolization is sometimes regarded as an indication but, once it has occurred, the situation cannot be retrieved by operating on the source. It is a moot point whether surgery after the event reduces the risk of further embolization but, once effective antibiotic treatment is started, embolization becomes uncommon.

5

CONGENITAL HEART DISEASE

About 1 per cent of babies are born with congenital abnormalities of the heart; many of these are localized abnormalities in otherwise apparently normal hearts, such as a defect in the atrial septum (ASD), persistence of the ductus arteriosus (PDA) or a localized narrowing in the aorta (coarctation). These are surgically curable. In more complex cases the abnormal development of the heart results in perhaps several coexisting abnormalities; a well known example is Fallot's tetralogy (see later) in which there is narrowing of the right ventricular outflow, a defect in the ventricular septum, an abnormal relationship between the aorta and the left ventricle, and right ventricular hypertrophy. Some of the components can be corrected surgically, but the heart remains abnormal. Finally, there are hearts that are lacking one or more of the fundamental components. If the functional anatomy cannot be corrected, the best that can be done may be a palliative operation; for example, increasing or decreasing the blood flow to the lungs. Notice the three words 'cure', 'correct' and 'palliate' that have been used and will be used in the sense outlined in this introduction.

Most cases of congenital heart disease are now diagnosed in infancy, or even *in utero* with the improving resolution of two-dimensional echocardiography. Some cases are evident at birth and most can be detected in the first weeks of life. If the condition is severe enough to reduce life expectancy or to produce limiting symptoms, an important question to be asked is 'can this be cured or corrected by surgery?' The timing depends on several factors. Other things being equal, an operation is easier and safer as the child increases in size. Some babies will not survive without urgent surgery, and some conditions deteriorate, so surgery must be performed early. For most cases where surgery plays a part in management, it is likely to be undertaken before school age. Congenital heart disease may first be detected by the obstetrician, paediatrician or family doctor but its management is largely in the hands of relatively few specialists. In this book we have taken the view that, just as the technical details of operations are not helpful except to those actually involved, there is no purpose in transcribing the subtleties of physical signs that may be elicited in some of these extremely rare conditions.

Typical presentations of cardiac disease in infancy are the mother's observation that the baby has difficulty in sucking and breaks off to pant, or that the baby becomes blue on crying. Murmurs may be heard but may appear at various times as the pulmonary vascular resistance, normally high *in utero*, falls and the flow of blood changes. In infancy the working diagnosis can often be made on probabilities, narrowed down on the basis of a few key features recognized by experience and rapidly confirmed by investigation. In childhood the history and examination are more helpful in diagnosis. Because not all patients with congenital heart disease can be 'cured', all practising doctors should be aware of a new population who have undergone surgery and have 'corrected' or 'palliated' abnormalities and live on into adult life, and may need further assessment and surgery.

There are various ways of organizing a chapter on congenital heart disease. Embryology helps us to understand some of the lesions but does not help a great deal in clinical classification. Some writers have felt that classification by presenting features (e.g. cyanotic versus non-cyanotic) has a certain logic in a problem-solving approach. Unfortunately the list of symptoms is limited (feeding poorly, seems chesty, not gaining weight) and fails to discriminate one case from another. Anatomy largely determines whether surgical cure or correction is possible, although the pulmonary vascular resistance may determine the outcome. The various conditions are therefore grouped in this chapter more or less by anatomical features, beginning with extracardiac lesions, then abnormalities of septation and valve lesions, ending with rare and complex congenital malformations. We have not listed everything that occurs.

Terminology

The terminology of congenital heart disease can be made bafflingly complex. We need not concern ourselves with this in too much detail but some explanation is helpful. In the normal heart we describe chambers as right or left, terms that relate only approximately to their anatomical position but are a shorthand for a statement about their functional connections, so the 'left heart' has come to mean those chambers that cope with the systemic circulation. In a heart that is abnormal in position and in which the chambers give rise to the wrong vessels, the ventricle is neither functionally nor anatomically on the 'left'. The modern morphologist uses the term 'left' ventricle to identify a chamber with recognizable structural characteristics of a left ventricle, irrespective of where it is or what it does!

'Dextrocardia' refers to a heart that is situated in the right hemithorax. More precise analyses of lateralization are suggested by the use of the term 'situs'. In situs solitus, the normal state, the right atrium and its cavae, the liver and the vertically running (eparterial) right main bronchus are where we expect them to be, on the right. They are all reversed in situs inversus (thoracic and abdominal situs virtually always agree). In some very rare cases there may be a form of symmetry with two 'right' atria, two superior venae cavae, a symmetrical bronchial tree, a central liver and no spleen. This is called asplenia syndrome or right-sided isomerism. In left-sided isomerism there is polysplenia. Both produce extremely abnormal hearts. Fortunately, to understand most forms of heart disease, description of well recognized patterns is sufficient.

Aetiology

There are three possible predetermining factors: intra-uterine infection, chromosomal abnormalities and genetic inheritance. The best known and most common example of intrauterine infection causing congenital heart disease (i.e. disease present at birth) is rubella infection in the first trimester. Rubella syndrome includes deafness, choroiditis and, in the heart, pulmonary valvular stenosis and pulmonary arterial stenoses. This condition should now be preventable. Chromosomal abnormality causing congenital heart disease is typified by the very high incidence (20 per cent) of atrioventricular septal defects in trisomy-21 (Down's syndrome). The best example of a genetically determined cardiac abnormality is bicuspid aortic valve, which appears to be an example of mendelian dominant inheritance. In most cases of congenital heart disease, however, the aetiology is unknown.

Persistent ductus arteriosus

The ductus arteriosus is a central feature of the fetal circulation. The pulmonary artery, the ductus itself and the descending aorta are a continuum, and are the route by which desaturated blood from the systemic venous circulation and the right heart reach the umbilical arteries and the placenta. The oxygenated blood from the umbilical vein runs in the ductus venosus, enters the right atrium via the hepatic vein and by streaming, and reaches the left heart through the ostium secundum (Fig. 5.1a).

The ductus arteriosus contains muscle in its wall; its closure is stimulated by a rise in oxygen tension and is inhibited by prostaglandins (PGE_1 is used therapeutically). As the lungs expand for the first time after birth and oxygen tension rises, there is powerful stimulus for the ductus to close, which usually happens within 12 hours of birth (Fig. 5.1b). Irreversible closure with obliteration to form the ligamentum arteriosum is complete in about 90 per cent of cases by 2 months of age. Spontaneous closure is uncommon beyond the first few months of life. 'PDA' is a standard abbreviation that is usually taken to mean patent ductus arteriosus but this is perhaps tautological and persistent ductus arteriosus is preferred by some.

Incidence and natural history

Persistent ductus arteriosus accounts for around 5–10 per cent of all congenital heart disease. It is one of the commonest forms of heart disease to occur as a consequence of rubella infection during pregnancy. It is twice as common in girls as in boys.

In about 30 per cent of cases PDA results in fatal congestive heart failure within the first year, the risk being highest in the first few months. Those who survive infancy, basically those with smaller shunts, have a risk of only around 1

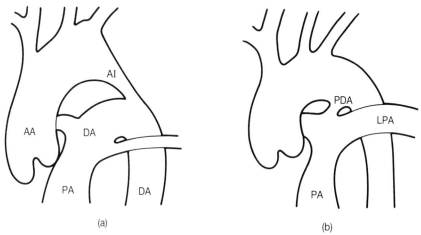

Fig. 5.1 (a) Relative sizes of the great vessels and the ductus arteriosus in the fetus. Oxygenated blood from the umbilical venous return passes from the hepatic vein, predominantly through the foramen ovale, and is ejected from the left heart to be distributed to the upper body. Desaturated blood passes through the right heart, out through the pulmonary artery (PA), bypasses the airless lungs, to pass via the ductus arteriosus into the descending aorta (DA). Note that the ductus arteriosus is large but the aortic isthmus (AI) and the right and left pulmonary arteries are relatively small. AA, ascending aorta. **(b)** Soon after birth the duct closes and the relative sizes of the great vessels gradually change to adult proportions. LPA, left pulmonary artery; PDA, persistent ductus arteriosus.

per cent per year. The risks later are of rising pulmonary vascular resistance and the development of Eisenmenger's syndrome (see later) which occurs in about 5 per cent; left ventricular failure in later life due to volume overload; and the development of endocarditis (more precisely, endarteritis) which is more common on a small PDA.

Presentation and diagnosis

In infancy, PDA is in the differential diagnosis of heart failure. It is one of the causes of a heart murmur discovered at routine medical examinations in childhood. At any age it may present for the first time as infective endocarditis. Heart failure or an incidentally discovered large heart may lead to the diagnosis in adult life.

The diagnostic clinical sign is the characteristic 'machinery murmur'. This results from the fact that throughout the cardiac cycle the systemic pressure is higher than the pulmonary artery pressure, so there is flow in systole and diastole. The pressure difference, however, varies cyclically, producing a rise and fall in the note reminiscent of the noise in a cotton mill or creamery where the various pieces of machinery were driven from a central steam engine through a system of shafts, wheels and belts which made a rhythmic humming noise. It is heard best in the left second space anteriorly, just below the clavicle. Similar murmurs, heard a little lower in the precordium, arise from a coronary arteriovenous fistula or an aortopulmonary window. If there is a big shunt the pulse may be collapsing. The heart may be large on x-ray, depending on the size of the shunt. Definitive diagnosis requires catheterization and aortography to confirm the diagnosis, to measure the size of the shunt through the PDA and to exclude associated abnormalities. The shunt is usually expressed as the ratio of the pulmonary to systemic arterial flows ($Q_P : Q_S$); in general, a ratio of less than $2 : 1$ is not associated with symptoms or a shortening of life expectancy.

Management

PDA can be cured surgically with an operation which is now one of the simplest in cardiac surgery. Ligation of a ductus was first performed by Gross in Boston in 1938, and now the ductus can either be ligated or divided between vascular clamps and oversewn. About 500 operations per year are performed in Britain, a rate of approximately 10 per million of the population. The perioperative mortality has been consistently under 1 per cent and, apart from sick neonates with other lesions, should be zero.

Operation may be life saving in those where PDA is the cause of heart failure in infancy. It may also improve the prognosis if the shunt is large (greater than $2 : 1$). It is debatable whether all cases of PDA should be subjected to operation. The only justification for operating on a small PDA with a shunt of, say, $1.5 : 1$ would be to reduce the already small risk of endocarditis. In the modern era of antibiotics, this is questionable dogma.

PDA may present particular problems in older patients because the ductus may calcify and the tissue can be very fragile. Sometimes ducts that have been ligated apparently recannulate. This may be due to incompleteness of the original operation. The duct can now be occluded with a balloon inserted percutaneously and this may replace surgery in many cases.

Coarctation of the aorta

Coarctation is a localized narrowing of the aorta at about the level of the entry of the ductus arteriosus. The external appearance is of waisting in the region of the aortic isthmus. It is less impressive than the true extent of the obstruction on the inside, where there is a shelf-like obstruction extending into the lumen from opposite the attachment of the ligamentum arteriosum. It is at least possible that this is an acquired lesion which develops due to the presence of contractile tissue in the aortic wall similar to, and in continuity with, that in the ductus. There is some evidence to the contrary, but there seems little doubt that the narrowness progresses in the first weeks of life. Intimal hyperplasia appears to progress. Apart from this typical form of coarctation, longer segments of tubular hypoplasia also occur. A more severe lesion which is probably unrelated is interrupted aortic arch, and sometimes stenotic aortic segments occur much more distally.

The residual lumen at the level of the coarctation may be extremely small, down to pinhole size. The distal aortic segment then receives the bulk of its supply through collaterals. The internal mammary artery and the periscapular vessels bypass the obstruction, and feed into the aorta through its intercostal branches, the highest of which is the third (Fig. 5.2). Coarctation is often

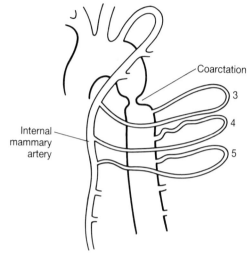

Fig. 5.2 The intercostal arteries (from the third down) become very much enlarged in coarctation. They connect the internal mammary artery, which arises well above the coarctation, to the aorta below it. The ribs are notched due to the increased size and tortuosity of the intercostal arteries. IVC, inferior vena cava; LA, left atrium; RA, right atrium; SVC, superior vena cava.

associated with persistent ductus arteriosus (PDA) and/or more complex congenital heart disease. A bicuspid aortic valve is associated in up to 40 per cent of cases but this is of no clinical importance in the majority. However, these valves can present with regurgitation or stenosis in later life and are prone to endocarditis.

Incidence and natural history

Coarctation represents a little over 5 per cent of cases of congenital heart disease. It is twice as common in boys as it is in girls. A minority develop severe heart failure in the first few weeks of life and die without surgical relief. Some develop heart failure later but the majority who survive infancy live through childhood without symptoms.

There is then a steady death rate through adult life at a rate of about 2 per cent per year. Left ventricular failure is the commonest cause of death but aortic rupture, endocarditis and subarachnoid haemorrhage also are causes of death in these patients. Subarachnoid haemorrhage is due to rupture of berry aneurysms of the circle of Willis. These may be an associated congenital abnormality, but hypertension in the upper half of the body increases the risk.

Presentation

Coarctation is among the causes of heart failure in infancy. It is one of the congenital heart lesions that can escape detection in infancy. It should be specifically considered and excluded in any new case of hypertension and in any case presenting with subarachnoid haemorrhage. It is a rare cause of 'endo-carditis'. It may be discovered incidentally on routine examination in childhood or adolescence or when a large heart is noted on chest x-ray, or left ventricular hypertrophy on ECG.

The most important and diagnostic sign is weakness and delay in the femoral pulses. This sign is elicited by palpating the right brachial pulse and the femoral pulse at the same time. The femoral pulse may be difficult to feel, or even absent, in coarctation. The brachial pulse should be palpated lightly so that the impulses are similar to the examining fingers – in a normal subject they are synchronous but there is a clear difference in coarctation. Hypertension in the upper limbs is expected but it should be taken in both arms to exclude an unusually sited coarctation.

Palpation over the back with the patient leaning forwards may reveal pulsation due to periscapular anastomoses. On auscultation there is a systolic murmur heard best over the back, and there may be a diastolic component in very tight coarctation. In addition, there may be evidence of a bicuspid valve.

The chest x-ray may show rib notching, sparing the first and second ribs and most marked in the third and fourth. The normal aortic knuckle is replaced by a double convexity due to the subclavian artery above and the poststenotic aortic dilatation below. Left ventricular hypertrophy on the ECG is usual, but until there is decompensation the heart size on x-ray is within normal limits.

In older subjects invasive investigation is usually performed. A pressure difference of 40 mmHg across the coarctation represents severe obstruction. The gradient is proportionally less severe and of rather different significance than that measured in aortic stenosis because in coarctation the distal segment can fill through collaterals and thus the pressure difference underestimates the severity of the stenosis.

Management

Any coarctation with a significant degree of obstruction should be operated upon. A substantial gradient is unequivocal evidence for intervention but even when that appears mild, say 25–30 mmHg, other factors such as proximal hypertension or left ventricular hypertrophy would be strong arguments in favour of surgery.

In infants and children the coarctation is resected and the aorta joined end to end, or the subclavian artery is used as a flap. In adults it may be easier to use a gusset to widen the aorta to a point well above and below the coarctation. Paraplegia is a rare but extremely worrying complication in these young, often asymptomatic, patients.

Hypertension may not regress, unfortunately. Residual hypertension may be brought out on exercise. The operation is therefore corrective but not always curative.

Atrial septal defect (ASD)

It is a relatively late step in phylogeny to have two separate circulations, each with its own pump, one dedicated to reoxygenation of the blood while the other delivers the oxygenated blood to the systemic circulation. Evolution has tackled this problem by septation of what was a single heart. The atria develop together, initially as a single chamber and later separate into two chambers, and it is by no means rare for things to go wrong. For some it is fascinating, and may help the memory, to relate congenital abnormalities to embryology; although this seems to work well for explaining the types of ASD, on the whole it is an armchair exercise. The heart disease is the real problem that concerns us – the embryology has been worked out to try to explain it, not the other way round.

Some atrial anatomy

The right atrium is the only one of the four cardiac chambers that is reasonably named in that it does lie to the right side of the midline and, both in health and in disease, contributes to the right border of the heart as seen on chest x-ray. It

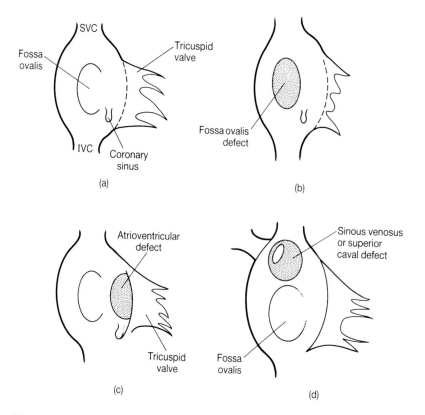

Fig. 5.3 The atrial septum viewed from the right. The fossa ovalis is a useful reference point (**a**). The commonest defect is in this area and is called a fossa ovalis (or ostium secundum) defect (**b**). A defect near the atrioventricular junction may be part of the spectrum of atrioventricular septal defects (**c**). If the defect is near the entry of the superior vena cava (SVC), it is commonly associated with anomalies of venous drainage into the atria. IVC, inferior vena cava.

receives venous return from the superior and inferior venae cavae and the coronary sinus, and passes it on, via the tricuspid valve, to prime the right ventricular pump, augmented by its own gentle contraction. The right atrial appendage (or the right auricle) has a characteristic blunt shape. The left atrium is a basically globular structure sitting symmetrically at the back, receiving the right and left superior and inferior pulmonary veins. Its appendage protrudes to the left and has a characteristic shape like a bent little finger.

Viewed from the right the septum has a smooth oval indentation called the fossa ovalis (Fig. 5.3a). The foramen ovale (which permitted placental venous return to stream through to the left heart) remains probe patent in about a quarter of adults. This is known as patent foramen ovale (PFO). It is kept closed by the slightly higher left atrial pressure, but under unusual circumstances it may open and in particular may permit paradoxical embolus if the right-sided pressures are high.

Types of atrial septal defect

There are three clinically important types of ASD. The most common form (80 per cent) is a hole, typically about 2 × 3 cm, in the fossa ovalis called simply a fossa ovalis ASD (or ostium secundum ASD to use embryologically based nomenclature) (Fig. 5.3b). About 15 per cent of examples of atrial septal defect are sited near the atrioventricular junction (Fig. 5.3c). These are still sometimes called ostium primum defects but are much better regarded as part of the spectrum of atrioventricular defects (see later) because the abnormality involves the atrioventricular valves and cannot be cured simply by suturing up the defect. The least common (5 per cent) involve the septum near the entry of the venae cavae, most commonly superior and are usually called sinus venosus defects (Fig. 5.3d). When these are high in the septum, they are typically associated with abnormalities of pulmonary venous drainage.

Incidence and natural history

As an estimate, ASD probably accounts for 10–20 per cent of congenital heart disease. It rarely causes problems in infancy and in general is very well tolerated for many years. However, the right heart and the lungs may have to handle many times the systemic cardiac output and in due course the volume load causes problems. A typical ASD is large enough to allow the pressures in the two atria to equalize and the flow is governed by the relative compliance of the two circuits. The thin-walled right ventricle and low-resistance pulmonary circulation will accept more flow than the thick-walled left ventricle and high-pressure systemic circulation. If as much blood flows through the ASD as through the mitral valve orifice (and this will occur with quite a small ASD) the resultant pulmonary artery flow is about twice that of the aorta: that is, the flow ratio $(Q_P : Q_S)$ is 2 : 1. Over the years the pulmonary vascular resistance rises due to development of pulmonary vascular disease, and the atria and the right ventricle dilate. Atrial fibrillation may supervene in middle life and by this stage the flow may reverse (Eisenmenger's syndrome), causing cyanosis.

Presentation

Although symptoms are mild, children with ASD may come to the attention of a doctor because of repeated episodes of chesty cough. Otherwise, they are likely to be picked up on routine examination, particularly at school medical examinations. Later, an abnormal chest x-ray may be noted. Cyanosis is rare in early cases but the associated anomalies of venous drainage may create partial or intermittent right to left shunting.

The signs are of a large pulmonary flow with a prominent right ventricular impulse over the precordium. Instead of the normal splitting of the second sound during inspiration, there is fixed splitting of the second heart sound because of the increased pulmonary artery flow throughout the respiratory cycle. There is a systolic murmur due to increased flow across the pulmonary valve. The low pressure flow across a large ASD does not create a murmur but there may be a detectable tricuspid flow murmur in diastole. End-stage disease has the features of right ventricular failure, which include peripheral oedema, ascites and hepatomegaly.

The chest x-ray shows a large heart with increased pulmonary vascular markings. The aortic knuckle is relatively small and the pulmonary artery is prominent. The ECG typically shows right bundle branch block pattern due to chronic right ventricular overload; the QRS axis is normal but towards the right. In an ostium primum or atrioventricular defect the ECG has a characteristic left axis deviation.

The important pieces of information that need to be gained by investigation in fossa ovalis ASD are the pulmonary artery pressure and the size of the left to right shunt. It is important to establish if there is an ostium primum ASD because the surgery for atrioventricular defects is altogether more complicated. Any associated anomalies, in particular of atrial venous connections, can be diagnosed.

Management

The question is whether surgical closure should be undertaken in all cases. In general, surgical closure of an ASD is recommended in all cases where the $Q_P:Q_S$ is $2:1$ or more. With a shunt of much less than that there is such a good outlook that it does not seem justified. In older patients, when the pulmonary artery pressure is already elevated, closure does not relieve symptoms or improve prognosis and should not be undertaken.

Surgical closure of ASD was undertaken in a number of ingenious ways in the early 1950s before cardiopulmonary bypass was available. They have all been superseded by cardiopulmonary bypass. The most successful and the one of most general interest was the use of hypothermia. The anaesthetized patient was cooled to 30°C in a waterbath. The chest was opened and the circulation arrested by occlusion of the superior and inferior venae cavae. At this temperature the brain is safe from ischaemic damage for several minutes and a fast, accurate surgeon could close the defect in 4–5 minutes! Very few units achieved really good results.

In the UK over 500 operations, with the support of cardiopulmonary bypass, are performed each year to close an ASD, with a mortality of under 1 per cent. The risks are small, so it is generally agreed that all but very small defects should be considered for surgical closure, which is, in most cases, a curative operation.

A simple fossa ovalis defect can be closed by direct suturing, which is curative. Large defects, atrioventricular defects (which are dealt with later) and those that involve the entry of the great veins must be patched to avoid distortion of important structures.

Ventricular septal defect (VSD)

The ventricular septum is anatomically part of the left ventricle in that it forms part of its circular cross-section. The right ventricle has a triangular cross-section. The three sides of the triangle are the convex curve of the septum which bulges into its cavity, and its anterior and diaphragmatic surfaces which meet each other at an acute angle are the 'acute margin' of the heart. The left ventricular side of the septum is smooth, as is the rest of the cavity, while the right ventricular side is heavily trabeculated.

Defects in the ventricular septum vary in size, site and number, and they may coexist with other cardiac lesions as part of a complex abnormality. In this section we concentrate on isolated VSD. Their size is important in determining the haemodynamic consequences and, therefore, symptoms and outcome. The pulmonary vasculature and the thin-walled right ventricle are very compliant compared with the systemic vascular resistance, so a relatively large volume of blood will pass through the VSD in preference to the aortic valve. The magnitude of the shunt is again expressed as a ratio of the pulmonary artery to aortic flow ($Q_P : Q_S$) and a value of over 2:1 is likely to be important. That means that the same amount of blood passes through the VSD as through the aortic valve, so the final output from the pulmonary artery is twice that from the aorta.

Their site is of less functional significance but of great surgical importance because it determines ease of closure and the risk of complications. They may be in the membranous septum, in which case they are near the conducting system, or in the muscular septum, when they are likely to be multiple, and, because of the trabeculations, they can be difficult to identify (Fig. 5.4).

Incidence and natural history

Ventricular septal defect is the commonest congenital abnormality present at birth, with an incidence of about 2 per 1000. A large proportion (probably more than 75 per cent of those detected in neonates) close spontaneously but only a minority (less than 25 per cent) present at a year will close.

The magnitude of the shunt increases in the first few days after birth with the natural fall in pulmonary vascular resistance and may reach over 4:1. Babies with large VSDs present in heart failure in the first few weeks of life. About 10 per cent die in infancy if not treated. Pulmonary vascular resistance tends to rise progressively in those with large shunts and becomes irreversible (Eisenmenger's complex); these patients die miserably in their teens and young adult

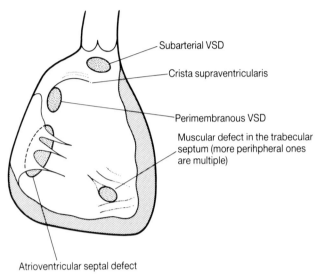

Subarterial VSD

Crista supraventricularis

Perimembranous VSD

Muscular defect in the trabecular septum (more perihpheral ones are multiple)

Atrioventricular septal defect

Fig. 5.4 The ventricular septum viewed from the right, showing the characteristic sites of ventricular septal defects.

life. Those with small VSDs are usually asymptomatic but are at risk from endocarditis.

Presentation, symptoms and signs

A large VSD is a cause of heart failure in infancy, presenting with tachypnoea and feeding problems. Moderate sized VSD may cause symptoms on exertion in later life. Small VSD is noisy and is readily detected but is asymptomatic, and safe apart from the risk of endocarditis. (This is the condition known as maladie de Roger.)

On examination the pansystolic murmur, sometimes associated with a thrill over the precordium, is the most striking physical sign. The chest x-ray shows increased pulmonary vascular markings and an enlarged heart in those with a significant shunt. Echocardiography and Doppler studies can also give useful information (see Chapter 6). Cardiac catheterization is justified if surgery is being considered, to measure the pulmonary artery pressure and check the size of the shunt.

Management

The decision has to be made as to whether surgical closure is required. In infancy, heart failure is managed and surgery is avoided in the hope that the VSD will close of its own accord, because the risks of operation for this condition in children under 1 year remain relatively high, around 15 per cent. In some cases a palliative operation is performed – pulmonary artery banding – to reduce the pulmonary flow and control the situation until the baby is larger. Symptomatic children and all with a pulmonary to systemic flow ratio $(Q_P:Q_S)$ greater than about 2:1 should undergo elective surgical closure. This is usually done before school age if the diagnosis has been made in infancy. The mortality is then under 5 per cent.

The operation requires cardiopulmonary bypass and became possible for the first time in the mid-1950s. The operation is ideally curative, provided the pulmonary vascular resistance has not risen. It is not always easy, however, and residual leaks, heart block and associated cardiac abnormalities are among the problems that make the results less than perfect in some cases. A little under 300 operations per year are performed in the British Isles, which is a rate of around 5 per million of the population.

Eisenmenger's syndrome

In three of the conditions already described – persistent ductus arteriosus (PDA), atrial septal defect (ASD) and ventricular septal defect (VSD) – the pulmonary circulation receives an excessive blood flow, several times that of the systemic circulation. In ASD, where the left to right shunt is in the low pressure part of the system, this is purely a volume load governed by the relative compliance of the two circuits. In PDA and VSD the pulmonary vasculature may be exposed to the full systemic pressure if the communication is large enough. If the pulmonary circulation is exposed to excessive pressure and increased flow the pulmonary arterioles hypertrophy, limiting the flow, and in time irreversible changes result. Eventually there is no net left to right shunt and the shunt may in fact reverse. When the resistances are nearly equal, shunt reversal happens, particularly during exercise when the peripheral vascular resistance falls, resulting in cyanosis. Pulmonary hypertension with a balanced or reversed shunt is known as Eisenmenger's syndrome.

The original description was of raised pulmonary vascular resistance in the presence of a large VSD, and strictly speaking this is Eisenmenger's complex. In some cases it appears that the normal reduction in pulmonary vascular resistance never occurs and irreversible pulmonary hypertension may be evident at presentation in even quite young children. Acquired pulmonary hypertension that develops over some years may be distinguished by the term Eisenmenger's reaction. For practical purposes, in adults and older children these distinctions are semantic.

Incidence and natural history

With time, the pulmonary vascular resistance rises in all large or moderate VSDs and these account for about a third of the cases. With large VSDs, irreversible changes are established in about half the cases by their 20s and most by their 30s. The median survival of these patients is only to the mid-30s although some patients tolerate the pulmonary hypertension well and appear to reach a stable state. Eisenmenger's syndrome is less frequent in PDA, which limits the pressure rather more and is very uncommon in straightforward fossa ovalis ASD. It is more common in women than in men.

Presentation and clinical features

The most striking feature is breathlessness. There may be a history of a murmur but usually these patients have not been symptomatic in childhood and the pulmonary vascular changes have developed insidiously. Other symptoms include haemoptysis, palpitations and fainting attacks. Cyanosis and clubbing are typical. If the underlying cause is a PDA, clubbing may be confined to the lower limbs and so-called differential cyanosis may be demonstrated.

The signs are those of pulmonary hypertension. There is elevation of the jugular venous pressure and a prominent right ventricular heave. There may be few clues as to the underlying lesion, as there is little left to right shunting and the diastolic murmurs may be quite or absent. There may be a pulmonary diastolic murmur due to pulmonary regurgitation, the Graham Steell murmur.

The ECG indicates right ventricular hypertrophy and the chest x-ray shows large central pulmonary arteries with peripheral pruning due to pulmonary vascular disease reducing pulmonary blood flow. Cardiac catheterization should be performed to prove the diagnosis and to confirm that there is no correctable underlying cause.

Management

Surgical closure of the defect, whether it is atrial, ventricular or arterial, should not be attempted. The situation is irreversible, the symptoms are not improved, the operation is likely to be complicated and the outlook is not improved. Some patients are made worse and die soon afterwards in right ventricular failure.

Medical treatment is supportive. Polycythaemia develops with an increase in viscosity, and some symptomatic relief may be obtained by venesection to reduce the haematocrit (packed cell volume). The combination of polycythaemia and right to left shunting puts these patients at risk of venous emboli reaching the systemic circulation, a condition called paradoxical embolism.

Atrioventricular septal defects

This is a spectrum in which there are abnormalities of both atrial and ventricular septation. In the past, arbitrary divisions into partial and complete defects or attempts to classify these lesions embryologically have led to a plethora of names; they are mentioned here so that it can be seen how they fit into what is best considered as a single condition, atrioventricular septal defects, albeit with a range of severity.

During development there is a common opening from the atria to the ventricles, which is called the atrioventricular canal by embryologists. The tissue outgrowths that form the atrioventricular valves and contribute to septation at the centre of the heart are called endocardial cushions. The terms 'endocardial cushion defect' and 'persistent' or 'complete AV canal' are synonymous and refer to this condition. At the milder end of the spectrum the only obvious septal defect is between the atria, low down, near the AV valves. This is commonly called an ostium primum ASD (it appears to be the remnant of the embryological ostium primum). It can also be thought of as part of the common AV canal and is therefore also known as 'partial AV canal'. It has been mentioned in passing among types of ASD but in fact there are often important abnormalities of the AV valves (Fig. 5.5) and the configuration of the septum is abnormal, so it is now regarded by surgeons and anatomists as part of the spectrum of atrioventricular septal defects because it shares their features and problems.

In its full form there is a low lying ASD, a high septal VSD and abnormalities of the two AV valves. There may be a single valve with shared leaflets bridging the deficient interventricular septum. In the normal heart the aortic and mitral valves are adjacent and in fibrous continuity; the left ventricle is conical with its entry and exit next to each other, and the mitral and tricuspid valves are attached to the septum at slightly different levels. All of these relationships are changed in hearts with atrioventricular septal defects. More detail of the morphology of this complicated and contentious subject is not appropriate here.

Incidence and natural history

This is a relatively uncommon form of congenital heart disease over all but it is present in 20 per cent of babies with Down's syndrome, and Down's children represent a fair proportion of all the cases.

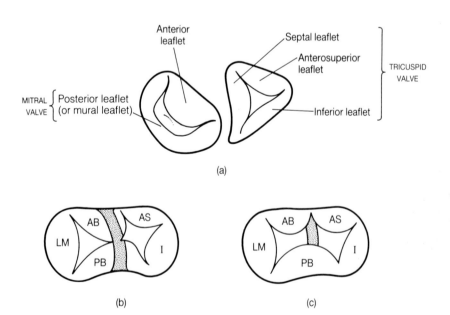

Fig. 5.5 (a) The relationships of the normal atrioventricular valves. **(b, c)** In atrioventricular defects where the orifices remain separate there is what appears to be a cleft in the anterior leaflet of the mitral valve. These components are seen to be quite distinct components of a common atrioventricular valve if there are defects in both **(b)** the atrial and ventricular septa, and **(c)** a common valve orifice. AB, anterior bridging; AP, anteroposterior; I, inferior; LM, left mitral; PB, posterior bridging.

Presentation

The milder cases with only an interatrial communication and without AV valve regurgitation are clinically indistinguishable from any other ASD. Those with VSD and severe mitral regurgitation are extremely ill and many die in infancy. Pulmonary vascular disease tends to progress rapidly and Eisenmenger's syndrome is frequent. The diagnosis can be made with confidence with two-dimensional echocardiography.

Management

Total surgical correction is possible but this cannot be regarded as curative. The valves present a considerable problem and have to be reconstructed and the two septal defects closed. In extremely sick infants, pulmonary artery banding to reduce the pulmonary blood flow may help control heart failure until the baby is larger and definitive repair may be attempted.

The mortality for attempted correction of severe lesions is still of the order of 15–20 per cent although better figures can be achieved by careful case selection. In surgery as exacting as this the best results are achieved by a few very experienced and talented surgeons. One of the debates has been whether it is justifiable to operate on these defects in Down's babies. They have a higher complication rate due to poor airway control and in any case do not have a very long expectation of life, for independent non-cardiac reasons. The ethical debate should include these facts as well as the emotional arguments.

Congenital abnormalities of the aortic valve

Several patterns of congenital abnormality occur in the region of the aortic valve. By far the commonest are the varying degrees of abnormality of the valve itself. There is a whole spectrum of abnormality (Fig. 5.6). The mildest form is failure of development of a commissure such that there is effectively a bicuspid valve. This occurs in about 1 per cent of otherwise normal hearts. It can be associated with coarctation. The most common form is absence of the commissure between the right and left coronary cusps, followed by absence of that between the right and non-coronary cusps. These are asymptomatic and do not cause aortic stenosis in infancy or childhood.

The next degree of severity is to have only one commissure, that between the left and non-coronary cusps. This usually results in some degree of obstruction as witnessed by a murmur and left ventricular hypertrophy. The most severe form has no proper commissures and varying degrees of thickening of the valve. The annulus may also be small. The worst cases present with heart failure in infancy.

Subvalvar aortic stenosis is due to a discrete fibromuscular ridge. The aortic valve is commonly abnormal in some way. Supravalvar stenosis usually takes the form of a shelf-like narrowing of the aorta at about the level of the commissures. The aortic valve is also abnormal in about a third of cases (Fig. 5.6).

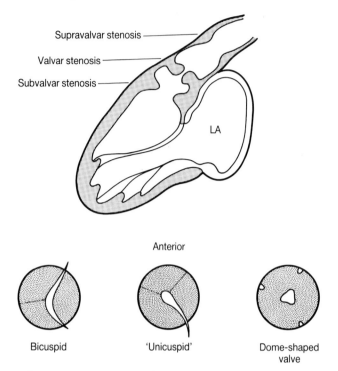

Anterior

Bicuspid   'Unicuspid'   Dome-shaped
                                                     valve

Fig. 5.6 Sagittal section of the heart, showing subvalvar, valvar and supravalvar aortic stenosis. The abnormal valve may have two rudimentary cusps, an eccentric comma-shaped orifice, or a central orifice in a doming valve. The first two tend to be tolerated at least through infancy and childhood. LA, left atrium.

Incidence and natural history

About 1 per cent of people have a bicuspid valve. In infancy, childhood and into adult life this usually functions normally. They do not have any gradient across the valve and subsequent comments about aortic stenosis do not refer to this group. They are at risk from endocarditis and then the valve becomes regurgitant. Otherwise it tends to thicken with time and those affected typically present in their 60s and 70s with aortic stenosis.

Congenital valvar aortic stenosis constitutes about 5 per cent of congenital heart disease. It is five times more common in boys than in girls. Some present in infancy with heart failure and these tend to have other abnormalities in the left ventricle or aorta. On the whole they do very badly. More commonly they present in childhood with a systolic murmur but few symptoms. The left ventricle hypertrophies and the degree of obstruction tends to progress. Sudden death is a fear for these asymptomatic children who want to run and play, but is rare apart from those with severe narrowing. Most cases of stenotic aortic valve disease detected in childhood have progressive thickening of the valve and the degree of obstruction becomes severe enough to need surgery by young adult life. They are otherwise likely to die suddenly or in left ventricular failure.

Subaortic stenosis presents in childhood or young adult life and may not be present or as severe at birth. The valve abnormalities associated with it may also be acquired due to the jet of blood hitting the valve cusps. They have a tendency to endocarditis. Supravalvar stenosis may form part of a congenital syndrome of infantile hypercalcaemia, elfin-like appearance and low IQ.

Presentation and clinical findings

Apart from those who present as infants in heart failure, most cases of congenital aortic stenosis are detected on routine examination in childhood. As systolic murmurs are common and many are innocent, the problem is to decide which murmurs require further investigation.

The history should be taken with a high index of suspicion, looking specifically for cardiac symptoms. The clinical signs of note include a systolic thrill, which would suggest significant obstruction as a cause of the murmur, and an ejection click, which is evidence of valvar stenosis. Unlike in adults, the character of the carotid pulse is not helpful. Clinical, radiological or ECG evidence of left ventricular hypertrophy would suggest that further investigation is needed. Initially this would be with two-dimensional echocardiography, and Doppler measurements will indicate the velocity of the jet through the valve and thus provide an estimate of the severity of the stenosis. Cardiac catheterization is sometimes necessary to document the gradient. A careful measurement of the left ventricular and aortic pressures on withdrawing the catheter may demonstrate the site of obstruction – below, at or above the valve (Fig. 5.7).

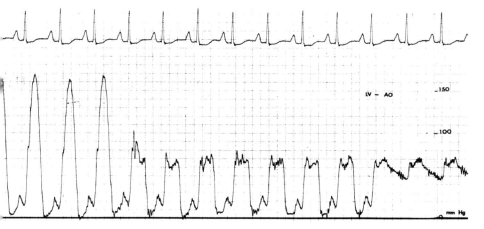

Fig. 5.7 Ventricular and aortic pressure traces from a catheter withdrawn from the ventricle into the aorta. The reduction in systolic pressure shows that the stenosis has been crossed before the diastolic pressure rises, indicating that the narrowing is below the level of the aortic valve. The pressure tracing at the point LV–Ao shows the transition in waveform shape at the level of the aortic valve; there is no difference in the systolic pressures at this level.

Management

Every effort is made to avoid operating on the aortic valve in childhood unless it is essential. Conservative operations to relieve the obstruction are not very satisfactory in that they relieve obstruction incompletely and may add regurgitation. Replacement may have to be with a small valve and may add the burden of anticoagulation. A gradient up to, say, 40 mmHg would be watched carefully. In severe stenosis with a gradient above 80 mmHg, surgery is essential. Cases falling between the two require careful judgement. Various dilatation techniques, transaortic and transventricular, have been tried and abandoned in the past, but the less invasive technique of balloon angioplasty may help to temporise.

Congenital aortic stenosis cannot be 'cured' and management may require a succession of manoeuvres, followed by valve replacement in later life.

Pulmonary stenosis

As with congenital disease of the aortic valve, the obstruction to right ventricular outflow may be subvalvar, valvar or supravalvar. These are usefully grouped together as right ventricular outflow tract obstruction (RVOTO). Subvalvar obstruction takes the form of muscular infundibular obstruction. Most commonly the valve itself is stenotic and typically it has a small central orifice with fusion of all three commissures. The pulmonary artery itself may be atretic.

Pulmonary stenosis of various types can occur in association almost any other combination of cardiac abnormalities, particularly Fallot's tetralogy.

Incidence and natural history

Pulmonary stenosis accounts for about 10 per cent of congenital heart disease and is a little more common in females. It varies widely in severity. It may present with severe hypoxia in the neonatal period and is fatal without treatment. The earlier it presents, the more severe the stenosis is likely to be. The severity progresses, partly because the valve does not grow with the child but also because secondary infundibular hypertrophy adds to the obstruction.

Presentation and clinical features

These patients are breathless, yet the lungs and left heart are protected so the usually argued mechanisms of breathlessness in heart disease cannot apply. The dyspnoea may be due to a limit to cardiac output imposed by the pulmonary stenosis. In many cases the foramen ovale persists and, as the right atrial pressure rises, blood shunts from right to left and there is cyanosis, at least on exercise. Dizziness on exertion and palpitations are other common symptoms.

The jugular venous pressure is raised with a prominent a wave as the right atrium contracts to fill a hypertrophied and therefore less compliant right ventricle. There is a systolic murmur of ejection type, loudest to the left of the sternum. Its length is proportional to the severity of the stenosis. An ejection click indicates that the obstruction is valvar.

Catheterization is usual to measure the gradient and to confirm the site. Associated abnormalities can also be demonstrated.

Management

Treatment is surgical. It is required urgently in sick infants, when it can be performed without bypass during a minute or so of inflow occlusion, achieved with tapes passed around the superior and inferior venae cavae. An incision in the pulmonary artery is controlled by a side-biting clamp which can be replaced to permit the circulation to be restored rapidly. In older and less critical patients it is performed on cardiopulmonary bypass. Asymptomatic cases with relatively small gradients can be safely left without operation.

Congenital abnormalities of the atrioventricular valves

The AV valves can be very abnormal in a variety of conditions, particularly the atrioventricular septal defects. It should be noted that the terms 'mitral' and 'tricuspid' must be used with caution in these very abnormal hearts. Isolated abnormality of the mitral valve (left-sided AV valve) is rare but includes some recognized types such as parachute valve, double orifice and cleft leaflets. These are not frequent enough to be considered further.

There are two well recognized forms of congenital heart disease involving the tricuspid valve that merit brief description: tricuspid atresia and Ebsiein's anomaly.

Tricuspid atresia

The right atrium has no AV valve. It communicates with the left atrium via an ASD and that empties via a left AV valve into a left ventricle. The right ventricle is typically hypoplastic and communicates with the morphological left ventricle by a VSD. The pattern of the disease presentation depends on whether or not there is pulmonary obstruction because this determines whether the lungs are under- or overperfused and, therefore, whether congestive failure or cyanosis is dominant.

In cases where the pulmonary circulation has been protected by an obstructive lesion, Fontan's operation in which a conduit is fashioned between the right atrium and the pulmonary artery offers some degree of correction.

Ebstein's anomaly

In 1866 Ebstein described this rare but quite distinct entity. The septal and posterior part of the tricuspid valve attachment is displaced from the atrioventricular junction down into the right ventricle. There is a wide spectrum of clinical consequences from death in infancy to virtually normal function.

The cases with severe tricuspid regurgitation present in infancy. Right ventricular function is usually abnormal and may lead to presentation in childhood. Cases that are haemodynamically satisfactory may have severe rhythm disturbances in childhood or adult life.

Fallot's tetralogy

Fallot's tetralogy is the most familiar of the complex congenital heart diseases. The 'tetralogy' comprises pulmonary stenosis, VSD, overriding aortic valve and right ventricular hypertrophy (Fig. 5.8). It is an instructive condition because the left to right shunt which one expects to occur with a VSD is limited by the coexistent obstruction to the right ventricular outflow. Superficially it might appear that any case where VSD coexists with pulmonary stenosis could amount to the same thing, but the relationship of the right ventricular infundibulum, the septum and the aorta presents a characteristic morphology. In an extreme form the aorta may be so malaligned in relation to the septum that it arises from the right ventricle, a condition called double outlet right ventricle (DORV).

The right ventricular outflow tract obstruction can be infundibular, valvar or at various levels in the pulmonary artery, or a combination of these. The VSD is typically large such that the right ventricle and left ventricle are at the same pressure. The aortic arch is right sided in 25 per cent of cases.

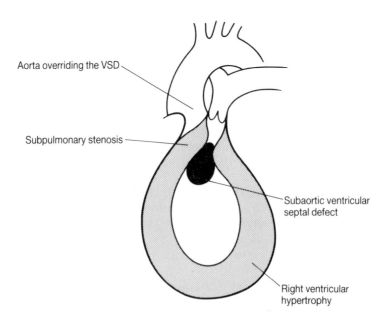

Aorta overriding the VSD

Subpulmonary stenosis

Subaortic ventricular septal defect

Right ventricular hypertrophy

Fig. 5.8 Fallot's tetralogy. The four features that make up the 'tetralogy' are narrowing of the pulmonary outflow (which may be any combination of infundibular hypertrophy, valvar stenosis and hypoplasia of the pulmonary artery), right ventricular hypertrophy, a defect in the ventricular septum and displacement of the aorta so that it straddles the septum.

Incidence and natural history

Tetralogy is the commonest cyanotic heart disease seen in children, and represents about 10 per cent of congenital heart disease. The natural history is related to the severity of the pulmonary stenosis. Before surgical treatment was feasible, about a quarter of babies with tetralogy died in the first year of life, and about half of the remainder died during childhood. The remainder then remained relatively stable but became polycythaemic with a tendency to thrombosis of the pulmonary arteries and at risk of cerebral thrombosis. Very few lived beyond 40. The natural history became very different when palliation by systemic–pulmonary artery shunts became possible.

Presentation and clinical features

The worst cases, those with pulmonary atresia or severe pulmonary stenosis, are obviously unwell in infancy. In the milder cases the pulmonary blood flow is adequate until infundibular hypertrophy develops and they become cyanosed in early childhood. The murmur of the VSD may be heard at examination at any time. If the diagnosis has not been made earlier, a characteristic history may be given by the parents of the child going blue on exertion and then getting relief by squatting. The explanation for squatting is that the child learns that, by increasing the systemic afterload, it can encourage a little more blood through the lungs and thus relieve its distressing hypoxia.

On examination there is cyanosis and clubbing. There is palpable right ventricular hyperactivity and a systolic murmur. The chest x-ray shows a boot-shaped heart and the ECG demonstrates right ventricular hypertrophy. The diagnosis can be made by two-dimensional echocardiography but, other than in sick neonates, cardiac catheterization is indicated.

Management

Treatment is surgical in other than the mildest cases, and 'total correction' is the objective in most cases. This has been possible only since cardiopulmonary bypass became generally available. The closure of the VSD involves a patch which must deviate from the line of the septum to accommodate the aortic root and, if there is very distorted anatomy, this amounts to an intracardiac baffle. The relief of the infundibular narrowing requires resection of muscle, but if the narrowing goes up to and includes the pulmonary valve, a transannular patch is required. About 200 such operations per year are performed in Britain and the overall mortality has remained close to 10 per cent. The risk is particularly high in the sick neonate and there has been a return to palliative shunting operations to temporize in these cases and perform definitive surgery at a later stage.

Systemic–pulmonary artery shunts

The objective of these operations is to palliate cyanotic congenital heart disease by diverting hypoxic arterial blood to the pulmonary circulation. The first, and still quite popular, shunt is the Blalock–Taussig operation in which the right subclavian artery (or left is there is a right-sided arch) is mobilized up to the vertebral artery, divided and anastomosed to the right pulmonary artery (Fig. 5.9). A modification is to interpose a synthetic (usually Gortex) graft. The Waterston anastomosis is between the back of the ascending aorta and the right pulmonary artery, and Pott's anastomosis is between the descending aorta and the left pulmonary artery.

Some cases of tetralogy remain very well palliated into adult life. The shunts themselves, especially Potts' anastomosis, add to the technical difficulties at reoperation.

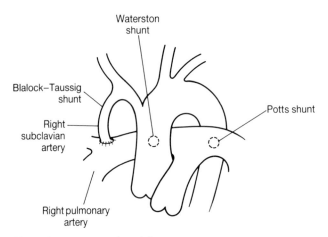

Fig. 5.9 Some examples of shunts.

Transposition of the great arteries (TGA)

In transposition of the great arteries (Fig. 5.10) the aorta arises from the right ventricle and the pulmonary artery arises from the left ventricle. If all else were as it should be, survival would be impossible because there would be two separate circulations. Existence is possible only because the circulations mix via an ASD, a VSD or a PDA, or some combination of the three. The presence, site and size of a VSD are variable and there may be stenosis of the origin of one or other great vessels.

One form, which adds to the potential confusion, is 'corrected transposition', in which not only are the ventriculoarterial connections discordant (to use the modern system of sequential chamber identification) but there is also atrioventricular discordance. The morphological right atrium, which collects systemic, desaturated blood, empties into a morphological left ventricle which in turn fills the pulmonary artery. The oxygenated blood from the left atrium enters a morphological right ventricle from which arises the aorta and it thus supplies the systemic circulation. Although the end-result may appear to be satisfactory in

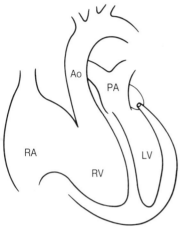

Fig. 5.10 Transposition of the great arteries – the aorta (Ao) arises from the right ventricle (RV) and the pulmonary artery (PA) from the left ventricle (LV). There must be an associated communication to support life which may be at atrial, ventricular or arterial level. RA, right atrium.

terms of the circulation, there is usually a VSD, often pulmonary stenosis, and there can be severe conduction abnormality.

TGA is the commonest condition to present with cyanosis at birth. Immediate palliation is by attempts to mix the circulation. Efforts are made to keep the ductus patent with prostaglandin (PGE_1) to permit some of the desaturated blood in the aorta to reach the lungs. In the catheter laboratory the atrial septum can be torn with a balloon pulled back through the patent foramen ovale (Rashkind's procedure) to maximize mixing at atrial level.

Diversion of the atrial blood, by ingenious methods of fashioning intra-atrial baffles, has been the mainstay of surgical treatment; two operations, Mustard's and Senning's, achieve this with relatively low risk. However, the longer term results are less certain, with the risk of the right ventricle not coping with the systemic load and problems with atrial baffles. These patients tend to return in adolescence with right heart failure and tricuspid regurgitation. The obvious solution of swapping the transposed great arteries is made difficult by the problem of reanastomosing the coronary arteries so that they receive arterial supply. This is now possible in selected cases.

Truncus arteriosus

As the name suggests, in truncus arteriosus a single great vessel leaves the heart. It gives rise to coronary arteries, pulmonary arteries and the arch arteries and arises over a large VSD, thus receiving blood from both ventricles (Fig. 5.11). It is rare, representing 2–3 per cent of congenital heart disease. Most babies die within a month. Those who survive the neonatal period are cyanosed and have rapidly progressive pulmonary vascular disease. Operations in early infancy have a very high risk but few babies survive to have a corrective operation at an older age.

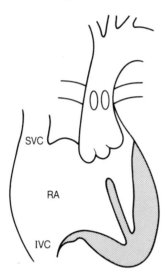

Fig. 5.11 Truncus arteriosus. There is a single great vessel leaving the ventricles. IVC, inferior vena cava; RA, right atrium; SVC, superior vena cava.

Total anomalous pulmonary venous drainage (TAPVD)

None of the pulmonary veins reaches the left atrium directly; they drain via one of the systemic veins (persistent left superior vena cava, the coronary sinus, a hepatic vein) to the right atrium. Survival depends upon the adequacy of venous mixing through the foramen ovale or an ASD. This is a rare condition, representing only 1–2 per cent of congenital heart disease. Nevertheless, it is of interest because it can be corrected with a good chance of cure.

Univentricular heart

A variety of morphological conditions can be included under this heading. There may be failure of septation of a heart that has the morphological features of both right and left ventricles. In other cases, one of the ventricles may be so underdeveloped as to be detectable only as a muscular pouch with no connection to any other chamber. The single functioning ventricle may then be recognized as being of right or left ventricular type. Septation is sometimes possible but is not always really successful.

Further reading

Julian, D. G., Camm, A. J., Fox, K. M., Hall, R. J. C. and Poole-Wilson, P. A. (Eds.) (1989) *Diseases of the Heart.* Bailliere Tindall, London.

6

CARDIAC ULTRASOUND EXAMINATION

Cardiac ultrasound

Echocardiography uses ultrasound to study the position and movement of intracardiac structures. Over the past 20 years it has developed into a major instrument of diagnosis in cardiology. The ultrasound waves are generated by materials with the property of piezo-electricity which undergo deformation when electrical potential is applied across them. A typical transducer will emit a beam of ultrasound of 2.5–5 MHz. The transducer emits ultrasound 3000 times a second; these impulses last approximately 1 us and are directed into the tissues to be studied. As the ultrasound passes through a homogeneous medium, its intensity is progressively reduced by absorption and scattering to an extent that depends on the characteristics of the material. When it encounters a change between two substances with different physical properties, such as blood and endocardium, or pericardium and epicardium, a proportion of the ultrasound waves is reflected (Fig. 6.1). The proportion reflected depends on the difference in density and the velocity of sound across the interface.

The reflected pulses return to the transducer after a time interval that depends on the depth of the structure from which they are reflected and the velocity of sound within the medium. Echoes from deeper structures return later than those from the more superficial ones; they can be selectively amplified to compensate for the attenuation that has occurred.

Cardiac ultrasound is used in two ways. It can examine a single region of the heart by demonstrating the change of position with time of structures along the line of a single beam (M, or motion, mode). Alternatively, a two-dimensional image can be generated using either a single crystal, which is mechanically oscillated through an arc, or multiple crystals, which are electronically operated. The two-dimensional technique is better for studying structure and anatomy. The advantages of ultrasound are many: it is painless and safe; it is reproducible; it does not depend on the introduction of any unphysiological substance such as contrast material; the equipment is portable and can be moved to the sick patient; and it is a relatively cheap investigation.

223

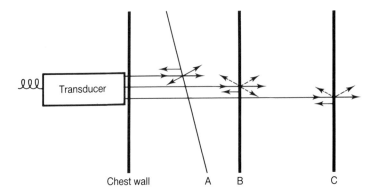

Fig. 6.1 Diagrammatic representation of ultrasound examination. The top beam, having penetrated the chest wall, encounters a structure, A, which is slightly more dense than the field on either side. The ultrasound beam will be reflected or refracted or will pass on through. In the second beam the events at the dense structure, B, are displayed. Because there is a marked change in density, more of the ultrasound is reflected and, as it is striking B at right angles, this will enhance the strength of the returning echoes. The lowest beam illustrates the attenuation that occurs as the ultrasound penetrates into the tissues; even though C is as dense as B, the returning echoes will not be so strong and will need to be enhanced electronically.

In conjunction with echocardiography the relatively newer technique of Doppler cardiography can give valuable extra information. Doppler ultrasound gives information about flow and function. The principle of Doppler cardiography makes use of the change in frequency that occurs when a wave is reflected from a moving rather than a stationary surface. The frequency is increased if the target is approaching, and reduced if it is moving away from, the source. This is best illustrated in everyday life by the consideration of the frequency of sound generated by a fast train approaching the platform of a station on which you are standing: as it approaches you the frequency of the sound increases, and then decreases as it passes you and disappears towards the horizon. The change in frequency depends on the frequency and velocity of the sound, the relative velocities of target and source, and the angle between the direction and motion of the ultrasound beam. With the aid of two-dimensional echocardiography to focus the Doppler beam accurately, it is possible to make observations in defined regions of the heart. Measurements can be made about the direction of the flow, the presence of abnormal flow together with the timing and velocity of blood flow.

Echocardiography

The heart can be studied by ultrasound from only a limited number of directions because the lung forms a barrier to ultrasound. In most adults it is possible to obtain satisfactory images from the parasternal position, from the apex, from the xiphisternal area and from the suprasternal notch.

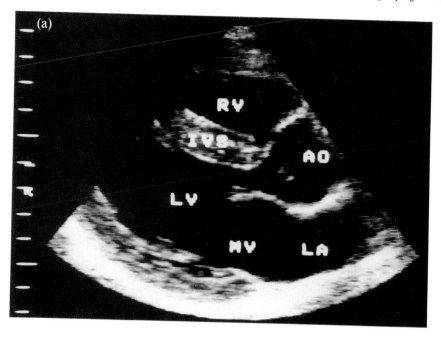

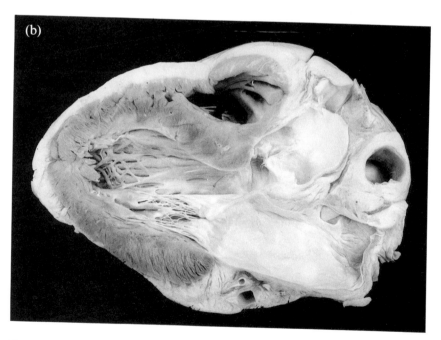

Fig. 6.2 (**a**) A two-dimensional echocardiographic examination using the parasternal long axis view. The chambers are labelled. (**b**) A section through the heart in the same plane. AO, aorta; IVS, intraventricular septum; LV, left ventricle; MV, mitral valve; RV, right ventricle.

Two-dimensional echocardiography

The parasternal long axis view is shown in Fig. 6.2, which demonstrates the relationship of the interventricular septum to the two ventricles. The superior aspect of the septum is continuous with the anterior wall of the aorta. The posterior wall of the aorta is continuous with the anterior leaflet of the mitral valve and the subvalve apparatus. Behind the aorta is the left atrium.

The transducer can be rotated through 90 degrees to obtain the minor, or short axis, view of the left ventricle (Fig. 6.3). At the level of the mitral valve this allows one to look into the mitral valve as though from below in the left ventricle; the mitral valve appears to open in diastole like a fish's mouth (Fig. 6.4).

The short axis view at a slightly higher level allows one to see the aorta in cross-section. The outflow tract of the right ventricle appears to wrap round the aorta with the tricuspid valve seen on the left side and the pulmonary valve on the right (Fig. 6.5).

All four chambers of the heart can be seen in the apical view (Fig. 6.6).

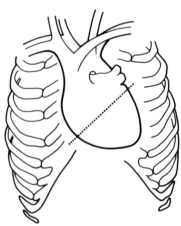

Fig. 6.3 A diagram of the short axis of the heart.

M-mode echocardiography

M-mode echocardiography is used to obtain a record of the motion of cardiac structures in a single direction. The technique was introduced earlier than two-dimensional echocardiography. It is performed almost exclusively from the left parasternal region, and four standard views of the heart are used (Fig. 6.7).

The first level demonstrates the aorta and left atrium (Fig. 6.8). The aortic root is shown as two parallel lines with the left atrial cavity behind it. The aortic root moves forwards during systole as the left atrium fills, and backwards during diastole following the opening of the mitral valve. Within the aortic root the aortic cusps are visible as a characteristic box-like configuration.

The second level is taken through the mitral valve (Fig. 6.9). The anterior leaflet has a characteristic M shape and a posterior leaflet is W shaped. The motion of the anterior cusp has several phases; with atrial systole there is a

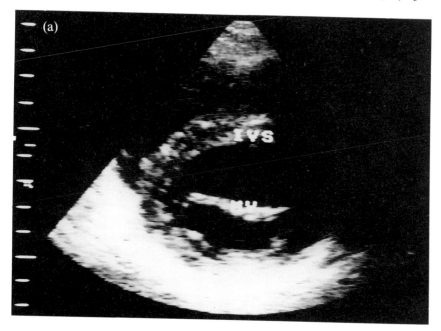

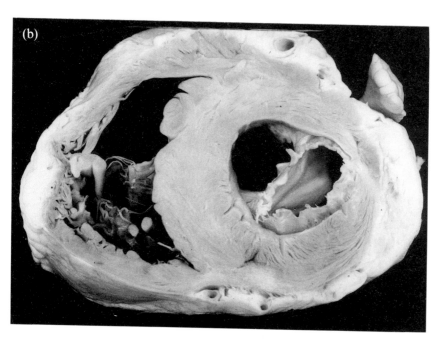

Fig. 6.4 (a) A two-dimensional echocardiogram using the short axis view of the mitral valve. (**b**) A section through the heart in the same plane. IVS, interventricular septum; MV, mitral valve.

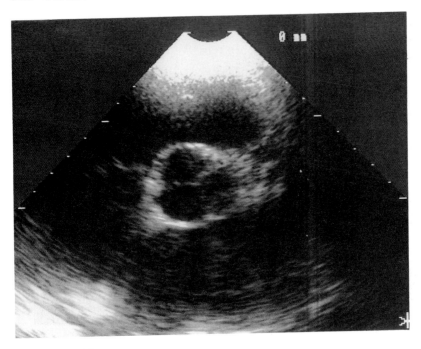

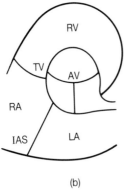

(b)

Fig. 6.5 (a) A two-dimensional echocardiogram using the short axis view of the aortic valve. **(b)** The diagram demonstrates the relationships of other structures to the aortic valve. AV, aortic valve; IAS, interatrial septum; LA, left atrium; RA, right atrium; RV, right ventricle; TV, tricuspid valve.

forward or opening movement (P) but at the onset of ventricular systole it has returned to the closed position (D). During ventricular systole the whole mitral valve is carried forwards as the ventricular volume drops. As ventricular filling starts the valve opens rapidly (O) and then during mid-diastole goes back to its closed position as the flow rate of the left ventricle drops (F). This mid-diastolic closure depends both on the normal physical characteristics of the cusps and on

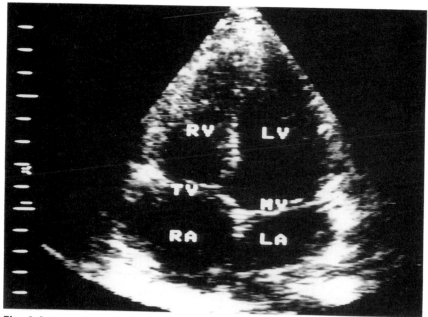

Fig. 6.6 A two-dimensional echocardiogram using the apical four-chamber view.

the flow pattern to the ventricle. The motion of the tricuspid valve is identical to that of the mitral.

The third level of examination is a transverse view across the left ventricular cavity, which allows left ventricular dimensions and wall movement to be measured (Fig. 6.10). It also allows measurement of the thickness of the interventricular septum and posterior wall.

There are some limitations to echocardiography. They include the inability to obtain information in a minority of patients, particularly those with chronic chest disease who have hyperinflated lungs. The resolution of the method is less good than that of standard radiology. The technique is very operator dependent and therefore requires a well trained person to obtain good and reliable information.

Associated techniques

Contrast echocardiography

Contrast echocardiography relies on the fact that cold fluid injected into the blood stream contains microbubbles. These bubbles can be seen passing through the heart. Abnormalities occur in the presence of a right to left shunt where the bubbles can be seen to pass directly into the left side of the heart. In a left to right shunt, contrast in the right heart chamber is washed out by contrast-free blood from the left side of the heart. In tricuspid regurgitation, contrast can be flushed into the hepatic veins.

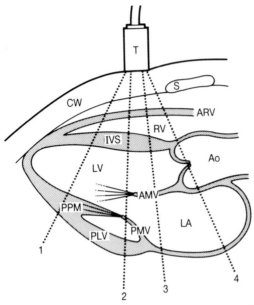

Fig. 6.7 Diagrammatic representation of the M-mode echocardiogram of the heart, showing the four standard views. The first view shows the aorta (Ao) and left atrium (LA); the second and third views are taken through the mitral valve; and the fourth view is taken of the left ventricle (LV). AMV, anterior leaflet of mitral valve; ARV, anterior wall of right ventricle; CW, chest wall; IVS, interventricular septum; PLV, posterior left ventricular wall; PMV, posterior leaflet mitral valve; PPM, posterior pupillary muscle; RV, right ventricle; S, sternum; T, transducer.

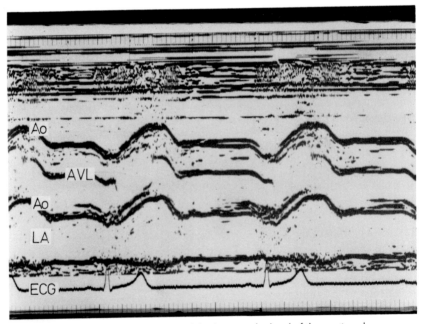

Fig. 6.8 M-mode electrocardiogram of the heart at the level of the aortic valve.

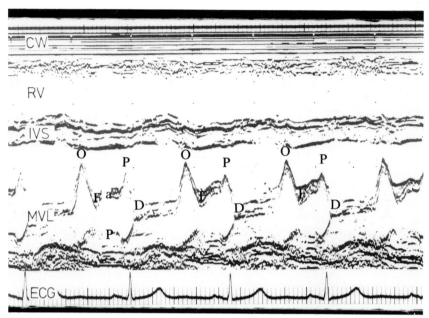

Fig. 6.9 M-mode electrocardiogram of the heart at the level of the mitral valve. a, anterior leaflet; p, posterior leaflet.

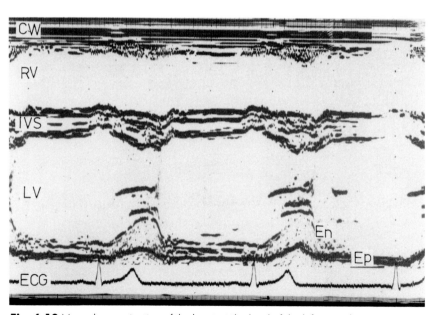

Fig. 6.10 M-mode examination of the heart at the level of the left ventricle.

Echo-phonocardiography

Echo-phonocardiography is the simultaneous recording of an M-mode echo-cardiogram, a phonocardiogram and, if required, a pulse wave and respiration recording. M-mode echocardiography is preferred in this technique because it allows a more leisurely examination of the timing of the ECG and heart sounds in regard to valve and wall movements. Figure 6.11 shows a simultaneous ECG phonocardiogram and echocardiogram. The closure of the mitral valve can be seen to correspond with the first heart sound and its opening to correspond with the opening snap.

Exercise echocardiography

Exercise echocardiography can be used to identify abnormal movement of segments of the left ventricle that has been made ischaemic by exercise. This technique has an equivalent sensitivity and specificity to exercise electro-cardiography.

Transoesophageal echocardiography

Transoesophageal echocardiography can be used in the patient who presents difficulties in obtaining good quality recordings because of chest disease. The close proximity of the oesophagus to the heart, and the absence of any intervening lung tissue, allows a transducer placed there to produce recordings of very high quality. It is a relatively new technique and suffers from the disadvantage of being uncomfortable for the patient.

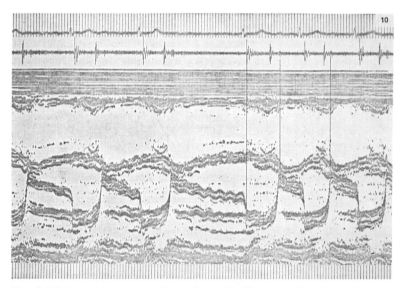

Fig. 6.11 An echo-phonocardiographic study illustrating the relationship between heart sounds and valve movements.

Doppler cardiography

An Austrian professor of mathematics and geometry, Johann Christian Doppler (1803–1853), is credited with the initial description of what has come to be known as the 'Doppler effect'. Doppler applied the principle to the shifts in light from stars but not directly to sound. It was Bays Ballot who, in the same century, applied this principle to sound. It was not until the peace following World War II that the benefits of the knowledge about sonar and radar circuitry were put to clinical use.

The technique evaluates blood flow by virtue of the ultrasound scattered by the red blood cells. The change in frequency between the emitted and the returned signal is called the Doppler shift. Normally, blood flow is laminar and red blood cells move at essentially the same speed as their neighbours. The Doppler shift recorded is therefore uniform. However, when blood flow becomes turbulent, such as in the presence of a narrowing of a vessel or stenosis of a valve, the red cells produce a variety of Doppler shifts at any instant in a cardiac cycle; this makes it difficult to predict accurately the precise extent of the narrowing.

Pulsed Doppler

In this mode there is one piezo-electric crystal which alternates as a transmitter and a receiver. A burst of ultrasound is emitted by the transducer which then receives the signals from the predetermined depth of interest (Fig. 6.12). The return signal is analysed for Doppler shifts for a very brief time period; accordingly, shifts in a frequency can be determined accurately at specific points along the beam.

The limitation of pulsed Doppler is its relatively slow sampling rates for high velocity flow.

Continuous wave Doppler

In this mode there are two piezo-electric crystals: one functions as a transmitter and the other as a receiver. Because the timing relationship between the emitted and received signal cannot be defined accurately, it is not possible to determine the depth of the recorded return signals. On the other hand, its very high sampling rates make it an ideal technique for high velocity flows such as occur in aortic stenosis (Fig. 6.13).

Clinical applications

Valvular stenosis

Blood flow through a stenotic valve has characteristic fluid–dynamic alterations. Proximal to the stenosis, blood flow is laminar. Within the stenotic orifice the velocity of blood flow increases in order to maintain the volume flow. It remains laminar until just distal to the stenosis, where it becomes turbulent and vortices of flow move in radial directions. The velocity of flow through a narrowed valve

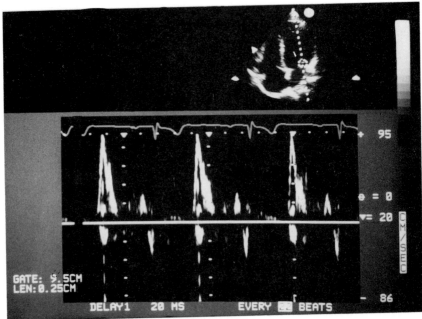

Fig. 6.12 Pulsed Doppler recording from just below the mitral valve in a normal patient. The position of the probe is seen in the four-chamber view in the top left of the picture. Flow towards the probe is recorded above the line. The ECG is shown at the top and is used for timing events. Normal mitral flow is in two phases; the first occurs when the mitral valve first opens in diastole. Flow then reduces almost to zero before the second phase, which occurs as a result of atrial systole.

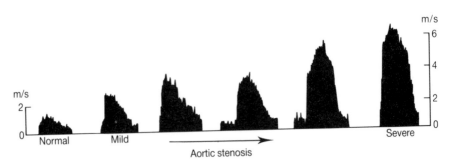

Fig. 6.13 Normal and varying degrees of severity of aortic outflow obstruction. All tracings are from the suprasternal notch. Calibration scales are the same in each continuous wave tracing. The site of the sampling probe is at the level of the aortic valve.

varies with the severity of the stenosis. If the stenosis is discrete the major determinant of the pressure drop is the peak velocity within the jet. Using a reliable simplification of the Bernoulli formula, the pressure difference across a stenosis can be determined by measuring the peak flow velocity in the stenotic orifice, squaring it and multiplying it by the constant 4. This method of non-invasive estimation of the gradient corresponds fairly well to the invasive measurement at cardiac catheterization.

Valvular regurgitation

Quantification of regurgitant lesions is more difficult than of stenotic lesions; in regurgitation there is a jet of blood flowing from a high pressure area into a low pressure. As a result there is a high velocity laminar jet of flow in the regurgitant orifice itself together with a flow disturbance in the chamber receiving the flow. To try to judge the severity of the valvular regurgitation, a technique termed flow mapping is used; it requires the use of pulsed Doppler. The sample volume probe is sited and sampled in different regions of the appropriate chamber; this enables a picture to be built up of the spatial relationships of the regurgitant flow. If the flow disturbance is present only in the plane just below the valve, mild regurgitation is present; if the flow disturbance is distributed widely, severe regurgitation is present. The size of the chamber into which the jet flows will have an influence on the flow characteristics. The introduction of colour flow Doppler has aided the assessment of the severity of regurgitant lesions.

Assessment of shunts of blood

Intracardiac shunts can be detected by demonstrating flow through an abnormal communication such as a ventricular or atrial septal defect. This can be particularly useful when the origin of a murmur is not clear clinically; this might occur, for instance, when a patient after a myocardial infarction develops a murmur. It is often very difficult to know whether this arises from an acquired ventricular septal defect or from the mitral regurgitation that may result from papillary muscle ischaemia or necrosis. The investigation can also be extremely useful in the neonate or the young child.

   Quantification of the shunt can be made by measuring and comparing the flows at appropriate different locations within the heart and great vessels. For instance, if there is a left to right shunt due to a ventricular septal defect, the pulmonary flow will be greater than aortic flow.

Further reading

Feigenbaum, H. (Ed.) (1986) *Echocardiography*. Lea & Febiger, Philadelphia.
Monaghan, M. J. (1990) *Practical Echocardiography and Doppler*. John Wiley, Chichester.

7

THE THORACIC AORTA

The aorta is conveniently demarcated at the diaphragm into the thoracic aorta above and the abdominal aorta below. Thoracic and abdominal aortic disease is often dealt with by different specialist teams, although practice varies from one country to another. This division may seem entirely arbitrary, but the truth is that, for historical reasons, the abdominal aorta (and the peripheral arteries) are handled by surgeons who were originally abdominal (or general) surgeons while thoracic surgeons handle the thoracic aorta. The abdominal aorta and peripheral vasculature are dealt with in Chapter 10.

Anatomy and structure

The thoracic aorta extends from the aortic valve to the diaphragm. It is usually considered in three parts which can be easily defined anatomically and which have important implications in terms of their pathology and, in particular, their surgical management.

The ascending aorta extends from the aortic valve to the origin of the brachiocephalic trunk. Its only branches are the right and left coronary arteries which arise a centimetre or so above the aortic valve in the respectively named coronary sinuses. Its first part, usually about 7–10 cm, lies within the pericardium; leakage from this part results in cardiac tamponade.

The arch of the aorta is the portion lying more or less horizontally, running obliquely backwards from just to the right of the midline in front, to reach the left side of the vertebral column. From it arise the three arch vessels, the brachiocephalic trunk, the left carotid and the left subclavian arteries (Fig. 7.1).

The portion of the aorta beyond the subclavian, opposite the ligamentum arteriosum, is called the isthmus and marks the beginning of the descending aorta which runs from there, on the left side of the vertebral column, to the diaphragm. It gives off paired intercostal arteries from the third rib onwards, a detail of anatomy that is important in the abnormal circulation associated with aortic coarctation.

The aorta has three histologically discrete layers. The outer layer, the adven-

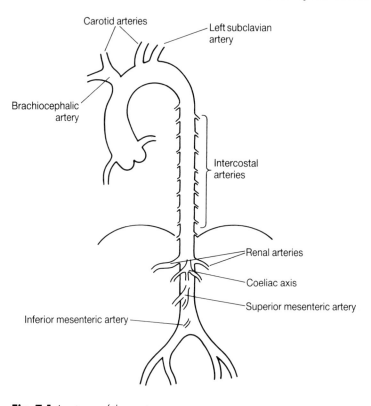

Fig. 7.1 Anatomy of the aorta.

titia, consists of a relatively thin layer of connective tissue. This is a discrete layer which can be dissected off by the surgeon and which can act as a life-saving, temporary containing layer after aortic trauma or dissection. The inner layer, the intima, is the layer in contact with the flowing blood. It is the layer in which atheroma develops. The bulk of the 2 mm or so of aortic wall consists of the media. This is a series of concentric layers of collagen and elastic tissue, nourished by vasa vasorum which penetrate its layers from the outside. There is no muscle in the aortic wall, so it plays no part in altering peripheral vascular resistance. The elastic content, however, permits it to expand in systole and recoil, so it is not just an inert tube. The pathological changes in this layer appear to be important in the condition called aortic dissection.

Function of the thoracic aorta

It is a mistake to consider the aorta simply as a passive conduit. It has important elastic properties and expands during systole. With the aortic valve closed during diastole the elastic recoil helps propagate onward flow.

Diseases of the thoracic aorta

The aorta may be congenitally abnormal. The commonest form is coarctation, which is a discrete narrowing in the region of the isthmus. A more generalized hypoplasia also occurs, but more rarely. These conditions are described in Chapter 5.

The acquired abnormalities of the aorta include aneurysm formation due to atherosclerosis, degenerative disease and tertiary syphilis. The aorta may also be involved in a process called aortic dissection, it is abnormal in Marfan's syndrome and various types of aortitis, and it may rupture due to major trauma. These will be described in turn.

Aneurysm of the thoracic aorta

Pathology

An aneurysm is a localized enlargement of an artery, which can be simply considered as a sac, in communication with its lumen. The wall of the sac consists of the layers of the aorta, although these are attenuated and abnormal due to disease of the arterial wall. A true aneurysm is lined by vascular endothelium although in reality the sac often becomes lined by thrombus. These are sub-divided and named according to their morphology. If they are longer than they are broad they are called fusiform. A more spherical 'blow-out' with a narrow neck is called a saccular aneurysm. (Small spherical aneurysms of the intracranial arteries are called 'berry aneurysms'; they are not dealt with in this chapter.)

Atherosclerosis is the usual cause of an artery dilating and forming a fusiform aneurysm. These aneurysms involve the descending aorta most commonly and are associated with hypertension. They lie next to the thoracic vertebra and can erode it and produce chronic pain. A minority extend as a continuous thoraco-abdominal aneurysm although, if the abdominal aorta is aneurysmal, it is much more commonly a localized abnormality with the aorta near the diaphragm being of near normal calibre. A classic cause of proximal, more saccular, aneurysms is tertiary syphilis. The media becomes weakened due to disease of the vasa vasorum and in time the aorta dilates. These aneurysms may erode the sternum.

If the aorta is injured, or ruptures due to disease, the blood may be contained by adventitia and surrounding structures. There is then a sac, communicating with the lumen but without a vascular endothelial lining; in fact, there may be very little aortic tissue in its wall. This is called a false aneurysm.

Aortic dissection is sometimes called dissecting aneurysm. In this condition the aortic media is abnormal and weak. The underlying histopathological change is called cystic medial necrosis and can be identified either side of the cleavage plane when sections of the aorta are examined. However, this is not a specific change but rather the evidence of aortic deterioration under a variety of circumstances. The intima tears and blood tracks up and down in a cleavage plain in the abnormal media. If this is contained by the adventitia the patient is left with a bulging aorta, appearing externally to be a fusiform aneurysm but internally having a double-barrelled structure. Because the sac is lined by abnormal media, rather than vascular endothelium, it does not fit into our definition so the term 'aortic dissection' is more precise than 'dissecting aneurysm', although both are used.

Clinical presentation of thoracic aortic aneurysm

History
Aneurysms may present with acute symptoms due to a sudden enlargement, leakage or rupture. They may cause a variety of chronic symptoms but, most commonly, they are asymptomatic and are detected incidentally.

A leaking thoracic aneurysm may cause severe pain, particularly in the back, and of course this is in the differential diagnosis of acute chest pain. There may be abrupt autonomic changes such as pallor and sweating, but if there is significant blood loss there is collapse due to sudden hypotension, and death may follow due to exsanguination. If the haemorrhage is contained, permitting survival, the site of the haematoma determines the symptoms, which can include stridor, haemoptysis, dysphagia or symptoms of superior vena caval obstruction. If an ascending aortic aneurysm ruptures into the pericardium, fatal cardiac tamponade follows.

The chronic symptoms include unremitting back pain due to thoracic vertebral erosion. There may also be symptoms due to compression of various structures and, in particular, hoarseness of the voice due to left recurrent nerve palsy.

An aneurysm may be detected on a chest radiograph taken for other reasons, such as the investigation of hypertension or as part of a routine preoperative screen. The aorta often looks abnormal in old age, due to elongation and therefore tortuosity. The distinction can usually be made with the aid of a good lateral and a penetrated posteroanterior film. Even if the aorta does look aneurysmal, it is worth asking the question 'What would we do about it?' before embarking on more elaborate investigations to prove the diagnosis.

Physical signs
There may be no abnormal physical signs. Erosion of the anterior chest wall occurs but is rare. The blood pressure may be raised, and chronic hypertension is probably a contributing factor in a high proportion of aortic aneurysms. A difference between the two arms should be sought, particularly if there have been acute symptoms. There may be bruits in the chest but these do not help in the diagnosis. Aortic stenosis may cause dilatation of the ascending aorta, which is a form of poststenotic dilatation rather than a primary aortic condition. The state of the aortic valve, whether stenotic or regurgitant, should always be considered if the ascending aorta is dilated.

Treatment

Hypertension should be controlled. The next question to be asked is whether there is a place for surgical treatment. This may be justified in an attempt to relieve severe pain. More commonly, operation is suggested for fear that the aneurysm may rupture and kill the patient. The question of operating on an asymptomatic patient to improve the prognosis must be considered most carefully. If the patient is elderly, we have to ask if the presence of an aneurysm is likely to significantly shorten enjoyable or useful life. If so, what are the chances of removing that hazard to survival and at what cost in terms of perioperative risk, complications and distress? The operative mortality for thoracic aneurysm surgery has remained over 20 per cent (United Kingdom Cardiac Surgical Register) so the wisdom and benefits of operating on these aneurysms remains questionable. There is, in addition, a substantial risk of paraplegia of around 15 per cent during surgery. The spinal cord receives some of its blood supply in a variable and unpredictable way from the artery of Adamkiewicz (or artery radicularis magna anterior), which is a branch of an intercostal artery between T9 and T12 in most people. In a minority it may arise as high as T5. It cannot be confidently identified intraoperatively. Ligation during surgery, or even temporary occlusion for a period of as little as 20 minutes, may result in irrecoverable paraplegia.

Aortic dissection

Pathology

There are two components to the gross appearance of aortic dissection, an intimal tear and a longitudinal split in the media.

The intimal tear is most commonly sited in the ascending aorta, 1–2 cm above the commissures of the aortic valve. It is usually more or less transverse or in a shallow spiral, and occupies about two-thirds of the circumference, predominantly the anterolateral (convex) aspect of the aorta. The second commonest site is just beyond the origin of the left subclavian artery in the aortic isthmus. The third site that is seen with any regularity is a tear in the arch of the aorta near the origin of the arch vessels.

The medial split or dissection runs from the tear for a variable distance, often in both directions. Usually about a third of the aortic circumference remains intact at any level and, as the dissection spirals along the aorta, it picks off side branches in a variable way. When the dissection involves the ascending aorta, it typically extends retrogradely to the aortic annulus, leaving the non-coronary cusp of the aortic valve unsupported and it may compromise the origin of the right coronary artery. The dissection may extend distally as far as the femoral arteries and any combination of arteries may be involved, some of which continue to fill from the false lumen.

Classification

It is useful to classify these cases, as the best management depends upon the site and extent of the dissection. The best known classification was proposed by DeBakey many years ago. He recognized that a tear in the ascending aorta with a dissection running all the way round the arch to involve the descending aorta was the most common and he called this type I. If the dissection stops at the arch vessels, it is type II. A dissection originating beyond the left subclavian artery is

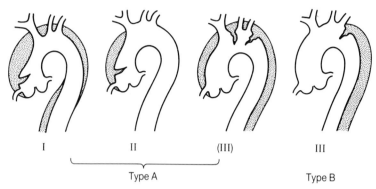

I II (III) III

Type A   Type B

Fig. 7.2 Classification of aortic dissections according to whether the ascending aorta is involved (type A) or not (type B). This is simpler than the DeBakey classification (types I, II and III). (Reproduced, with permission, from T. Treasure, 1986, *Dissection of the Thoracic Aorta*, Recent Advances in Surgery, vol. 12, Churchill Livingstone, Edinburgh.)

called type III. Not all cases fit easily into this classification and for most surgical purposes it is simpler to consider whether the ascending aorta is involved or not (Fig. 7.2). If it is, the dissection is almost universally fatal without surgery. If the process is confined to the descending aorta the prognosis is more favourable.

Predisposing causes

A healthy aorta cannot be split in this way. The aortic media in these cases has a characteristic but non-specific histological appearance (cystic medial necrosis) which is also associated with normal ageing. It has even been suggested that cleavage of the layers is the first event and the intimal tear is a secondary consequence, although this seems a little unlikely because the tear is found at angiography, at surgery and at postmortem if the search is adequate. The likely explanation is that the intimal tear can progress to dissection only in a vulnerable aorta.

There are several well recognized predisposing causes. The most characteristic is Marfan's syndrome in which it results from a specific aortic pathology. Hypertension is very commonly associated with dissection, particularly in cases involving the descending aorta. There is a clear association with bicuspid aortic valve disease, and it is of interest that the dissection originates at the convexity of the aorta just where the excentric jet impinges. It may occur in pregnancy; although this is extraordinarily uncommon, it is even rarer otherwise in women of childbearing age, so the relationship is a real one.

Clinical picture

History
Dissection of the aorta produces a sudden, severe, tearing pain in virtually all cases. Although it is listed along with myocardial infarction in the differential diagnosis of chest pain, the onset and nature of the pain are characteristic and

dramatic, and usually readily distinguishable. Later there may be involvement of the right coronary artery, with resulting inferior ischaemia, and the distinction may be more difficult. The pain may be in the chest or the back, and a sensation of tearing down into the abdomen is virtually pathognomonic.

Physical signs

There is usually collapse with pallor and sweating, and death may follow within a few minutes or hours as the aortic adventitia stretches and gives way. In those who survive the initial event, the blood is contained within the aortic adventitia and surrounding tissues, little or none is lost to the circulation, and the arterial pressure is often dangerously high.

All the pulses should be felt and documented. The dissecting flap can extend or move within the aorta and obstruct the aortic branches. Absent or weak pulses, which vary from time to time and particularly if different sites are affected, are typical of dissection. The blood pressure may differ in the different limbs. The immediate diastolic murmur of aortic regurgitation should be specifically listened for because it is strong evidence in favour of the diagnosis of aortic dissection. Evidence of ischaemia in one or more vascular territories should also be sought. Hemiplegia, due to cerebral vessel involvement, and paraplegia, due to impairment of spinal cord supply, are serious complications. Lower limb, renal and mesenteric ischaemia may all occur.

Investigations

A plain chest x-ray is an important preliminary investigation although in an elderly patient the aortic outline is often exaggerated due to elongation and increased tortuosity. It should be as near to a standard posteroanterior (PA) film as can be achieved, to get the best chance of diagnostic information. Widening of the mediastinum, loss of definition of the aortic knuckle and fluid in the left chest are the features to look for to support the diagnosis.

If the clinical features and preliminary investigations support the working diagnosis of aortic dissection, the admitting team have to decide if surgical intervention should be considered. If so, this may involve moving the patient to a specialist cardiac surgical centre and a phone call at this stage is sensible if intervention is being considered because if it is discounted, the management can be simplified and elaborate investigations can be avoided. The possible means of confirming the diagnosis are angiography, either by intra-arterial injection or by digital subtraction, or computed tomography (CT). Echocardiography supports the diagnosis if a flap can be detected in the ascending aorta. Transoesophageal echocardiography, if available, is valuable. Magnetic resonance imaging (MRI) will show the aorta well but is unlikely to be a practical option in most units for some time to come.

Management

Control of the blood pressure is vital and should be started immediately, whatever subsequent decisions are made about investigation, transfer or surgery. A vasodilator such as nitroprusside should be given by infusion, supplemented with a β-blocker. Arteriolar vasodilatation will reliably reduce the mean pressure but the shearing force of the pressure change (dP/dT) should also be reduced by β-adrenoceptor blockade. An arterial cannula to measure the pressure and a bladder catheter to monitor the urine flow permit the pressure to be reduced to the limits of tolerance as judged by renal and cerebral function. Reduction of arterial pressure to levels as low as 80–90 mmHg systolic may be tolerated and may permit the condition to stabilize.

Operative treatment is generally advised in cases where the ascending aorta is involved (types I and II) because the natural history is so awful due to severe aortic regurgitation, involvement of the cerebral and coronary arteries, and sudden deterioration due to rupture into the pericardium and death from cardiac tamponade. Surgery is usually best avoided in dissection confined to the descending aorta (type III) where conservative management has about 60 per cent of success, which is no worse than operative treatment (Fig. 7.3). Neurological impairment, other than transient episodes, or established renal failure, are contraindications to operation, as the chances of a good outcome then become remote. Extreme old age and intercurrent illness are relative disincentives for the same reason.

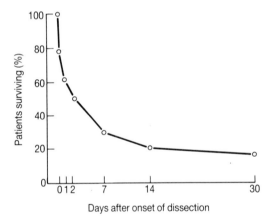

Fig. 7.3 Proportion of patients surviving with time from dissection (type A). (Data from Anagnastopoulos, 1972.) (Reproduced, with permission, from T. Treasure, 1986, *Dissection of the Thoracic Aorta*, Recent Advances in Surgery, vol. 12, Churchill Livingstone, Edinburgh.)

If operation is undertaken, it must be in a cardiac surgical unit and will require facilities for cardiopulmonary bypass. The aortic valve can usually be conserved and the simplest operation that will restore the continuity of the aorta is the most likely to succeed (Fig. 7.4).

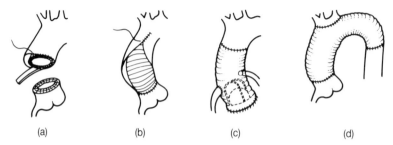

(a)   (b)   (c)   (d)

Fig. 7.4 Technical options in the surgery of type A dissections. (**a**) The dissection is being repaired with reinforcing strips of Teflon. In (**b**), (**c**) and (**d**) it is replaced to varying degrees. (Reproduced, with permission, from T. Treasure, 1986, *Dissection of the Thoracic Aorta*, Recent Advances in Surgery, vol. 12, Churchill Livingstone, Edinburgh.)

Marfan's syndrome

Marfan's syndrome is an autosomal dominant inherited abnormality of connective tissues. Those with the condition fully expressed are tall, with disproportionately long arms, such that their span exceeds their height. The digits and metacarpal bones are disproportionately long. They tend to be pigeon chested and to have a high arched palate. They are usually short sighted but, in addition, often have poor vision due to a strong tendency for the lens to dislocate. Abnormalities of the cardiovascular system are common, including dissection of the aorta and regurgitation of the aortic and, less frequently, the mitral valve. The abnormalities related to the aortic root are responsible for the early death of the majority of these people. Less severe forms, without Marfan habitus, may still have abnormalities of the aortic roots, leading to aortic valvar regurgitation and dissection of the aorta.

Aortic pathology

The aortic root shows a marked tendency to dilate in Marfan's syndrome, due to an inherent abnormality in the tissues of the aortic wall. The annulus, the sinuses of Valsalva and the proximal aorta are most severely involved. Progressive aortic regurgitation is common, and aortic dissection is the most common cause of death.

Management

Patients with Marfan's syndrome should be monitored for evidence of aortic root dilatation. Two-dimensional echocardiography is a most useful investigation for this purpose. Routine treatment with β-blockers reduces the force of contraction of the heart (dP/dT) and may reduce the rate of deterioration of the aorta and thus prolong life.

If the aortic regurgitation becomes severe, if the root enlarges progressively or if the patient survives an episode of acute dissection, surgery is necessary. This is made difficult by the quality of the aortic tissues, which hold sutures poorly.

Takayasu's disease

This is an arteritis that affects the aortic arch, narrowing its branches. Thrombosis and distal embolization may occur. It occurs at a much younger age than the other forms of arteritis, affects women more than men and is unusual in involving the aorta rather than the distal vessels.

Traumatic aortic rupture

In victims of motor accidents, air crashes and falls from a height one of the common lethal injuries is rupture of the aorta. This has a particular, characteristic, pattern. In most cases it is rapidly fatal, or the combination of other injuries does not permit survival, but in those who survive to reach hospital there is a chance of surgical cure (Fig. 7.5).

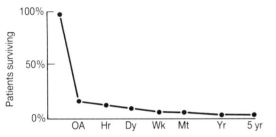

Fig. 7.5 Proportion of patients surviving with time from a traumatic aortic rupture. OA, on arrival. (Data from L. F. Parmley, T. W. Mattingley, W. C. Manion and E. J. Jahnke, 1958, Non-penetrating traumatic injury of the aorta. *Circulation* **17**, 1086–1101.)

Pathology

The aortic rupture occurs just beyond the left subclavian artery in nearly half the cases. There is typically a transverse tear of half or more of the aortic circumference. This is believed to occur, and so consistently at this site, because the descending thoracic aorta is relatively fixed, by its paired segmental, intercostal arteries and its retropleural position, to the vertebral column. The heart, with the ascending aorta, swings forward as the body as a whole is brought to an abrupt halt by the impact and the tear occurs at the junction between the mobile and immobile parts (Fig. 7.6). The Greek origin of the word (*aerein*, to rise) indicates that the aorta was seen as something which held up or suspended the heart. If the tear is full thickness the overlying visceral pleura will not contain the haematoma for long and the victim exsanguinates into the left hemithorax. If the aortic adventitia remains intact, it contains the aortic blood for a variable period of time. The majority rupture completely within some hours but a small minority survive with a well contained false aneurysm which can be evaluated more electively.

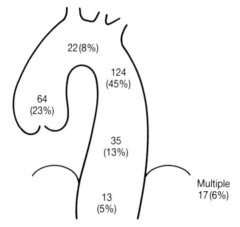

Fig. 7.6 Relative frequency of the anatomical sites of traumatic aortic rupture. (Data from L. F. Parmley, T. W. Mattingley, W. C. Manion and E. J. Jahnke, 1958, Non-penetrating traumatic injury of the aorta. *Circulation* **17**, 1086.)

Multiply injured patients

In multiply injured patients urgency dictates that we must depart (with due caution) from the logical and time-honoured process – history, examination and investigation lead to complete diagnosis and definitive treatment. There must be a routine that permits urgent resuscitation, a rapid diagnostic process and emergency treatment to be started, and for all three to proceed in parallel. No specific system or particular problem should be allowed to dominate the management of the patient as a whole. The investigation and operation for suspected ruptured aorta come high in the list of priorities but restoration of oxygenation and circulation with attention to the central nervous system are of paramount importance.

Sometimes this pattern of aortic rupture occurs in someone who has walked away from an accident, a situation that is particularly difficult because the index of suspicion will be low.

Diagnosis of aortic rupture

Clinical signs are not always helpful in making the diagnosis. If it is suspected, a very critical examination of all the peripheral pulses should be documented. There may be weak or absent femoral pulses, or the left arm pressure may be lower than the right. Sometimes there is a murmur due to turbulence at the site. The neurological state of the lower limbs should be observed and recorded.

A chest x-ray is the single most important investigation and, if at all possible, a good quality PA film should be obtained. The management hinges upon this information, but the surgical team should be prepared to accompany the patient to the radiology department so that other aspects of resuscitation and diagnosis may continue. An emergency casualty film taken supine often suggests a widened mediastinum but if a good chest x-ray remains suspicious, the diagnosis must be proven. This can be done by aortography in most radiology departments, digital subtraction angiography or CT in some, and by cine-angiography in cardiac units. Transoesophageal echocardiography, where available, may be valuable. Which test to use and, if the patient has to be transferred, whether this should be before or after investigation, depend on his overall state, the local facilities and the distance away from a unit that might offer a better chance of a successful operation.

Management

In principle, the operation is simple. The aorta is clamped above and below, and the tear is repaired. In practice, the mediastinum is the site of a massive haematoma which obliterates all landmarks, the circulation may tolerate poorly the alteration in peripheral resistance involved in clamping, the tissues may take sutures badly and the central nervous system remains at risk. Some patients are better managed with hypotensive measures (see 'Aortic dissection', earlier in this chapter) until the patient's state and the surgical team are more auspicious.

8

PERICARDIAL DISEASE

Normal pericardium

The normal pericardium consists of a fibrous and a serous component. The fibrous pericardium is a relatively unyielding membrane that is fused with the central tendon of the diaphragm below and with the pulmonary artery, aorta and pulmonary veins above. It may extend up these vessels for several centimetres. The serous pericardium, in which the heart is invaginated, has a parietal and a visceral layer; the latter is called the epicardium and covers the surface of the heart and origins of the great vessels. The pericardial cavity is a potential space which normally contains a small volume of fluid. The cavity becomes enlarged in the presence of pericardial disease as a result of an increase in the volume of fluid, and its capacity may then become considerably increased.

The normal pericardium is not essential to life. Both layers can be removed without any apparent ill effect. It is probable that the presence of a normal pericardium limits the stroke volume during exercise and prevents inappropriate distension of the ventricular myocardium; this may become important in the patient with chronic heart failure.

Congenital abnormalities of the pericardium are uncommon and are usually associated with additional anomalies of the heart and great vessels.

Acquired pericardial disease

Pericardial disease can be considered in two distinct ways: firstly, in terms of the aetiology and, secondly, in terms of the physiological and clinical disturbances that are produced.

Aetiology

The diseases that affect the pericardium are displayed in Table 8.1.

Table 8.1 Diseases affecting the pericardium

Acute idiopathic pericarditis	
Infections	Viral
	Bacterial
	Toxoplasmosis, amoebiasis
	Nocardiasis
	Echinococcal
Inflammatory	Postcardiotomy
	Dressler's
With systemic disease	Connective tissue disorders
	Rheumatic fever
	Uraemia
	Hypothyroidism
Neoplastic	Primary
	Secondary
Haemorrhage	Trauma
	Aortic dissection
	After myocardial infarction
Drug induced	

Acute idiopathic pericarditis occurs predominantly in young adults. A viral aetiology can be implicated in approximately half the cases, the commonest virus being the Coxsackie B. There can also be evidence of associated myocardial involvement. The typical clinical features are chest pain, influenza-like symptoms, palpitation and a skin rash. The condition is usually self-limiting.

Bacterial infections of the pericardium may be due to blood-borne infections or by direct extension from the lungs or pleural space. It is not usually an isolated event and occurs most commonly in the patient with overwhelming disease.

Tuberculous infection of the pericardium is usually secondary to infection elsewhere. The infection may present as an acute pericarditis, a pericardial effusion or as constrictive pericarditis. Treatment consists of antituberculous therapy; the addition of steroids will reduce the likelihood of constriction later. Surgery may be necessary if tamponade or constriction occurs.

Fungal pericarditis is uncommon but infections with actinomycosis, coccidiomycosis and histoplasmosis have been reported. Pericardial involvement in hydatid disease is recognized in areas where the disease is endemic.

A substantial proportion of patients may develop evidence of acute pericarditis after myocardial infarction. This will present as a friction rub. The associated pain or discomfort must be differentiated from that of further myocardial ischaemia. Pericarditis may occur also as part of Dressler's syndrome; this occurs in about 3 per cent of those sustaining a myocardial infarction and typically presents between 2 weeks and several months after the event. It is usually a self-limiting febrile illness accompanied by pericardial and/or pleural pain together with evidence of inflammation of other serosal surfaces; it will usually respond to indomethacin or aspirin, although occasionally steroids are required. High levels of anti-heart antibodies may be found.

Pericarditis occurs in about 10 per cent of patients with acute rheumatic fever. It usually presents with the features of an acute pericarditis or the development of a pericardial effusion.

Pericardial involvement occurs with connective tissue disorders such as rheumatoid arthritis and systemic lupus erythematosus.

In chronic renal failure the patient may present with pericardial pain and a pericardial rub. These manifestations will subside with the treatment of the renal failure.

Hypothyroidism may present with a pericardial effusion which is typically silent. The effusion does not need treatment and will subside when thyroid replacement therapy is given.

Malignant involvement of the pericardium may be due to primary tumours of the pericardium such as a mesothelioma or sarcoma. More commonly the tumour is metastatic. The patient may initially present with an arrhythmia. Tamponade or pericardial constriction may develop subsequently.

Radiation to the mediastinum may cause a pericarditis.

Haemorrhage into the pericardium can cause tamponade. This may occur with a dissection of the ascending aorta. It may also occur as a result of direct trauma such as a penetrating wound or after heart surgery.

Drugs such as procainamide or hydralazine can occasionally cause pericarditis; this subsides when the drug is withdrawn.

Syndromes associated with pericardial disease

Pericarditis

Clinical features

The chest pain of pericarditis is usually retrosternal in position and sharp or rough in character. It is often aggravated by movement or deep inspiration. It can be modified by position, often being relieved by sitting up and leaning forwards. It can mimic angina pectoris and can be made worse by exertion. It can be associated with dyspnoea but usually because inspiration is painful and the patient adopts a different pattern of breathing. The onset of the pain is usually sudden but may be preceded by several days' malaise and other non-specific symptoms.

The main abnormality on examination is the presence of a pericardial rub. This is a superficial scratchy noise, best heard with the diaphragm of the stethoscope. The sound can be mimicked by rubbing the hair above your ear with your finger tips. The rub may be audible all over the precordium; it may be so soft as to be heard in only one small area and may be made louder by moving the patient into different positions; it is usually louder down the left sternal edge. In patients in sinus rhythm the rub has several components corresponding to atrial and ventricular systole and diastole. As a result of this cadence it can sometimes be mistaken for the murmurs of mixed aortic valve disease. Some patients are actually aware of the relationship of the heart action to the pain associated with the rub and describe the different components of the pain. Rubs are typically evanescent. Irregularity of the pulse due to a supraventricular arrhythmia is common with acute pericarditis.

Investigations

The typical ECG abnormalities consist of symmetrical elevation of the ST segments with the concavity upwards (Fig. 8.1). This occurs in most leads except aVR and is typically most pronounced in standard lead II. In contradistinction to the ST segment changes of a myocardial infarct, there is no reciprocal ST depression nor are there any pathological Q waves. In the early stages of the illness the T waves are upright; over the next 2–3 weeks they may become inverted. In the subacute phase the ST segment elevation is absent and the T waves are inverted; this may lead to a mistaken diagnosis of myocardial ischaemia. If there is a large pericardial effusion the PQRST complexes may be of low voltage (Fig. 8.2).

A chest x-ray may show enlargement of the heart shadow but it is difficult to determine whether this is due to pericardial fluid or an enlargement of a cardiac chamber.

Echocardiography is the investigation of choice for detecting a pericardial effusion. M-mode echocardiography displays the pericardial fluid as an echo-free space between the epicardial and parietal pericardium posterior to the left ventricle but not extending behind the left atrium where there is no potential space. Two-dimensional echocardiography gives more anatomical information

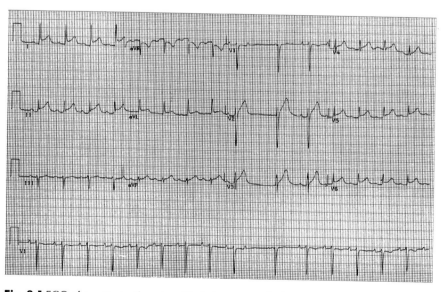

Fig. 8.1 ECG of a patient with pericarditis. It shows sinus rhythm with an atrial premature beat. The QRS complexes are normal and there are no Q waves. There is ST segment elevation in most leads without any ST segment depression. The ST segment is concave upwards.

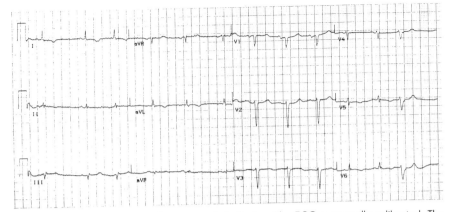

Fig. 8.2 ECG of a patient with a pericardial effusion. The ECG is normally calibrated. The PQRST complexes are of small voltage. There are quite widespread ST segment and T wave abnormalities.

about the distribution of the fluid and is very helpful if the effusion is loculated (Fig. 8.3). The amount of fluid present can be quantified approximately. The volume of fluid gives no indication of the haemodynamic effect; a very small volume of fluid can produce life-threatening tamponade whereas a large effusion may be entirely symptomless. The critical determinant is the speed at which the fluid accumulates and its effect can only be judged clinically.

Cardiac catheterization is rarely required but can sometimes give helpful information if the echocardiogram is technically impossible. The presence of fluid can be determined best by positioning the venous catheter on the lateral wall of the right atrium; normally this thin-walled chamber corresponds to the border of the cardiac silhouette. If there is fluid in the pericardium, the catheter tip will be separated from the border of the heart by the fluid. If there is pericardial constriction present, the diastolic pressures in the two ventricles will become virtually identical (Fig. 8.4); the high venous pressure will be recorded with its characteristic waveform.

Treatment

Acute idiopathic pericarditis is usually a self-limiting process which requires symptomatic treatment only. Occasionally, life-threatening pericardial tamponade can develop. Because of the likelihood of an associated myocarditis it is advisable to rest the patient until the pain and symptoms have completely subsided. The supraventricular arrhythmias can be treated with digoxin but may be persistent and troublesome until the pericarditis subsides. If the pericarditis is due to Dressler's syndrome or the postcardiotomy syndrome it will usually respond to aspirin or indomethacin; occasionally, steroids may need to be used. If the pericarditis is part of a more generalized disease the treatment will need to be appropriate for that disease.

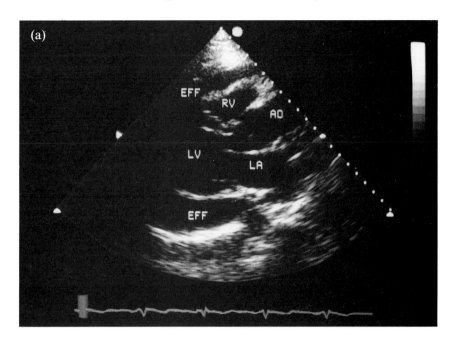

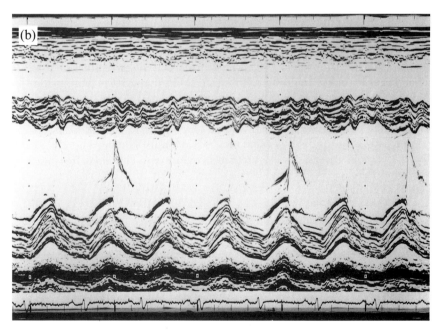

Fig. 8.3 (**a**) Two-dimensional echocardiogram, demonstrating a large posterior pericardial effusion. This is most marked behind the ventricles and becomes smaller behind the left atrium, where the pericardium is firmly attached to the pulmonary veins. Ao, aorta; EFF, pericardial effusion; LA, left atrium; LV, left ventricle; RV, right ventricle. (**b**) The M-mode displays the echo-free space behind the ventricle.

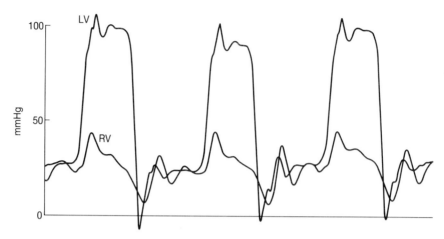

Fig. 8.4 Simultaneous pressure recordings from the right (RV) and left (LV) ventricles. The scale is shown in mmHg. The diastolic pressures in the two ventricles have become almost identical as a result of the increased pericardial pressure.

Pericardial tamponade

Tamponade is a French word of German origin meaning compression of the heart. Pericardial tamponade is a complication of a pericardial effusion. The pericardial pressure becomes high enough to interfere with the ventricular filling. The volume of fluid required to cause cardiac compression varies. If the fluid has collected slowly, in excess of 2 litres may be present; but if it has collected rapidly, a few hundred millilitres may lead to cardiac tamponade.

A number of compensatory mechanisms maintain cardiac output as the pericardial pressure rises and compromises the cardiac output. A sinus tachycardia develops because the stroke volume is relatively small and fixed, and an adequate cardiac output will depend on the heart rate. The peripheral vascular resistance also increases, so the arterial pressure is maintained in spite of a reduction in flow.

The patient with pericardial tamponade will have evidence of a reduced cardiac output. The skin may be cold and sweaty and the pulse volume small. There will be a sinus tachycardia. The patient will have the physical sign of a paradoxical pulse; this sign is characteristic of tamponade and implies severe embarrassment of the circulation (Figs. 8.5 and 8.6). In the normal person there is a slight reduction in arterial pressure or pulse pressure with inspiration; this reduction in systolic pressure does not exceed 10–15 mmHg. The patient with a paradoxical pulse will have a reduction of greater than 15 mmHg with inspiration and the pulse may actually disappear. This may be felt best in the femoral artery. The paradoxical pulse is thus an exaggeration of the normal. The paradox that Kussmaul described is 'the pulse in all arteries, in the presence of regular and continuing heart motion, becomes very small or disappears entirely in regular intervals defined by inspiration and returns immediately with expiration'.

The sphygmomanometer is used to measure the amount of paradox; in

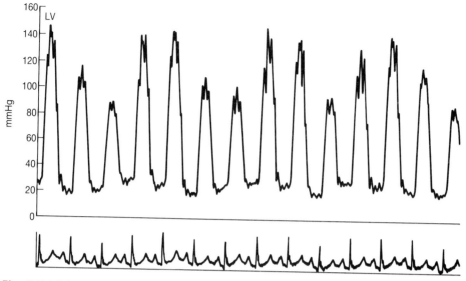

Fig. 8.5 A left ventricular pressure tracing of a patient with acute tamponade. The diastolic pressure is elevated. With inspiration there is a drop of 30–40 mmHg in systolic pressure.

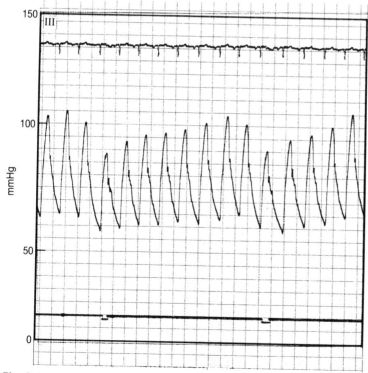

Fig. 8.6 An arterial tracing from a (different) patient with acute tamponade. There is a 30 mmHg drop in the systolic pressure with inspiration.

essence, two pressures are recorded – the systolic pressure on expiration and that on inspiration. With the patient breathing quietly the cuff is blown up to a level to occlude the systolic pressure. It is then possible to allow the cuff to deflate slowly and record the systolic pressure on expiration. Several respiratory cycles will be necessary to record the systolic pressure. As the patient inspires, so the Korotkoff sound will disappear; the cuff is now deflated until the systolic pressure can be recorded consistently on inspiration as well as on expiration. The difference in the two systolic pressures gives the degree of paradox. It is important to avoid asking the patient to take deep breaths, as this will tend to produce a Valsalva manoeuvre which will modify the arterial response.

The abnormality of right atrial filling in pericardial tamponade is reflected in the jugular venous pulse. The pressure is raised and may be difficult to see. The waveform is normal. In the patient with only mild tamponade the venous pressure may be only slightly elevated but the pressure will rise with inspiration.

Differential diagnosis

A myocardial infarction involving the right ventricle may present with a paradoxical pulse and a raised venous pressure; the history and ECG should enable the correct diagnosis to be made. Other causes of a paradoxical pulse include heart failure, pulmonary embolus and bronchial asthma in which the paradoxical pulse is caused by the changes in intrathoracic pressures. The clinical presentation should enable the distinction to be made between these conditions.

Treatment

Pericardial tamponade requires emergency treatment by means of pericardial aspiration. This can be performed with local anaesthesia at the patient's bedside by a skilled operator. It is not without risk and full resuscitation apparatus should be available. Pericardial aspiration (pericardiocentesis) is usually performed from the xiphoid approach. The aspiration needle is attached to the V lead of an ECG machine which is isolated electrically from the patient; this helps the operator determine when the tip of the needle strikes the epicardium and produces the ST segment changes of the 'current of injury pattern'. This procedure will relieve the acute emergency. The patient will need to be watched for a recurrence of tamponade. Should it recur, further aspiration may be necessary; alternatively, a pericardial window (pericardiotomy) can be created surgically. This also enables some histology of the pericardium to be obtained.

Constrictive pericarditis

The essential feature of constrictive pericarditis is the presence of compression of the heart which results in a syndrome characterized by a high venous pressure, oedema and ascites. There may also be myocardial involvement due to atrophy and fibrosis of the subepicardial layer of the ventricular wall. Calcification may be present and this may be in the form of plaques or as an almost complete shell around the heart.

Pathophysiology

Pericardial constriction prevents ventricular filling in late diastole. Early diastolic filling and pressure are normal (Fig. 8.7). Because the pericardium is indistensible the normal volume causes a marked increase in the filling pressure. This is reflected in both right and left atrial pressures, as both sides of the heart are usually involved symmetrically. The increase in venous pressure may be considerable and will lead to hepatic distension, ascites and peripheral oedema (Fig. 8.8). The stroke volume will be limited and cardiac output is therefore maintained by means of the heart rate.

Clinical features

In severe cases the venous pressure may be very high and in excess of 20 cm of blood above the sternal angle. There will be a marked y descent, reflecting the normal early diastolic pressure in the ventricles (Fig. 8.9), and contrasts with the venous wave in tamponade where the filling pressure is high throughout diastole.

The precordial impulse is not usually palpable. The heart sounds are soft; an early diastolic sound is frequently present – it occurs earlier than a third sound and is termed a pericardial knock. The liver is enlarged and ascites is often present together with peripheral oedema; the patient may also be jaundiced. It is easy to see how a mistaken diagnosis of cirrhosis is often made; the important

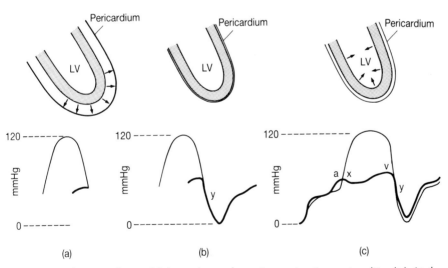

Fig. 8.7 Left ventricular and left atrial waveforms in constructive pericarditis. (**a**) At the beginning of diastole the left ventricle (LV) is beginning to fill; there is initially no problem with filling and the high left atrial pressure falls rapidly when the mitral valve opens (the rapid y descent). (**b**) The ventricle is now impeded by the thick, resistant pericardium and can distend no more. Blood continues to arrive in the atrial cavity and the pressures therefore rise. (**c**) Ventricular systole commences, starting from a high pressure. Systole itself is unimpeded. The V wave of the atrial pulse is produced in the usual manner but at a higher pressure. Similar events occur on the right side with similar diastolic pressures but lower systolic.

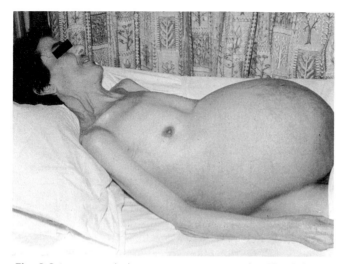

Fig. 8.8 A patient with chronic constrictive pericarditis. The abdomen is grossly distended with ascites and the venous pressure is markedly elevated. The patient also has peripheral pitting oedema. (Picture by courtesy of Dr A. Hollman.)

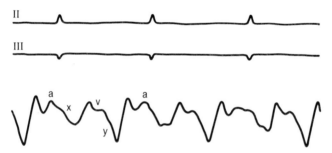

Fig. 8.9 Tracing of venous pressure in a patient with constrictive pericarditis. The characteristic sharp y descent is well shown.

distinguishing feature is the venous pressure. Although a paradoxical pulse can sometimes be present, it is absent in 75 per cent of patients with chronic constrictive pericarditis.

The clinical features of this condition are often muddled with those of acute tamponade. The two conditions are different in so many respects that, as long as the underlying pathophysiological basis is understood, they cannot be confused.

Investigations

The chest x-ray may show a normal or a slightly enlarged heart due to the pericardial thickening, but the lung fields are clear. An important finding is calcification of the pericardium. There may also be evidence of pulmonary tuberculosis. The ECG may show a number of rather non-specific features, which include atrial fibrillation, low voltage complexes, T wave flattening and, occasionally, right ventricular hypertrophy. An echocardiogram may show pericardial fluid or thickening but may be unhelpful. Cardiac catheterization will confirm the considerable elevation of the right and left atrial pressures and similarity of the ventricular filling pressures. Angiography will demonstrate the pericardial thickening.

Differential diagnosis

Cirrhosis of the liver can easily be confused with this condition. The high venous pressure in constrictive pericarditis and its absence in cirrhosis should enable the correct diagnosis to be made. Heart failure may also be incorrectly diagnosed; the lung fields can be clear in both conditions although crepitations or evidence of pleural fluid will point the clinician towards heart failure. Another helpful distinction is the ability of the patient with constrictive pericarditis to lie down flat in spite of the high venous pressure! Very different from the patient with heart failure.

A restrictive cardiomyopathy may present a very similar picture and will sometimes be very difficult to distinguish from constrictive pericarditis. So difficult sometimes is this distinction that, in spite of investigations that include cardiac catheterization and angiography, surgery has to be performed to explore the pericardium and, if necessary, to perform a pericardiectomy.

Treatment

The treatment is surgical and should be recommended whenever the exercise tolerance or evidence of fluid retention cannot be controlled by moderate doses of diuretics. The temptation to treat the signs with strong diuretics must be resisted; these signs all result from the high filling pressures that are necessary to maintain an adequate cardiac output. To produce an abrupt reduction in filling pressure may be dangerous and cause hypovolaemic shock.

The operation itself may be long and difficult, as the calcification may extend down into the ventricular muscle and need to be dissected out. The traditional approach is through a left anterior interspace thoracotomy, which provides excellent access to the left ventricle but is difficult should cardiopulmonary bypass be required. Some surgeons prefer the median sternotomy. Not only the parietal pericardium but also the adherent epicardium must be removed. Because of the high risk of pericardial tears and of excess blood loss the procedure is performed with the immediate availability of cardiopulmonary bypass. The results of surgery are usually very good. If a tuberculosus aetiology is suspected, chemotherapy is usually started prior to the operation.

Further reading

Fowler, N. O. (Ed.) (1985) *The Pericardium in Health and Disease*. Futura, New York.

9

CARDIAC SUPPORT, ARTIFICIAL HEARTS AND TRANSPLANTATION

Attempts to support temporarily or completely replace organ systems have been made with varying degrees of success, but among the organs of the body that are vital for continued survival the one that has the simplest, and conceptually most reproducible, function is the heart.

Support of the heart can be considered under three circumstances:

1. Planned temporary support to permit surgery – a period of hours at most.
2. Support of a sick patient while awaiting recovery or while preparations are made for surgery – a period of days.
3. Permanent support or replacement of the heart – for life.

Support of the cardiovascular system during surgery

Cardiopulmonary bypass was first used successfully in the Mayo Clinic in 1953 and is now very well established. It is employed in about 20 000 operations per annum in the UK and probably more than 200 000 in the USA. The methods are quite standardized. The patient is fully heparinized, usually with an initial intravenous bolus dose of 3 mg/kg (1 mg = 100 units, i.e. over 20 000 units for a typical adult) which is replenished at intervals either according to results of clotting studies or according to a set protocol. The patient's blood is drained out through pipes positioned in the right atrium or separately into the superior and inferior venae cavae. It is passed through an oxygenator which removes carbon dioxide and replenishes its oxygen content. The blood may have the gas mixture bubbled through it or remain separated from it by a membrane. The oxygenated blood is pumped back into the arterial system, usually through a cannula of about 1 cm in diameter in the ascending aorta (Fig. 9.1) at a flow to match the expected cardiac output. The pressure is governed by the patient's peripheral vascular resistance, which can be influenced pharmacologically. The distribution of flow is hard to determine but, fortunately, autoregulation is maintained to a large extent even under these very artificial circumstances. The gas content can also be adjusted but the oxygen consumption cannot be directly influenced.

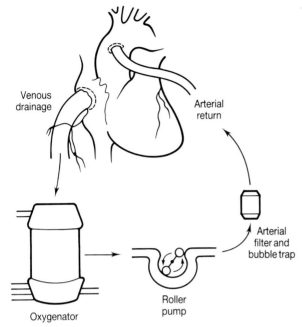

Venous
drainage

Arterial
return

Arterial
filter and
bubble trap

Roller
pump

Oxygenator

Fig. 9.1 The principal components of the bypass circuit.

Bypass is tolerated remarkably well by the body although it is a very imperfect system. Interactions between the blood and artificial surfaces cause activation of platelets, clotting cascades and the inflammatory system. Flow from the pump never has the pulsatility of the heart's own output with its abrupt rise in pressure. Probably a combination of these effects results in imperfect perfusion of the microcirculation, which can be detected as organ damage particularly in the lungs, liver and brain. Nevertheless, the intrinsic risks of cardiopulmonary bypass have become very small, provided the bypass time is relatively short, ideally within 2 hours. Thereafter the damage to organs is progressive; eventually this alone would prove fatal. Therefore, cardiopulmonary bypass cannot be regarded as a means of supporting the failing ventricle.

Temporary support of the failing heart

It should be remembered that cardiopulmonary bypass is used by the surgeon to permit total access to a still, blood-free heart. Attempts to extend the use of total bypass to longer term cardiac support has not been successful. It is more useful to decide which part of the system has failed and to support that, perhaps only partially.

Intra-aortic balloon counter-pulsation

This is a well established method of assisting the left ventricle for a period of hours or days. It can be used for up to 2–3 weeks but it is a mistake to use it unless there is reason to expect improvement in left ventricular performance, or surgical correction of the underlying problem. There must be some output from the heart, as the device is capable only of augmentation.

The principle is simple and therefore appealing. A cylindrical balloon of up to 40 ml volume, at the end of a catheter, is threaded up from the femoral artery to lie as high as possible in the descending aorta (Fig. 9.2). It can be inflated and deflated abruptly with a low viscosity gas such as helium or carbon dioxide, from an external pump. The pump is triggered from the patient's electrocardiogram or arterial pressure; the balloon is timed to inflate as soon as the aortic valve has closed as judged by the position of the dicrotic notch. This displaces its volume of blood, creating a second pressure wave, and causes retrograde flow available to perfuse the coronary arteries as their resistance falls during diastole. The balloon is collapsed as close to aortic valve opening as possible, thus reducing the afterload and perhaps even sucking blood out of the heart.

The system works best with sinus rhythm but timing is also straightforward with electrical pacing of the heart. Irregular rhythms are much more difficult to manage. Balloon augmentation is less satisfactory in the presence of aortic regurgitation and is not usually employed under these circumstances. The balloon can be positioned very quickly by percutaneous techniques or introduced as a surgical manoeuvre. Low level heparinization is usual. There can be

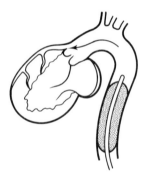

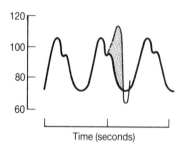

Time (seconds)

Fig. 9.2 The balloon positioned in the descending aorta can be abruptly inflated and deflated, timed from the ECG. The diastolic pressure is augmented, aiding coronary flow.

serious problems with damage to the aorta or compromise to the blood supply to the leg but these are avoidable with modern equipment and careful technique.

Extracorporeal membrane oxygenation (ECMO)

This system is applicable when the cardiac function is adequate but the lungs have failed, and is therefore for pulmonary rather than cardiac support. It is an extension of bypass techniques but, provided cardiac output is adequate, requires only venous cannulation. It has had very limited success over years of trying and is mentioned here only for completeness.

Left ventricular assist device (LVAD)

For over 20 years there have been attempts to make devices, either implantable or sited externally, that will support the heart, and in particular the left ventricle. In this particular context we are discussing temporary support, a means of holding the patient until cardiac function recovers or a more permanent solution can be found. The commonest approach is to implant a device with a chamber through which the blood flows, with non-return valves at the inflow and outflow connections, a principle similar to the left ventricle. A membrane is driven to and fro across the chamber by a gas pumped through drive lines from the outside. The outflow is connected to the aorta, and the inflow to either the left atrium or the left ventricle. There are many permutations, none of which has become standard. Few patients in this category have recoverable ventricular function so the whole philosophy depends upon holding the patient until a more permanent solution, at present a donor heart, becomes available.

Permanent cardiac support or replacement

This subject is in the process of rapid change and those who are interested in an up-to-date account of the subject should consult current journals rather than textbooks. Nevertheless, some principles are becoming established.

Anyone writing about cardiac surgery in 1950 would have done well to predict the course of events over the ensuing years. From that viewpoint there were several possibilities. The techniques of profound hypothermia and circulatory arrest were well established and some people considered the extension of these techniques as the way of the future. Cross-circulation from a relative was used successfully by Lillehei and colleagues from 1954 and seemed at that stage at least as likely to succeed as the early heart–lung machines. Perhaps a pharmacological approach with a metabolic blocker might have been considered and there were certainly those who thought that cardiac surgery had gone as far as it could, and perhaps should, go. Of the possibilities, it would have been impossible to predict that extracorporeal circulation with a machine would be used with great success in hundreds of thousands of cases each year.

Similarly, if we now try to look at the future of total cardiac replacement we cannot predict whether we will still rely on human hearts; if so, will their availability change with time due to evolution of ethical considerations or methods of tissue preservation? Will we instead use animal hearts, thanks to progress in immunology? Or will totally implantable mechanical hearts become as practical a consideration as the electronic pacemaker?

Cardiac transplantation

Throughout the 1960s Shumway, in Stanford, California, was working on an experimental programme of cardiac transplantation but Christiaan Barnard performed the first human transplant recorded, in South Africa, in 1966. Over the next few years many centres tried one or two transplant operations but there were few who survived more than a month or so and attempts were largely abandoned although Shumway continued to work steadily at the problem until he achieved success. Meanwhile, in Britain, there was a moratorium on cardiac transplantation throughout the 1970s. During the 1980s cardiac transplantation increased dramatically. Organ procurement and preservation, case selection and the management of rejection have all been important factors in its development.

Indications and case selection

The ideal case should have severe, intolerable and permanent impairment of cardiac function. The commonest indications are end-stage ischaemic damage to the left ventricle and people with dilated cardiomyopathy. The condition must be so severe, on the best available medical treatment, that the relief obtained would be appreciated in spite of the burden of immunosuppression, monitoring of rejection and the associated morbidity that accompanies transplantation at present. If the pulmonary vascular resistance is already raised the normal right ventricle of a donor heart cannot cope, and this is an absolute contraindication to simple orthotopic heart transplantation. Associated pathology such as impaired renal function, hepatic dysfunction, cerebral impairment or diabetes usually exclude the patient. As with all new procedures, there will be a tendency to extend the indications to include more and more desperate cases until a realistic balance is learned by experience. Age is a consideration but the age limit is a flexible one and has gone up with increasing confidence in the technique and the use of immunosuppression. With a limited supply of organs, younger patients (say, under 55) will tend to have preference because as a group they are more likely to enjoy the greatest benefit. Finally, considerable psychological resilience and determination are required.

   The donor must be declared brain dead. There are clearly defined criteria that must be met and the diagnosis must be confirmed by two senior doctors, one of whom must not be involved in the care of the patient. The donor should be healthy in other respects, free from significant infection and preferably under 45 years of age. The politics and ethics involved in encouraging potential donors, their families and the doctors who look after them are key factors that will influence the availability of hearts for transplantation in the future. Once a potential donor has been identified a recipient with a compatible blood group is chosen. More refined tissue matching has not been found to influence outcome. The donor heart is taken as a planned procedure in an operating theatre. If kidneys and other organs are to be used the initial dissection is performed while these are perfused by the heart. The donor is heparinized, the aorta is cross-clamped and cold hyperkalaemic cardioplegic solution is infused into the coronary arteries and the heart is excised. If kept cold (4–6°C) and electrically silent it will beat well on reperfusion several hours later; distant organ procurement is therefore possible.

Meanwhile the recipient has been called into hospital and prepared for surgery. These patients maintain a state of readiness, often carrying a radio-pager so that they will not miss any chance of a heart. Once the availability of a suitable heart is certain the recipient is taken to theatre, anaesthesia is induced and preparations are made for cardiopulmonary bypass. The heart is replaced orthotopically. The donor and recipient hearts are not excised in the same way but rather with incisions that conserve tissue on the donor heart and the recipient's vessels to give the surgeon as much flexibility as possible with his suture lines. Thus there are typically two sinoatrial nodes in the recipient's body.

Methods of immunosuppression vary considerably but the use of cyclosporin has been a major advance responsible for great improvements in results. Steroids, azathioprine and antithymocyte globulin are also used for maintenance or for treatment of acute rejection.

Heart–lung transplantation is indicated for patients with end-stage lung disease but also for those where the pulmonary vascular damage is so severe that heart transplantation alone is not possible. In the former group the heart itself may be healthy and used in turn as a donor heart.

Permanent artificial heart

The possibilities for permanent artificial hearts include an orthotopic device that would replace the left and right ventricles (a total artificial heart) and heterotopic devices along the lines of the ventricular assist devices described earlier, which might permanently replace the function of the left ventricle. In the short term both have been achieved but the problem of freeing the patient from an external source of power has not been overcome. The major problem persists of compatibility of the device with the blood so that it will work in the circulation without clotting up or throwing off systemic emboli. At the time of writing these devices are experimental and the way ahead is not clear.

Permanent biological support

Cardiomyoplasty

The latissumus dorsi muscle can be transformed by appropriate electrical stimulation from a fast twitch skeletal muscle to a slow twitch muscle that behaves like the heart. It can be mobilized on a neurovascular pedicle and wrapped round the heart and triggered to contract with it to augment its systolic force. This has now been used in over 100 patients but remains experimental.

Aortic counter-pulsation

An alternative use of the trained latissimus dorsi is to wrap it round the aorta, timed to contract in diastole, acting rather like the intra-aortic balloon already described. This is theoretical rather than of present practical application. Nevertheless, the appeal of an approach that avoids foreign materials and the inherent problems of infection and thromboembolism, and is free from the risks of rejection, is very attractive.

10

DISORDERS OF THE PERIPHERAL ARTERIES, VEINS AND LYMPHATICS

DISORDERS OF THE PERIPHERAL ARTERIES

Oxygenated blood is delivered to the tissues of the body by a branching system of vessels, the arteries. They are subject to primary vascular pathology, they may be involved as part of a systemic disease, or they may become obstructed by embolism as a result of disease elsewhere. Partial or complete failure to deliver blood, which is what the word ischaemia means, is the commonest manifestation of arterial disease.

Impaired circulation to the limbs

Acute occlusion of a major limb artery

In acute vascular occlusion, obstruction may be due to extrinsic compression, to disease of the artery itself or to obstruction within its lumen, most commonly resulting from thrombosis. These may coexist, and one may lead to another. This coexistence is not infrequently the case in acute vascular occlusion associated with limb injuries; fracture of an adjacent bone may obstruct arterial flow due to direct pressure, distortion of the artery or direct puncture of its wall. Intimal damage and subsequent thrombosis may cause ischaemia to persist after the external compression is relieved. Direct sharp injury to the artery may also result from a stab wound, or when the artery is punctured either to sample blood or inadvertently by a drug addict. Acute intraluminal occlusion may be caused by an embolus. The heart is the most likely origin of the embolus; the typical and commonest causes are atrial fibrillation in association with mitral stenosis, mural thrombus following myocardial infarction, vegetations from endocarditis and cardiac myxoma. It is difficult to distinguish clinically between arterial embolism and acute thrombosis that has occurred on an atheromatous plaque in a diseased but previously unoccluded artery. Finally, peripheral ischaemia may be seen as a result of extremely poor cardiac output. Subsequent resuscitation may result in survival with ischaemic damage to the toes and feet.

Clinical presentation

Acute ischaemia results in a pale, painful limb. If flow is not restored, paraesthesia and then anaesthesia and paresis follow. When arterial occlusion is the result of trauma, attention may be focused on the injury and the vascular problem may be overlooked until the ischaemic damage is irreversible. A history of pre-existing heart disease, in particular episodes of palpitation or chest pain, whose significance may not have been appreciated, should be specifically sought in taking the history.

Physical findings

The affected limb becomes white and cool, compared with the normal side. The pulses are absent. There is tenderness in the muscle initially. Sensibility is altered at the extremity first, anaesthesia supervenes and the muscles become paralysed. Physical examination should include a careful check for arrhythmia or cardiac murmurs that would point to a source of embolism.

Investigations

Acute ischaemia is a surgical emergency. Undue delay will result in progressive distal thrombosis and irreversible limb ischaemia, despite adequate disobliteration of the original occlusion. As soon as the diagnosis of acute occlusion due to thrombosis or embolus has been made, the patient should be heparinized. Where there is reasonable doubt whether the occlusion is embolic or thrombotic, an arteriogram is essential, which may be performed on the operating table for expediency.

Treatment

Disobliteration is most likely to be successful if an embolus has lodged at a large bifurcation such as the lower aorta or the common femoral artery. In an acutely ischaemic lower limb, absence of arterial pulsation below the femoral or popliteal artery is an indication for operation. If the popliteal pulse is palpable, indicating that the occlusion is more distal, embolectomy is less likely to have a dramatic effect in relieving the problem. Distal occlusions are managed by heparinization, while awaiting the development of adequate collaterals. Acute occlusion in the upper limb is better tolerated as far as viability of the limb is concerned and embolectomy is less likely to be technically successful, so judgement should be exercised.

Embolectomy of the arm can be performed through the brachial artery, and the leg through the common femoral artery. Both procedures can be done under local anaesthetic, using an embolectomy catheter (Fig. 10.1). A postoperative on-table arteriogram should be performed to ensure that all the embolus has been removed. The embolus should be sent for histological confirmation of the diagnosis. Occasional fragments of myxoma or cardiac vegetations are retrieved and the diagnosis is made in this way.

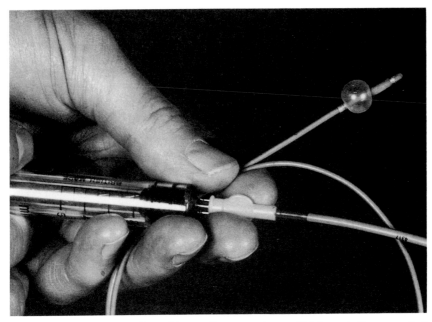

Fig. 10.1 Embolectomy catheter. This is a Fogarty catheter which has a balloon near its tip. It can be passed into an artery, to beyond occluding thrombus, with the balloon deflated. The catheter is then withdrawn with the balloon inflated, extracting the embolus.

If the acute occlusion is due to thrombosis on a pre-existing atheromatous narrowing, the passage of an embolectomy catheter is deprecated because inevitable trauma to the atheromatous plaques may further compromise the collaterals. If thrombosis is suspected at the outset, an arteriogram must be done. Sometimes this will demonstrate that an urgent bypass graft can be undertaken, if the run-off is adequate. More often there will be extensive occlusion of the arteries and small peripheral vessels, in which case thrombolysis should be attempted. The arterial catheter is advanced under radiological control into the thrombus and a low dose of streptokinase (5000 u/hour) is injected. Further arteriography is performed to monitor the progress of clot lysis. The low dose of streptokinase used minimizes systemic effects but monitoring the coagulation system is essential.

Any artery that has been traumatized must be repaired. This may be possible by suturing the defect, although a vein patch is usually necessary. Arterial spasm should never be accepted as the cause of arterial insufficiency unless damage to the artery has been conclusively excluded.

After embolectomy the patient should be treated to prevent recurrent embolization, which may require long-term oral anticoagulation. An underlying cardiac cause should be assessed and managed appropriately.

Chronic occlusion of a major limb artery

Atherosclerosis is a ubiquitous condition in developed countries. Endothelial cells are damaged, usually at sites of turbulent blood flow. Platelets adhere to the damaged surface and liberate platelet-derived growth factor (PDGF). PDGF stimulates synthesis of extracellular components of the artery wall, such as collagen. In addition, endothelial cell damage permits lipid infiltration of the arterial wall, and the resulting fibrolipid plaque narrows the arterial lumen. If the atheromatous plaque ulcerates through the overlying endothelium, platelets become adherent to the arterial wall and the resulting thrombus will further narrow, or completely obliterate, the artery. Endothelial cells contain prostacyclin, which normally inhibits platelet aggregation. Smoking markedly increases the incidence and severity of atherosclerosis by restricting prostacyclin synthesis. Atherosclerosis is also more common in diabetic patients.

Clinical features

The patient initially experiences pain in the lower limb muscles on exercise. This symptom is known as intermittent claudication, derived from the Latin verb *claudicare*, to limp; it is most important in the recognition and assessment of peripheral vascular disease. In the majority of cases the pain is a gripping, cramp-like sensation in the calf muscles and is due to atherosclerotic narrowing of the superficial femoral artery as it runs deep to the adductor muscles in the thigh. In about 30 per cent of patients the principal lesions are in the iliac arteries, and these patients experience buttock claudication. Bilateral iliac artery disease leads to the Leriche syndrome,* which, in men, consists of buttock claudication and impotence. The pain is brought on by walking and may bring the sufferer to a halt, to wait until the pain has eased before he can continue. The pain comes on sooner on walking up an incline or carrying a load, but may be avoided by adopting a leisurely pace.

Some patients do not present until the ischaemia is at a very advanced stage and causing pain at rest. Rest pain may be particularly severe in bed at night.

The patient will usually find that he has to get out of bed and walk around to relieve the pain. Indeed, some patients will have had to sleep sitting in a chair for several months. Finally, in its most advanced form, the skin and underlying tissues undergo ischaemic necrosis, a condition known as gangrene. Gangrene usually begins at a pressure point, such as the heel or the outside of the foot. The pressure impairs the marginal capillary circulation and the skin ulcerates. Healing requires additional blood flow that cannot occur in the ischaemic foot; the ulcer does not heal but instead progressively enlarges.

Physical findings

At rest, the leg may appear healthy, unless there is already gangrene. The superficial veins on the dorsum of the foot may be collapsed or fill slowly. If the

---

* René Leriche (1875–1956) described his syndrome while Professor of Clinical Surgery in Strasbourg. He later became Professor of Medicine, Collège de France, Paris.

ischaemic foot is elevated, it will become pale and, if then lowered over the edge of the bed, red due to a reactive hyperaemia (Buerger's sign*).

Skin necrosis should be carefully looked for on the foot. The most important feature of the examination is palpation of the pulses, as this enables the site of the occlusion to be localized. If neither femoral pulse can be felt the aorta is probably thrombosed immediately beyond the renal arteries, whereas an absent femoral pulse on one side indicates unilateral iliac artery occlusion. If the femoral pulse is present but the popliteal and foot pulses are not palpable, the occlusion is probably in the superficial femoral artery. When feeling the pulses, a thrill, due to turbulence, may be present. Such turbulence denotes irregularity of the vessel wall. The turbulence may be audible with a stethoscope as a bruit, even if it cannot be felt.

Investigations

The full blood count should be measured, as anaemia will aggravate intermittent claudication. Polycythaemia increases blood viscosity, which will also impair lower limb blood flow. Because lower limb ischaemia is usually a feature of diffuse arterial disease, an ECG should be performed. The blood sugar and lipid profile may give information about predisposing factors.

Blood flow is usually normal in the resting limb, unless there is extreme ischaemia with rest pain, but flow does not increase normally with exercise.

Even in the absence of a palpable pulse, arterial flow can be detected with a Doppler probe.† This works on the principle that a sound wave that strikes a target moving towards an observer is reflected with an increase in the frequency shift (Fig. 10.2). The Doppler probe can be placed over an artery, such as the dorsalis pedis artery, and a sphygmomanometer cuff placed proximal to the probe. It is possible to measure the pressure in the cuff at which flow ceases (ankle pressure). If the ankle pressure is less than 40 mmHg, the foot is critically ischaemic. Alternatively, the ankle and brachial pressures can be compared. Normally the ankle pressure should be more than 90 per cent of that measured in the brachial artery.

In patients in whom arterial surgery seems appropriate, the anatomy of the vessels must be displayed by arteriography. The arteriogram must confirm the site of the occlusion and demonstrate that there is an adequate artery beyond the occlusion into which the bypass graft can be anastomosed. This is known as the 'run-off' (Fig. 10.3).

Treatment

Most patients with intermittent claudication will improve spontaneously if they stop smoking and take daily exercise to the limit of their tolerance. This improvement is due to the development and enlargement of collateral arteries,

---

* Leo Buerger (1879–1943) was a surgeon in New York; he described this sign in 1910.

† Christian Johann Doppler (1803–1853), Professor of Experimental Physics, formulated the Doppler principle.

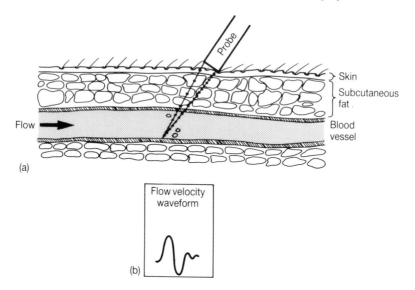

(a)

(b)

Flow velocity
waveform

Fig. 10.2 (a) A sound wave travelling towards an object (e.g. red blood corpuscle) moving towards the source of the sound wave will be reflected with an increased frequency. This shift in frequency can be recognized as an audible recording or can be printed out in graphic form (**b**). Flow in large arteries is initially forward, there is then a transient reverse flow as the aorta dilates and finally a final forward flow due to the elastic recoil of the aorta. (Flow velocity waveform.)

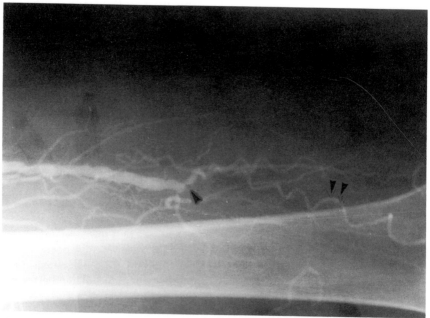

Fig. 10.3 Superficial femoral artery occluded at adductor canal (single arrow). There are numerous well developed collaterals (double arrow).

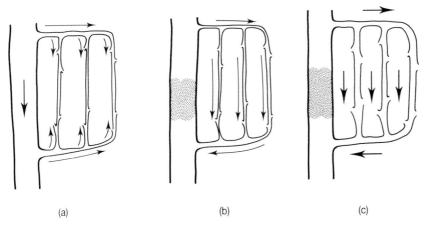

Fig. 10.4 The development of collateral circulation. (**a**) Normal flow down a patent artery. (**b**) The main artery is occluded and the collaterals are poorly developed. However, these channels will enlarge and to some extent compensate for the occlusion in the main vessel (**c**).

which, to some extent, take over the role of the major occluded artery (Fig. 10.4).

Conservative treatment is inappropriate for those who present with intolerable rest pain, gangrene and for the 15 per cent of claudicants who deteriorate despite conservative measures. In these patients, if the blockage is only short or incomplete, it may be possible to dilate the artery under radiological control with a balloon catheter placed across the area of disease (Fig. 10.5). This technique is developing rapidly. More cases are becoming suitable for non-operative reopening of narrowed or occluded vessels as laser and other devices are added to the treatment armamentarium.

When transluminal balloon dilatation is not feasible, it may be possible to perform a bypass graft. If the occlusion is in the aorta or iliac artery, a Dacron prosthetic tube is usually employed. If the occluded artery is below the inguinal ligament, the results, using the patient's own saphenous vein, are substantially superior to a prosthetic tube, which should be used only if the vein is unavailable. Because of the unidirectional valves in the long saphenous vein, the vein has either to be dissected out of the leg and reversed or the valves must be destroyed (*in situ* vein bypass). The development of prosthetic grafts has enabled the ingenious surgeon to route the arterial flow through extra-anatomical pathways: for instance, by the axillofemoral route in the presence of an aortic occlusion, or a femoral-to-femoral cross-over for unilateral iliac occlusion (Fig. 10.6). Long-term graft patency is dependent upon many factors, which include whether the patient has continued to smoke and the state of the distal vessels before the operation. However, the 5-year patency figures for a prosthetic aortobifemoral graft are roughly 80 per cent; for a femoropopliteal saphenous vein bypass graft 65 per cent; and for a femoropopliteal prosthetic bypass graft 40 per cent.

Some patients present with necrosis due to ischaemia. The toes are dusky and become black. If they remain uninfected they desiccate, a condition called dry

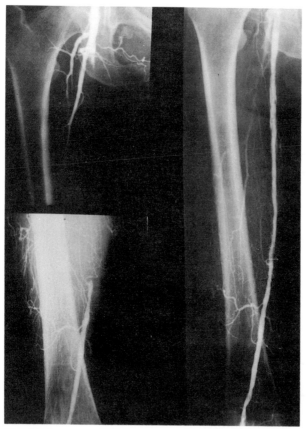

Fig. 10.5 A successful balloon dilatation of the superficial femoral artery, demonstrating the initial long obstruction and subsequent successful recanalization

gangrene, and eventually demarcate and drop off. If infected, the condition is called wet gangrene. This will rapidly threaten the patient's life, and unless the circulation can be restored the limb must be amputated. Even if the limb is not infected, it is usually extremely painful and prevents sleep. Sleep deprivation, particularly in the elderly, causes severe confusion; an amputation has to be reluctantly recommended. Gangrene often commences at an area of pressure on the foot such as on the heel or on the sides of the forefoot. Great care must be taken to prevent the occurrence of infection in any patient with an ischaemic foot.

In patients with lower limb ischaemia, the gangrene may be confined to the foot or a part of the foot. The arterial occlusion that caused the gangrene will be in a major proximal artery, resulting in severe ischaemia of the whole limb. If a local amputation of the gangrenous toe or forefoot is performed, the amputation will not heal and the skin closure over the stump will break down. In order to achieve healing, the amputation for ischaemic gangrene must be performed fairly high on the leg. If possible, the knee joint should be spared, but about 25 per cent of

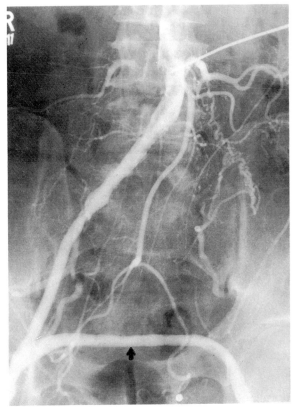

Fig. 10.6 An occluded left iliac artery and femoro-femoral cross-over graft (arrow).

amputations are mid-thigh. Amputations are undertaken in patients with widespread arterial disease and only 50 per cent of these are still alive 2 years after an amputation. Wherever possible, the amputee is fitted with an artificial limb and, with the aid of physiotherapy, will learn to walk well. Unfortunately, after they are discharged, many patients leave their new artificial leg in the corner of the house and make do with a wheelchair existence. The home environment can be modified to facilitate the amputee. The occupational therapist will be able to recommend domestic aids, such as handrails for the bath and toilet and ramps for the wheelchair.

Impaired circulation to the brain

The word 'stroke' comes from old English and has been used to describe the sudden onset of illness since the seventeenth century with, from earlier times, the implication of an act of God. By usage it includes focal or lateralized neurological deficit, of potentially serious nature, of abrupt onset, with or without alteration of consciousness. The word conveys the sudden, unheralded nature of the condition without pretending to know the exact aetiology and serves as well as the no more precise term, cerebrovascular accident, or its abbreviation CVA. The underlying cause may be thrombosis on pre-existing vascular disease, embolism of platelet aggregates from atheromatous plaques in the internal carotid territory or intracerebral haemorrhage.

Stroke is a major problem among the elderly. The incidence in the developed nations for those over 70 years of age is 20 patients/1000 population per year. In a third of these patients the stroke is confined to the internal carotid territory. Among those suffering a stroke, one-third will die, one-third will be seriously disabled and incapable of a future independent existence, while the remaining third will make a satisfactory recovery.

With established stroke there is no place for surgical intervention to restore blood supply. The vascular surgeon is more interested in those with episodic ischaemia, in whom the risk of a subsequent stroke may be reduced.

Clinical features

Some patients experience sudden weakness of a limb, difficulty in speech or blindness (amaurosis fugax), but make a complete recovery within a day. These short-lived episodes from which there is complete recovery are termed transient ischaemic attacks (TIAs) and are probably due to platelet emboli that temporarily occlude a cerebral or retinal artery. The patient with amaurosis fugax characteristically describes the symptom as a curtain coming across the field of vision.

Physical findings

By definition a stroke is a neurological event that has residual signs beyond 24 hours. The characteristic patterns are those of right and left hemiplegia. A motor deficit affecting the upper and lower limbs and the face on the side opposite to the cerebral lesion is typical. A homonymous hemianopia is common. Loss of speech is usual with a right-sided stroke (left-sided cerebral lesion). The findings after a stroke are dependent on the extent of neurological damage. The focus of treatment is on rehabilitation, as the underlying cause will not influence the outcome from that event.

On the other hand, if a patient presents more than 24 hours after a TIA, there should be no evidence of residual neurological deficit. Occasionally, the patient may experience amaurosis fugax during the interview, in which case it may be possible, with the ophthalmoscope, to see small, clear platelet emboli travelling along the retinal arteries.

Some patients will be found to have a carotid bruit. It is important to establish that the bruit does arise from the carotid artery and is not conducted upwards from a diseased aortic valve. Treatable causes of recurrent embolism such as mitral stenosis or cardiac myxoma should be considered, and one should be particularly alert to this possibility in a relatively young patient.

Investigations

If a stroke is to be prevented after a TIA, it is important to establish first if the patient has significant disease of the carotid arteries. Initial investigations should be non-invasive. It is possible to visualize the carotid arterial plaque with an ultrasound probe and to assess the size of any stenosis. In addition, carotid blood velocity can be measured by a Doppler probe. The greater the stenosis, the higher the arterial velocity. These two techniques can be combined in the Duplex scanner, which images the carotid artery, measures the cross-sectional area of the artery and the volume flow at any point along the carotid artery in the neck.

If the non-invasive techniques suggest that there is a carotid arterial disease, particularly where there is a stenosis, reducing the cross-sectional area of the artery by more than 75 per cent, the patient should have an arteriogram.

The arteriogram is preferably performed by digital vascular imaging (DVI). In DVI the contrast is injected intravenously rather than intra-arterially. Despite dilution, sufficient contrast can be detected in the arterial tree to enable high quality images of the carotid to be obtained, by computer. If DVI is inadequate or unavailable, a carotid arteriogram or a four-vessel arch aortogram will be required.

Treatment

If a patient presents after an established stroke, surgical intervention is inappropriate. The aim of the surgical team is to be able to identify those patients who are at risk of experiencing a major stroke, due to an operatively correctable lesion. The two principal syndromes that have been implicated as predisposing to the development of a stroke are transient ischaemic attacks (TIAs) or the asymptomatic carotid bruit.

Transient ischaemic attacks are usually adequately controlled by antiplatelet agents, principally aspirin. Carotid endarterectomy is restricted to those patients who continue to have TIAs despite aspirin, or in whom aspirin is contraindicated (e.g. active duodenal ulcer). In an endarterectomy, the artery is opened lengthways across the diseased segment and the abnormal intima and luminal portion of the media are separated and removed. In an attempt to protect the brain while the carotid artery is clamped, most surgeons insert a shunt to maintain internal carotid flow while they perform the endarterectomy.

Even greater controversy surrounds the indications for carotid endarterectomy in patients who have an asymptomatic carotid bruit. Some American surgeons have recommended a prophylactic carotid endarterectomy to patients prior to other major surgery or operations requiring cardiopulmonary bypass such as coronary artery surgery. In reality the risk of intraoperative stroke during cardiopulmonary bypass is no greater in those with asymptomatic bruits than in those without (1–2 per cent) and the risk is at least as great from the surgery of carotid endarterectomy itself. The relationship between asymptomatic carotid bruit, with or without operation, and the occurrence of subsequent stroke is so unclear that most neurologists are very conservative in its management.

There are some patients with chronic cerebral ischaemia who have major disease of their internal carotid arteries that is too extensive for an endarterectomy. An operation in which the superficial temporal artery is mobilized, passed through a craniotomy and anastomosed to the middle cerebral artery (external carotid–internal carotid bypass, or EC–IC) has been pioneered but has very limited applications and questionable benefit.

Impaired circulation to the bowel

The abdominal viscera are supplied by three arteries, the coeliac artery and the superior and inferior mesenteric arteries. Occlusion may be acute, due to thrombosis or embolus, or chronic with gradual narrowing of the arterial lumen. Intestinal ischaemia may occur also following portal vein thrombosis.

Clinical presentation and findings

Patients with acute intestinal ischaemia experience severe abdominal pain of quite sudden onset, often with diarrhoea that may contain blood. There may be a discernible source for an embolus, such as atrial fibrillation or a recent myocardial infarct. When the patient is examined initially, the symptoms appear to be out of proportion to the findings. This is a characteristic feature and the severity of the condition may be underestimated. However, if the diagnosis is not appreciated and appropriate treatment instigated, the ischaemic bowel will perforate, causing generalized peritonitis and the physical findings will change dramatically.

Chronic intestinal ischaemia is a rare condition. These patients experience very severe abdominal pain after meals and therefore avoid food and lose weight. They have the appearance of 'emaciated misery'. They often have evidence of other peripheral arterial disease and there may be an abdominal arterial bruit.

Management

Occasionally, the diagnosis of acute mesenteric ischaemia is suspected sufficiently early that there is time to undertake an arteriogram and even lyse the occlusion with intra-arterial streptokinase. Unfortunately, the clinical presentation is vague and more often than not the diagnosis is not appreciated until there is obvious peritonitis. Faced with massive intestinal infarction, there is little the surgeon can do except remove the necrotic bowel, exteriorize the viable ends as abdominal wall fistulae so that they can be observed, and commence intravenous feeding. The viable bowel can be reanastomosed at 10–14 days, and patients can survive surprisingly well despite the loss of almost their entire small intestine.

Patients in whom the diagnosis of chronic intestinal ischaemia is being considered should be carefully screened as gastric, pancreatic and colonic lesions are more commonly the cause of severe abdominal pain than chronic intestinal ischaemia. The diagnosis is confirmed by mesenteric arteriography, and at least two of the three major intestinal arteries have to be severely diseased before this diagnosis can be seriously considered.

Ischaemic colitis

The right and transverse colon receive arterial supply from the superior mesenteric artery while the left colon is supplied by the inferior mesenteric artery. The anastomoses between the two at the splenic flexure is characteristically poor. If the blood supply from either artery is reduced, the splenic flexure is typically the most vulnerable site.

Clinical presentation and findings

The patient characteristically presents with pain in the left side of the abdomen, fever and diarrhoea, which may contain blood. Usually, the symptoms resolve in a few days but occasionally the ischaemia segment narrows as an ischaemic stricture or it may even perforate.

Management

On sigmoidoscopy or colonoscopy, the rectum is normal (unlike ulcerative colitis) but there are oedematous blebs due to submucosal oedema, surface ulceration or even rigid strictures in the region of the splenic flexure. A barium study may show 'thumbprinting' (Fig. 10.7) from the early stages, which is due to

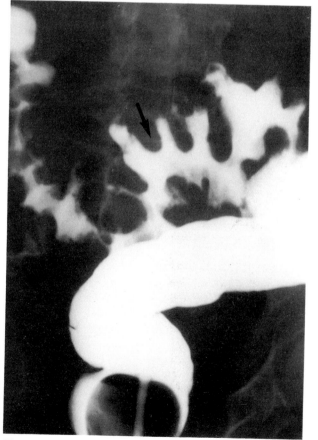

Fig. 10.7 Barium enema examination showing thumbprinting due to ischaemic colitis (arrow).

submucosal oedema. This usually resolves but occasionally may progress to an ischaemic fibrotic stricture (Fig. 10.8).

Usually, the symptoms resolve without treatment, but an operation may be necessary if a stricture causes intestinal obstruction or if the ischaemic episode progresses to gangrene.

Impaired blood supply to the kidneys

Renal artery stenosis is an interesting but very rare cause of serious hypertension. Stenoses in the renal artery may be due to atheroma but in a minority of patients, particularly young women, there is fibromuscular dysplasia (Fig. 10.9). The renal artery develops luminal ridges due to medial thickening by fibromuscular tissue. The intervening areas are thin and contain abundant smooth muscle cells. The aetiology remains obscure but the conditions may involve other vessels, particularly the internal carotid artery, the coronary artery and the coeliac artery.

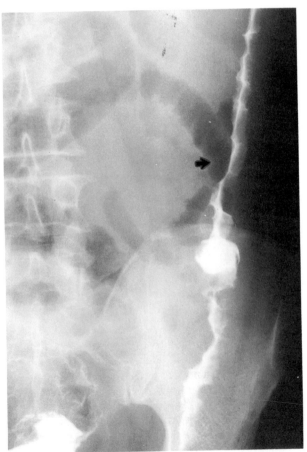

Fig. 10.8 Barium enema showing a long ischaemic stricture of descending colon (arrowed).

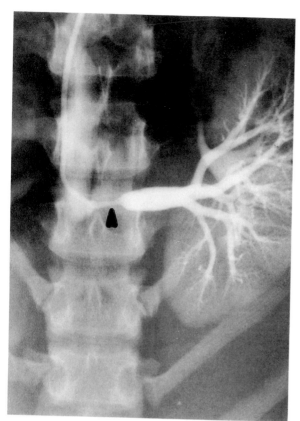

Fig. 10.9 Arteriogram demonstrating a tight renal artery stenosis (arrow).

The diagnosis can be checked by measuring the renal vein renin levels. Renal stenosis is preferably treated by transluminal balloon dilatation, but where this is not possible an endarterectomy of the diseased segment is undertaken. If the renal arterial disease is unilateral, nephrectomy on the affected side may be the most appropriate surgical treatment.

Aneurysms

An aneurysm is a dilatation of an artery. A true aneurysm is due to disease of the arterial wall and is lined by vascular endothelium. A false aneurysm may occur if the artery is damaged, blood leaks out and a haematoma is formed contained by surrounding tissues. There may be a central cavity but of course no endothelial lining. Aortic dissection is a better term than the alternative, 'dissecting aneurysm'. In this condition there is a dilated portion due to blood tracking outside the true lumen, into a false lumen, contained by the dissected layers of the media. The definition of aneurysm is thus confusing, but an all-embracing definition is 'a sac in communication with an artery'.

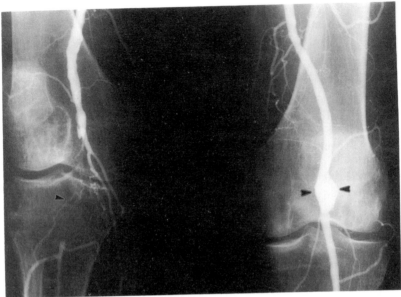

Fig. 10.10 Arteriorgram showing a popliteal aneurysm (double arrow). The popliteal artery on the contralateral side has previously thrombosed (single arrow).

The dilated aneurysmal wall may weaken and then rupture. This is particularly likely to occur with an abdominal aortic aneurysm. The greater part of the lumen of the aneurysm contains clot, which may break away to cause a distal embolus, or the lumen may thrombose. Acute thrombosis of an aneurysm may occur with distal ischaemia and is particularly frequent with popliteal aneurysms (Fig. 10.10).

Clinical presentation and findings

Major abdominal aneurysms may present with abdominal pain that frequently goes through to the back. They may be asymptomatic and noticed incidentally by the patient or the doctor as a pulsatile intra-abdominal mass. These aneurysms may only come to light when the patient collapses with hypotension due to acute blood loss into the abdomen. Ruptured abdominal aortic aneurysm is one of the more common causes of sudden death.

Peripheral arterial aneurysms may present as a pulsatile swelling, or as a cause of acute ischaemia when they thrombose. Occasionally, they may cause pressure symptoms on the surrounding nerves or veins.

Investigations

An aneurysm can easily be measured by ultrasound or computed tomography (CT). The larger the aneurysm, the greater is the risk of complications. Any abdominal aneurysm whose horizontal diameter exceeds 5 cm should be resected if the patient's cardiac state is satisfactory. The risk of an aneurysm rupturing increases markedly if it exceeds 6 cm.

Management

An abdominal aortic aneurysm is resected and a Dacron prosthesis inserted. The operation for an elective aneurysm is relatively safe with an operative mortality in the range 5–8 per cent. However, about 10 per cent of abdominal aneurysms are associated with extensive retroperitoneal fibrosis. These inflammatory aneurysms are extremely hazardous to resect and many surgeons favour treating them with steroids. If the aneurysm has ruptured prior to presentation, the mortality is about 50 per cent for those who reach hospital.

Any peripheral aneurysm liable to thrombose is ligated immediately above and below, and a vein bypass inserted to redirect the flow round the occluded aneurysm. A false aneurysm must be treated by removing the surrounding clot and repairing the arterial defect, either by suture or a vein patch.

Small vessel disease

Raynaud's phenomenon

Patients with Raynaud's phenomenon* develop painful extremities, usually the fingers, on exposure to cold. The fingers become blue or white in the cold and then bright red and painful as they are warmed. The condition may be primary (Raynaud's disease), for which there is no apparent cause except for an accentuated digital artery spasm in response to the cold. In primary Raynaud's, necrosis of the end of the digits does not occur. Raynaud's phenomenon may be secondary to a collagen disease, particularly scleroderma. It may be secondary to cryoglobulinaemia or the use of vibrating tools such as a drill or chain saw.

It is important to exclude other causes of cold cyanotic hands; for instance, pressure on the subclavian artery from a cervical rib or occlusion of the major artery by atheroma.

This symptom is initially managed conservatively. Affected patients should keep their hands and feet warm. Specific vasodilators such as nifedipine are helpful. Those with severe symptoms from primary Raynaud's phenomenon can expect excellent short-term improvement from a sympathectomy, but the symptoms tend to recur after a few months, although they are usually less incapacitating.

Disseminated intravascular coagulation (DIC)

This process is triggered by a wide variety of stimuli, including septicaemia and advanced malignancy. There is a widespread deposition in the microcirculation of altered fibrinogen and platelets, with consumption of coagulation factors and platelets. The commonest presentation is bruising and oozing from venepunc-

---

* A. G. Maurice Raynaud (1834–1881), physician in Paris. He described the phenomenon in 1862.

ture sites. Occlusion of the microcirculation may be the predominant feature, in which case the patient presents with skin necrosis, despite patent major vessels; 'dead digits – patent pulses'. DIC is treated by identification and correction of the disease process. The patient may have to be supported with platelets and clotting factors until the underlying disease is treated. The role of anticoagulant treatment is controversial.

Cold injury

The injury produced by exposure to cold depends upon the severity of the hypothermia, its duration and the environmental conditions. The injury includes tissue freezing (frostbite) and non-freezing cold injuries (trench foot and chilblain). If the ambient skin temperature falls below 4°C, ice forms with cellular dehydration and platelet aggregation. There is tissue necrosis. Such patients, when rescued, must have all wet and constricting clothing removed and the frozen part rewarmed rapidly. Damaged tissues are protected to prevent infection and necrotic tissue is allowed to demarcate prior to amputation.

Trench foot occurs when a limb is subjected to combined cold and wet although the ambient temperature remains above freezing. There is often profound vasospasm of the skin vessels, resulting in superficial gangrene, but no deep tissue destruction. The injured limb should be rewarmed; if profound vasospasm persists, sympathectomy may be helpful.

Diabetes and foot ulceration

Patients with diabetes are more vulnerable to the development of atherosclerosis which, as in the non-diabetic, may progress to ischaemic foot ulceration. In addition, a small proportion develop a characteristic diabetic ulcer on the sole of the foot, despite an apparently normal blood supply.

It has been demonstrated that these necrotic ulcers occur as a consequence of underlying diabetic neuropathy. The neuropathy results in paresis of the flexor muscles and the intrinsic muscles of the foot, and a disproportionately large part of the body weight is transmitted through the metatarsal heads rather than the hallux. Furthermore, the sensory loss prevents the patient appreciating that there is a developing foot ulcer.

A diabetic neuropathic foot ulcer is often associated with deep-seated sepsis, and extensive resection of the infected tissue is necessary before the ulcer will heal.

Arteriovenous malformation (AVM)

An arteriovenous communication or fistula may occur between an artery and a vein due to congenital malformation or as a result of trauma. Traumatic communications develop through a haematoma if the two vessels have been injured adjacent to each other. In addition, arteriovenous fistulae are created deliberately, for certain therapeutic procedures such as renal dialysis.

The arterial flow causes dilatation and tortuosity of the veins. If the fistula is large and of acute onset, it may cause heart failure. Congenital AVM may cause overgrowth in a developing limb, and usually has multiple intercommunications.

A pulsatile swelling may be present if the lesion is superficial and there is a continuous bruit. Pressure on the artery proximal to the fistula causes the swelling to diminish in size, the bruit to cease and the pulse pressure to return to normal.

The congenital fistulae are difficult to eradicate because of multiple communications and, unless unsightly, are best left alone. However, if the feeding artery is suitable, it may be possible to offer temporary control by thrombosing the principal fistulous communication under radiological control.

The acquired fistulae tend to enlarge and, as there is usually only a single communication between the artery and vein, it is normally possible to isolate the fistula and repair it operatively.

DISEASES OF VEINS

The systemic venous system returns blood to the right heart. A combination of the pumping action of muscles on the deep veins and the presence of unidirectional valves in most veins ensures that flow is towards the heart, in spite of the effect of gravity (Fig. 10.11).

Venous disorders affecting the lower limb are extremely common and of great importance; knowledge of the basic anatomy of the venous system is a prerequisite to understanding the pathology and clinical features of venous disease. The veins are divided into a deep and a superficial system (Fig. 10.11). The superficial veins drain into two constant vessels, the long and short saphenous veins; the long saphenous vein enters the femoral vein at the saphenofemoral junction and the short saphenous vein enters the popliteal vein in the popliteal fossa. In addition, their major tributaries communicate with the deep system by perforating veins that penetrate the deep fascia. Valves prevent reflux of blood into the superficial veins when the calf muscles contract.

Venous thrombosis

Superficial thrombophlebitis

Thrombosis of superficial veins with surrounding inflammation occurs quite commonly. This may be initiated by local trauma or inflammation. The area is tender, red and oedematous but the process is self-limiting and usually innocent. It does not spread to the deep system, treatment is for symptomatic relief and anticoagulation is not indicated.

Occasionally, a succession of superficial veins are involved at different sites, a condition called thrombophlebitis migrans. This may be the harbinger of occult abdominal malignant disease, particularly carcinoma of the pancreas.

Deep venous thrombosis (DVT)

Thrombosis of the deep veins of the lower limb and the pelvis is a serious and potentially lethal condition. Predisposing factors are immobility, heart failure,

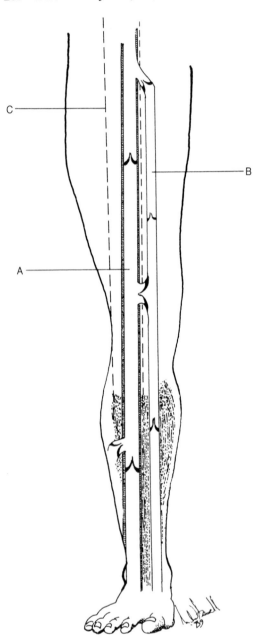

Fig. 10.11 The venous drainage of the legs depends on two venous networks: the deep (A) and superficial (B) systems. They are separated by the deep fascia (C). They communicate principally at the saphenofemoral junction and saphenopopliteal junction. In addition, there are numerous perforating veins that run between the long or short saphenous vein, perforate the deep fascia and join the deep venous system. A series of valves ensures that the venous blood runs from the superficial to the deep system. Contraction of the muscles that surround the deep veins propels blood back towards the heart.

cigarette smoking, oral contraceptives, age, obesity, trauma and surgery. Any elderly patient confined to bed is at risk but it can affect young, fit men with no more immobility than that imposed by a trans-Atlantic flight. Dissection of the deep veins of the calf has shown the presence of thrombi in about 60 per cent of surgical patients who have come to necropsy. Detection by scanning the legs after administration of radioactive-labelled fibrinogen shows accumulation (i.e. evidence of deep vein thrombosis) in over 20 per cent of all surgical patients. It therefore represents a very common condition, particularly when there has been local surgery, trauma and immobility such as in those undergoing pelvic or hip operations. Thrombosis is promoted by three factors first proposed by Virchow* in 1856:

1. Change in the vessel wall
2. Change in the blood flow
3. Change in the constituents of the blood

The importance of the triad endures although more is now known about the interplay of local and systemic effects on the vascular endothelium, the abnormalities of the venous circulation and the changes in clotting factors and platelet function that accompany trauma, illness and surgery. Local trauma on the calf or pelvic veins may accompany injury or surgery is this area but local pressure on the calf veins may occur during any operation or sojourn in bed. Venous stasis from absence of a muscle pump action is one factor but elevation in venous pressure due to heart failure may also be important. Hormonal factors are also important, as indicated from the increased incidence in women, particularly those taking oestrogen as a contraceptive.

Clinical diagnosis

The clinical recognition of venous thrombosis is notoriously difficult. The patient may present with a massively swollen blue leg (phlegmasia cerulea dolens) due to an iliac vein thrombosis. Less often, a major venous thrombosis may cause spasm in the adjacent artery, in which case the leg is white (phlegmasia alba dolens). Thrombosis of a deep calf vein may cause a little swelling of the calf with tenderness with pain on dorsiflexion of the ankle (Homans' sign†) but this sign, although routinely taught, has been discredited. DVT may be associated with pyrexia but there are so many other causes of pyrexia in a bedridden or postoperative patient that fever is non-specific and diagnostically unhelpful. In many instances of subsequently proven venous thrombosis the patient has been entirely symptom free. Conversely, patients who are thought clinically to have a DVT often have normal venograms.

Investigation of venous thrombosis

Ultrasound is of value in detecting venous thrombosis that extends into the

---

* Rudolph Ludwig Karl Virchow (1821–1902), pathologist, Berlin.
† John Homans (1877–1954), Professor of Surgery, Harvard University, Boston. He described calf pain on dorsiflexion as a sign of deep vein thrombosis.

inferior vena cava. Thrombosis of the iliac veins or lower limb veins can be demonstrated by venography but this is a more troublesome investigation and its interpretation is not always straightforward. Venous thrombosis can also be detected if there is an alteration in the Doppler flow pattern of blood through the femoral vein. During the active process of thrombosis, fibrinogen is taken up into the clot and if the fibrinogen has previously been labelled with a radioactive marker (^{131}I), sites of active thrombosis can be detected. This is a research tool and of little value in clinical practice. Unexpected venous thrombosis, particularly in patients with a family history of venous thrombosis, warrants measurement of antithrombin III, protein C and protein S levels because congenital deficiencies of these proteins render a patient susceptible to venous thrombosis.

The subsequent course depends on the site of venous thrombosis. If an iliac vein has become occluded, subsequent lysis of the thrombus, through the action of plasmin, may be incomplete; this leaves the patient with permanent venous obstruction, resulting in a cyanosed tense leg, which hurts on exercise (venous claudication). In time, some develop lower limb ulceration. Thrombi in the more distal veins are usually lysed completely. Unfortunately, in the process the venous valves may be destroyed. The perforating veins may also be affected. The normal flow of blood from superficial to deep systems is reversed and superficial veins and their tributaries are subjected to high pressures. Varicosities of the superficial veins develop. The capillaries leak fibrinogen, which polymerizes to form insoluble fibrin clot in the interstitium and acts as a barrier to the diffusion of oxygen and other nutrients to the dermal cells. The tissues become pigmented and thickened and very susceptible to minor injury and ulceration.

Venous ulceration is most severe above the medial malleolus, where several prominent perforators are located. Long-standing ulceration may be complicated by haemorrhage that may be fatal. Elevation of the limb or local pressure is all that is required to save life from venous bleeding but a drive to hospital sitting up in a car may result in exsanguination.

A long-standing venous ulcer may become malignant (Marjolin's ulcer*).

Pulmonary embolism

The most feared complication of a deep venous thrombosis is a pulmonary embolus. Usually, the thrombus remains adherent to the wall of the vein and subsequently lyses. In some cases, thrombus breaks free into the venous circulation and may travel to the pulmonary circulation where it may become impacted in a major pulmonary arterial branch or, if the embolus is small, it will impact in a peripheral branch. Thrombi in the femoral, iliac or other major veins are more dangerous than the small distal thrombi. A peripherally lodged pulmonary embolus presents as acute pleuritic chest pain, breathlessness and minor haemoptysis. The major pulmonary embolus causes acute circulatory collapse and may be responsible for sudden unexpected death. Pulmonary embolism is discussed in Chapter 3.

* René Marjolin (1812–1895), surgeon, Paris.

Prevention of deep venous thrombosis

It is possible to reduce the risk of DVT and death from pulmonary embolism if preventive measures are taken in those identified as being at greatest risk. Low dose heparin (5000 units subcutaneously 12-hourly) given with premedication and continued until the patient is mobilized reduces the incidence of DVT and, probably, the risk of death from pulmonary embolism. Venous stasis can be reduced if patients wear compression stockings while on the operating table and postoperatively until they are mobile.

DVT is treated by oral anticoagulation for 3 months to prevent extension of the thrombus and to minimize the incidence of long-term venous hypertension and ulceration. Fibrinolytic drugs may, if introduced early, turn out to be a more effective treatment than anticoagulation.

Established chronic venous insufficiency is helped by the use of a graduated elastic compression stocking. The maximum pressure is exerted at the ankle and this promotes venous return towards the heart on exercise. Patients (especially those with ulceration) should sleep with the foot of the bed raised 20–25 cm. Whenever possible, they should rest with their legs elevated. Chronic ulcers heal with bedrest and elevation but break down again with monotonous regularity. They may be helped by ligation of incompetent perforating veins in the vicinity of the ulcer (Cockett's operation*), combined if necessary with skin grafting of the ulcerated area.

Attempts to bypass venous obstruction and to repair damaged valves have not been successful.

If a patient is experiencing repeated pulmonary emboli, despite being adequately anticoagulated or where there is a contraindication to anticoagulation, an umbrella filter can be passed into the inferior vena cava via the internal jugular vein. Screening facilities are necessary to ensure that the filter is released distal to the renal veins. The filter is wedged in the distal inferior vena cava with the intention of preventing further embolus reaching the lungs.

Varicose veins

There are no valves in the iliac veins or the inferior vena cava so, in the upright position, a considerable hydrostatic force, about 40–50 mmHg, is exerted on the valve at the saphenofemoral junction. If the valve fails, pressure is exerted on the valve below, which in turn may fail, eventually resulting in incompetence throughout the length of the long saphenous vein. The resulting head of pressure, reaching in excess of 100 mmHg, causes the poorly supported superficial veins to become tortuous and dilated. Weakness of the valve at the saphenofemoral junction may be an inherited tendency. Varicose veins may also be secondary to previous DVT that has damaged the valves of the perforating veins, such that, on exercise, blood flows from the deep system to the superficial, causing localized varicosities.

Varicose veins are prominent and unsightly, but by themselves are rarely

* Frank Bernard ('Ace') Cockett (contemporary), retired consultant surgeon, St Thomas's Hospital.

symptomatic. Pigmentation, eczema and ulceration are features of pre-existing damage to the deep veins and not a consequence of varicose veins, except in a few cases (less than 5 per cent).

Where there are incompetent valves at the junction of the deep and superficial veins the varicosity may be in the form of a large 'blow out'. At the sapheno-femoral junction this is called a saphenovarix, which may be confused with a hernia.

Physical examination

To determine whether the saphenofemoral vein is competent the patient lies down and the leg is elevated to empty the veins. A tourniquet is then applied around the upper thigh and the patient is asked to stand up. If the sapheno-femoral valve is incompetent, when the tourniquet is removed, blood can be seen to run down filling the varicosities. If the varicosities are secondary to perforating vein incompetence, they will gradually fill despite the tourniquet remaining in place. A cough by the patient will generate a pressure wave detected as a thrill by the examiner's fingers if the saphenofemoral junction is incompetent.

Treatment

Treatment may be desired for cosmetic reasons because, in general, varicosities are harmless. They are, however, very unsightly and some sufferers have considerable discomfort.

Treatment depends upon the type of varicosity. If the saphenofemoral junc-tion can be demonstrated to be competent the varicosities can be diagnosed as secondary to incompetence of the perforators. They can then be treated by injection sclerotherapy. In this procedure the perforating vein is accurately localized by identifying the defect in the deep fascia with the finger tip and demonstrating that pressure upon it controls the varicosity and stops it refilling as the leg is put down. A small amount of sclerosant is injected into it and the vein controlled with a localized pad under a pressure bandage to encourage throm-bosis of the perforating vein. To prevent the thrombus extending into the deep veins the patient is encouraged to take regular exercise. Early recanalization is prevented by bandaging the leg.

If there is saphenofemoral incompetence, injection sclerotherapy will not succeed. The saphenous vein and other tributaries should be ligated and divided at the junction with the femoral vein (Trendelenburg ligation*). Previously the whole long saphenous vein was stripped at the same time but this rather barbaric procedure is probably unnecessary and certainly prevents the vein from being used later as a bypass graft for coronary or femoropopliteal bypass surgery.

---

* Friedrich Trendelenburg (1844–1924), Professor of Surgery at Bonn and, later, Leipzig.

Venous gangrene

This is due to extensive thrombosis of peripheral veins. The arterial pulses are normal. It usually affects the toes and forefoot.

Anticoagulation is used to prevent extension of the process. When the gangrenous area has demarcated it will usually be fairly superficial and can be removed. The deeper layers are pink and healthy and suitable for skin grafting.

Leg ulcers

Leg ulcers are extremely common and affect about 5 per cent of people over 70 years of age. There are many causes although we are most familiar with venous ulcers (Table 10.1). However, many patients with venous ulcers also have impaired arterial circulation which delays healing.

Table 10.1 Causes of leg ulcers

Traumatic
Including accidents and local injections

Vascular
Deep venous insufficiency
Arterial due to chronic arterial insufficiency or arteritis (e.g. rheumatoid and irradiation)
Lymphatic

Metabolic
Diabetes mellitus
Necrobiosis lipoidica diabeticorum

Haematological
Polycythaemia
Leukaemia
Sickle cell anaemia
Thalassaemia
Spherocytosis

Dermatological
Pyoderma gangraenosum
Chilblains

Infections
Tuberculosis (lupus vulgaris and erythema induratum)
Bacterial
Syphilis (gumma)
Fungal

Malignant
Basal cell carcinoma
Squamous
Melanoma

Miscellaneous
Frostbite
Self-inflicted
Insect bites

Klippel–Trenaunay syndrome*

This rare syndrome is a pure venous congenital malformation in association with bone and soft tissue hypertrophy. The arteries and capillaries are normal. The condition affects predominantly the lower limbs and perineum but the face and mucosal surfaces may also be involved. It is present from birth but becomes manifest in the second decade. Both the deep and superficial venous systems may be involved. The veins dilate enormously and become varicose. In order to try to improve the cosmetic appearance, where possible, the soft tissues and abnormal veins may be excised.

THE LYMPH NODE AND LYMPHATICS

The lymphatic system drains the extravascular compartment and returns the fluid and proteins to the venous system. The smallest lymphatic vessels in the tissues are closed, permeable tubes similar to blood capillaries. Like veins, the lymphatic vessels have valves that allow the flow of lymph to be directed centrally. The major vessels of the lymphatic system are the cisterna chyli, which is important in the absorption and transport of dietary fats, and its continuation, the thoracic duct, which terminates in the left brachiocephalic vein at the junction of the internal jugular and the subclavian veins. In every 24 hours the thoracic duct returns to the circulation a volume of fluid equal to the total plasma volume and containing over 50 per cent of the total circulating plasma protein.

Acute lymphangitis

Superficial infection may travel from an extremity of a limb along the superficial lymphatics. In these patients it presents as one or more tender red streaks in the skin, corresponding to the inflamed lymphatics. The draining lymph node is also frequently tender and enlarged.

The limb should be rested and the appropriate antibiotic prescribed.

Lymphoedema

This condition is due to interstitial oedema because of failure of the lymphatic system. Lymphoedema may be primarily due to congenital abnormality of the lymphatic vessels, which may be absent (aplasia), diminished (hypoplasia) or dilated and tortuous (hyperplasia). In each case, there may, in addition, be fibrosis of the lymph nodes. Primary lymphoedema is predominantly seen in women and is usually initially recognized in their teens. It may be familial (Milroy's disease†). If the diagnosis is made before 35 years of age, it is called lymphoedema praecox, and if over 35 years, as lymphoedema tarda.

Alternatively, the lymphatic system may be damaged by infection, particularly with filariasis (*Wuchereria bancrofti*). The lymph nodes may be

* Maurice Klippel (1858–1942), neurologist, Salpêtrière, Paris. Paul Trenaunay (b.1875), physician, Paris.
† Terence John Milroy (1855–1942), Professor of Medicine, Omaha, Nebraska.

obstructed by tumour, which may be either a primary lymph node malignancy (lymphoma) or secondary spread. Finally, primary lymphoedema may follow radiotherapy; for instance, following treatment for breast cancer or if the nodes have been excised in the operation known as block dissection. A combination of node excision and radiotherapy is a particularly potent cause of lymphoedema. Secondary lymphoedema implies normal lymphatics unable to cope with an excess accumulation of fluid as in cardiac failure, nephrotic syndrome or venous hypertension.

The swelling may develop rapidly or, in the case of primary lymphoedema, rather gradually. The limb is uncomfortable but there is no acutely painful episode. The oedema initially pits readily, but as the tissues become more fibrotic, pitting becomes harder to elicit. The skin of the lymphoedematous leg may become hyperkeratotic.

The diagnosis is generally made by exclusion of other causes of generalized oedema (cardiac and renal) and local causes due to venous obstruction. The diagnosis can be confirmed by lymphangiography.

The initial treatment of lymphoedema is by the use of a compression stocking or armlet. This may be combined with a pneumatic compression boot, for use when the patient is at rest. In a patient with localized lymphatic obstruction it may be possible to perform a lymphovenous anastomosis using the operating microscope. Where this is not possible in patients with normal deep lymphatics but an inadequate superficial system, it may be feasible to excise the oedematous subcutaneous tissue and apply split skin grafts to the exposed deep tissues.

Lymphangioma

Capillary lymphangioma consists of small subcutaneous vesicles, due to localized clusters of lymph sacs. These sacs do not communicate with the lymphatic system. Cavernous lymphangioma (or cystic hygroma) is a similar but considerably larger subcutaneous lymphatic cyst. The defect is congenital and is usually recognized at birth, although it may not become apparent until later. It is usually sited near the root of the neck or axilla.

Brilliant transillumination is a characteristic finding in lymphangioma. The capillary lymphangioma should be excised as extensively as is possible compatible with primary skin closure. Any cysts not excised may resolve spontaneously. The cavernous variety may be difficult to excise because these lymphatic cysts are closely adherent to important nervous and vascular structures. They are probably preferably treated by drainage, and subsequent fibrosis often prevents reaccumulation

Lymph fistula

This is usually seen following operations that have inadvertently divided a major lymphatic pathway. It is most commonly seen after a groin exploration. The clear lymph drains quite profusely initially, but usually ceases spontaneously after a few days and re-exploration is rarely necessary.

The thoracic duct may also be a source of a lymphatic leak, in which case it is the fat-containing chyle that accumulates in the chest, a condition known as chylothorax. This may happen spontaneously in intrathoracic lymphoma. It also occurs after surgical dissection, particularly for resection of an oesophageal carcinoma, after operations on the aorta or after dissection in the root of the neck for sympathectomy. Copious quantities of milky fluid drain with loss of dietary fat, circulating proteins and lymphocytes. In about half the cases reoperation is required to find and secure the leak.

Enlarged lymph nodes

Lymph nodes commonly enlarge during an acute or chronic infection. In the acute infection, the regional lymph nodes may be painful with characteristic lymphangitis. The lymphadenopathy may resolve if an appropriate antibiotic is administered. If the area becomes fluctuant, which indicates the development of an abscess, formal operative drainage is necessary. Lymph nodes will also enlarge if there is infection by a variety of viral agents. Infective mononucleosis is characterized by painful enlargement of lymph nodes. There is a characteristic increase in the mononuclear count and there are specific serological tests. Lymph node enlargement is also a feature of the acquired immunodeficiency syndrome, in which case the human immunodeficiency virus antibodies will be elevated.

Chronic inflammation in which suppuration does not occur is commonly caused by tuberculosis in the neck and lymphogranuloma inguinale in the groin. Tuberculous lymphadenitis has become much more prevalent in Britain recently among Caribbean and Asian immigrants. The painless node is clinically indistinguishable from a malignant node, but, when examined histologically, there are characteristic giant cells with caseation. Tubercle bacilli may be isolated by culture.

Lymphogranuloma inguinale results from a *Chlamydia* infection contracted by sexual intercourse. The primary lesion consists of small vesicles on the genitalia. Some 3–6 weeks later the inguinal nodes enlarge and subsequently break down and sinuses form. In the female, lymphatic spread from vulva to the perirectal tissues may result in a rectal stricture. The diagnosis is confirmed by the detection of antibodies by microimmunofluorescence.

Tumours

Lymph nodes are a common site of both primary and secondary malignant disease. Primary tumours are classified as either Hodgkin's disease or malignant lymphoma (non-Hodgkin's lymphoma). Hodgkin's disease commonly presents as a painless enlargement of a peripheral lymph node. In more than 80 per cent of the patients the cervical nodes are the site of first manifestation. In malignant lymphoma, lymphadenopathy is again the commonest mode of presentation. However, the enlarged lymph nodes are present in various different lymphatic node areas.

Most carcinomas, and also melanomas, metastasize readily to the regional draining lymph nodes. Lymph node enlargement may be the initial presentation of certain carcinomas such as a primary gastric carcinoma, presenting as enlarged nodes near the termination of the thoracic duct (Virchow's node*). If the metastases present in the cervical region, the commonest primary is in the head or neck. Involvement of the supraclavicular nodes suggests a primary within the thorax, abdomen or breast. A variety of tumours may present as disease in the axillary or inguinal nodes. Malignant melanoma is an example of a tumour that may present with nodal metastases although the primary has not been identified.

Patients who are suspected of having a malignant lymph node should first have a careful examination to search for the primary. In addition to clinical examination of the breast and abdomen, an ENT examination should be performed. If no primary is identified, they should be admitted for operative excision. Their subsequent management will depend upon the histopathology.

---

* Rudolph Ludwig Karl Virchow (1821–1902), pathologist, Berlin.

11

HYPERTENSION

Definition

The blood pressure of the population is a continuously distributed variable (Fig. 11.1). There is therefore a problem of the definition of 'high blood pressure'. This is compounded by the fact that the actual measurement of the blood pressure may produce the defence or alerting reaction in the patient which will cause a spuriously high reading. To allow for this, it is usual to take the pressure on several occasions; this will allow the subject to become familiar with the surroundings and with the examiner. Furthermore, the blood pressure varies widely during the day and night, and also varies with the activities of the subject at these times.

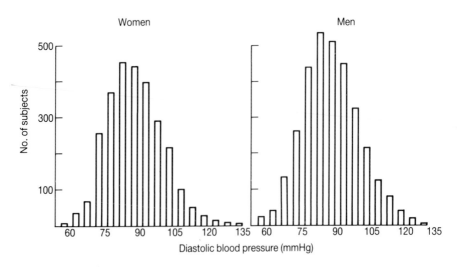

Fig. 11.1 Frequency distribution of diastolic blood pressure.

Technique of measurement

The blood pressure is usually measured in the arm by an indirect method using a sphygmomanometer (Fig. 11.2). In a narrowed blood vessel the flow of blood is speeded up through the narrowed segment of vessel and gives rise to turbulence. This is the basis of the Korotkoff sounds* described in 1905. There are five phases of Korotkoff sounds, of which only the first, fourth and fifth are now used. Korotkoff phase I is the level at which consecutive beats produce sounds that are heard as the cuff is being slowly deflated; these sounds are of short duration, and give way to sounds or murmurs of longer duration which Korotkoff described as phase II. Phase III is due to an augmentation of phase II, causing by an increasing volume of blood passing through the partially constricted artery. Phase IV is the pressure at which the loud sound muffles to become softer. Phase V is the total disappearance of any sound.

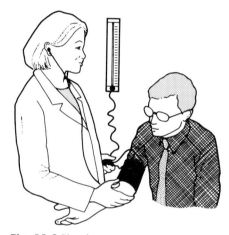

Fig. 11.2 Blood pressure measurement using a sphygmomanometer.

Errors in the technique of measurement can produce incorrect blood pressure readings which may have serious consequences. Therefore, only an observer who is aware of the factors that lead to false readings should measure the blood pressure. Particular attention needs to be paid to the following points:

1. The subject must be helped to relax and should be in either the lying or sitting position.
2. The cuff round the arm should be at the level of the heart in order to reduce baseline error.
3. The cuff should be of sufficient size to occlude the brachial artery effectively. The cuff consists of an inflatable bladder within a restrictive cloth sheath. Provided the sheath is long enough to wrap round the arm and be easily secured, the length of the sheath is not important. It is the length and

---

* Nikolai Sergeyevich Korotkoff (1874–1920), a Russian pioneer vascular surgeon working in the Military Medical Academy in St Petersburg.

width of the inflatable bladder that are crucial. The length of the bladder is one determinant of the area of pressure that is applied to the artery. If the bladder is too short, the blood pressure will be overestimated. The bladder should nearly or completely encircle the patient's arm. For normal or lean arms a 35 cm bladder is recommended; for large or muscular arms longer bladders, up to 42 cm, are needed (Fig. 11.3). Unfortunately, a lot of commercially made bladders are only 23 cm long. With these shorter bladders it is very important that the centre of the bladder is positioned over the artery. The width of the bladder is also important because it determines the length of the artery to be occluded: too narrow a bladder leads to overestimation of the pressure. The width should be at least 40 per cent of the circumference of the arm. In adults the recommended widths for lean, normal and obese arms are from 12 to 15 cm.

4. The cuff needs to be applied smoothly and neatly to prevent any herniation of the bladder.

5. While palpating the artery, the cuff is blown up until the arterial pulse can no longer be felt. The palpation serves two purposes: firstly it avoids patient discomfort caused by inflating the cuff higher than necessary. Secondly it prevents the examiner missing the auscultatory gap that occurs in some patients. In this situation, as the cuff is deflated, the Korotkoff phase I sound disappears only to reappear at a lower level. If initially the cuff is inflated only to a pressure that lies within this auscultatory gap, no sound is generated and the systolic pressure will then be recorded to be much lower than it actually is!

6. The mercury column should be lowered at a rate of about 2–3 mm/s.

7. There is still debate as to what should be defined as the diastolic pressure. The options are to use phase IV, the change from a loud to a muffled sound, or to use phase V, the disappearance of the sound. Phase IV tends to record pressures that are a few millimetres higher, and phase V records pressures a

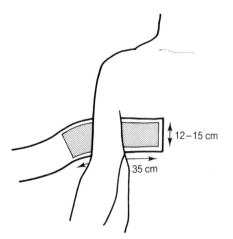

12–15 cm

35 cm

Fig. 11.3 The cuff and bladder dimensions that are required for the accurate estimation of blood pressure in a normal or lean adult.

few millimetres lower, than the true intra-arterial pressure. Since doctors and nurses are about equally likely to record one rather than the other, and since it is rarely stated which is being used, the authors are of the view that both should be recorded. Thus a blood pressure might be recorded as 140/90/85; this at least means that everyone else knows what is being recorded!

8. A common source of error is caused by the observer's digit preference. This tends to a preference for numbers ending in 0 or 5 and usually below the correct reading. This error can be eliminated by use of a sphygmomanometer where the mercury is not seen until after the pressure has been recorded; alternatively, the scale or zero is randomly altered and the correction made later. The bias can also be avoided by recording to the nearest 2 mmHg.

9. The error caused by parallax when viewing the top of the mercury column can be eliminated by correct positioning of the column of mercury. The height of the column above the patient does not matter since it is a closed system.

10. The equipment must be in good working order (Fig. 11.4).

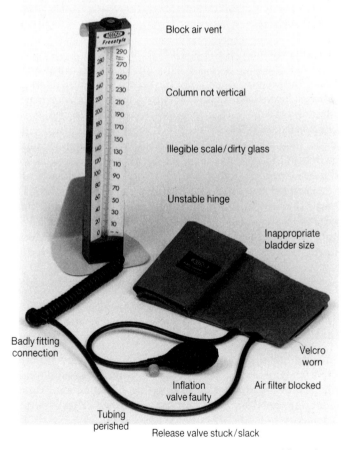

Fig. 11.4 A sphygmomanometer, identifying common problems that interfere with its reliable performance.

11. In most patients in whom sustained increase in blood pressure is being assessed, at least two auscultatory measurements should be made in both the lying and the standing positions. If these readings do not agree within 10–15 mmHg of each other, a further reading should be taken after a few minutes.
12. Blood pressure should be measured in both arms in all patients with a raised blood pressure when they are first being assessed. A recording in both arms and the leg is necessary if a coarctation of the aorta is suspected.

The size and nature of the problem

In a prospective study of a community living in Framingham, Massachusetts, 37 per cent of the men and 51 per cent of the women who died of cardiovascular disease had been noted previously to have an elevated blood pressure on at least three occasions. The mortality of such subjects was more than double those who had a normal blood pressure. Similar increases in the risk of death can be seen in data from life insurance companies. The consequences of the actual level of blood pressure will depend not only on the measured arterial pressure but also on both risk factors such as age, race, sex, glucose intolerance, smoking habits and cholesterol levels.

Hypertension is not a disease or abnormality in the same sense as pneumonia or osteoporosis. The disease processes associated with a high arterial pressure are the consequences of the ensuing damage to the arterial vessels or to target organs such as the kidneys, brain or the heart. Death due to hypertension may be directly caused by the increased stress on the vessels, resulting in such conditions as cerebral haemorrhage or aortic dissection. Alternatively, it may cause heart failure, due to the increased work required of the heart, or renal failure, due to direct damage to the kidneys. These conditions are largely preventable by the recognition and treatment of the moderate or severe hypertension. Unfortunately, the large majority of deaths related to hypertension are caused by coronary artery disease. There is little proof that treatment of the elevated blood pressure actually reduces the likelihood of this complication.

Some trials of the treatment of mild hypertension (diastolic blood pressure phase V, 90–105 mmHg) have produced evidence that treatment will reduce some of the complications. This has far-reaching implications, since 15–20 per cent of the adult population in developed countries might be candidates for treatment!

Aetiology and classification

If a cause for an elevated blood pressure is not found, it is termed essential hypertension. About 95 per cent of patients with hypertension in the community will have essential hypertension. In a small proportion of patients a primary renal, vascular or endocrine cause for the hypertension is found. This hypertension is then called secondary.

Benign and malignant hypertension

The term 'benign' is a misnomer and should not be used. It was introduced to contrast with a malignant form of hypertension. This, at the time, was a very appropriate term since, untreated, the vast majority of patients with malignant hypertension died within 6–12 months of the diagnosis being made. Since the discovery and introduction of effective drug therapy the prognosis has been radically improved. A better term to use nowadays is 'accelerated hypertension'. The cause of the change from a stable form of hypertension to the accelerated form is not well understood. There appears to be a change in the ability of arterioles to resist the raised arterial pressure, with a consequent insudation of plasma and fibrin into the vessel wall, a rapid rise in the peripheral resistance and a fall in tissue perfusion. The pathological hallmark is the appearance of hyalinization of the arterioles, the so-called fibrinoid necrosis.

Secondary hypertension

The main causes can be conveniently considered under four headings:

1. Vascular causes; these include coarctation of the aorta and renal artery stenosis.
2. Endocrine causes; these include Cushing's syndrome, Conn's syndrome (or primary aldosteronism) and phaeochromocytoma. The oral contraceptive pill can also cause hypertension.
3. Renal causes; these include any renal affliction, but most commonly nephritis, chronic pyelonephritis, polycystic kidney or a diabetic kidney.
4. Hypertension in pregnancy; pre-eclamptic toxaemia.

The clinical features that suggest the presence of secondary hypertension are shown in Table 11.1. Despite the relative rarity of secondary hypertension, it is important to recognize the condition and to treat the underlying cause as well as the blood pressure.

Table 11.1 Clinical features that suggest a secondary cause of hypertension

History	Examination
Known to have renal disease	Delay in femoral pulse
On oral contraceptives	Oedema
Thirst, nocturia or polyuria	Palpable kidneys or bladder
Dysuria or haematuria	Uraemic features
Excessive consumption of analgesic	Features of Cushing's syndrome
Extreme weakness	Abdominal bruits
Taking drugs such as steroids,	Neurofibromata
monoamine oxidase inhibitors or	
containing liquorice	

Essential hypertension

This is a diagnosis of exclusion. The vast majority of patients with this condition are treated by the primary care physician and only about 2–3 per cent are referred to hospital outpatients.

Aetiology

Essential hypertension is a multifactorial condition. Some of the factors involved are:

1. Family history. A family history is common. Genetic factors are important; the number of genes involved is probably small.
2. Salt intake. There is some influence of salt intake upon arterial pressure. The relationship is complex and the details are not yet fully elaborated.
3. The sympathetic nervous system. A number of drugs used in the treatment of hypertension act via the autonomic nervous system. The contribution of overactivity of the autonomic nervous system in essential hypertension is controversial.
4. Age. In 'civilized' populations, blood pressure rises with age in contradistinction to some 'primitive' societies. In males this happens steadily whilst in women it only starts to occur after the menopause.
5. Structural change in small arteries. Adaptive changes in the arterioles can be demonstrated in animals; relatively small changes in the wall thickness can have pronounced effects on the resistance to flow and thus on the arterial pressure. These changes may well be reversible.
6. Baroreflex sensitivity. There is a diminution in baroreflex sensitivity with increasing age and with increasing arterial pressure. Whether these changes are the cause or the result of the hypertension is not known.
7. Psychological factors. There is a clear relationship between mental or emotional stress and a temporary rise in blood pressure. However, there is little evidence for a sustained elevation due to stress. The concept of cardiovascular reactivity is discussed further in Chapter 13. The development of behavioural techniques for the treatment of hypertension is also considered in Chapter 13.
8. The kidney. The renin–angiotensin–aldosterone system is of great importance in the control of blood pressure.
9. Natriuretic hormone. A circulating natriuretic hormone could, by inhibiting sodium transport in cells other than renal tubules, alter the sensitivity of arterioles to vasoconstrictive influences.
10. Antidiuretic hormone. The evidence of an important role for antidiuretic hormone in essential hypertension is controversial.
11. The role of endothelin, a potent vasoconstrictor peptide secreted by the endothelium, is yet to be determined.

Pathology

The pathology of essential hypertension reflects the combination of adaptive and degenerative changes in the heart and circulation. The heart may initially appear normal. With time there develops the gradual hypertrophy of the left ventricle. In the small arteries and arterioles there is thickening of the muscular media (Figs. 11.5 and 11.6). Over time the changes in the heart and the blood vessels become more marked and the potential for reversal of the changes becomes less. In the heart there are several changes that affect its performance: the larger muscle fibres increase the volume of tissue between the capillaries and therefore the blood supply becomes a little more tenuous; the increased muscle thickness reduces the compliance and increases the filling pressure; the coronary arteries develop atheromatous disease. These factors all contribute to the development of hypertensive heart failure.

The mechanism of production of the generalized arterial lesions is not well understood; two important factors are the high arterial pressure and the related increased lipoprotein deposition in the vessel wall. The consequences of this medial and intimal hypertrophy is most important in the kidney and brain (Fig. 11.7). In the kidney the lesions may impair blood flow and contribute to the development of renal failure. In the brain, small Charcot–Bouchard micro-aneurysms develop. They occur commonly in the region of the thalamus and the white matter around the corpus striatum, are up to 1 mm in size and are the cause of cerebral haemorrhage which is such a tragic complication of this condition.

The appearance of hyalinization of the arterioles, the so-called fibrinoid necrosis, corresponds with a change in the ability of arterioles to resist the raised arterial pressure, with a consequent insudation of plasma and fibrin into the vessel wall, a rapid rise in the peripheral resistance and a fall in tissue perfusion with the development of microinfarcts in the retina and kidney (Fig. 11.8).

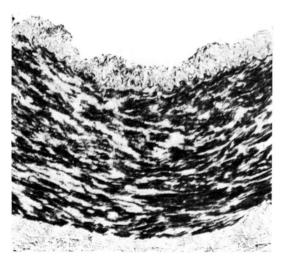

Fig. 11.5 Section of hypertrophied radial artery, from a case of systemic hypertension in a young subject, showing hypertrophy of the media. (Smooth muscle appears black.) ×140 (Reproduced, with permission, from J. R. Anderson (Ed.), 1985, *Muir's Textbook of Pathology*, 12th edn, Edward Arnold, London.)

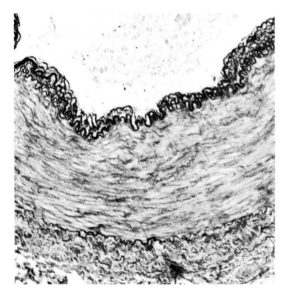

Fig. 11.6 Another section of the same artery as in Fig. 11.5, showing increase of elastic tissue formed by replication of the internal elastic lamina. (Elastic tissue appears black.) ×120 (Reproduced, with permission, from J. R. Anderson (Ed.), 1985, *Muir's Textbook of Pathology*, 12th edn, Edward Arnold, London.)

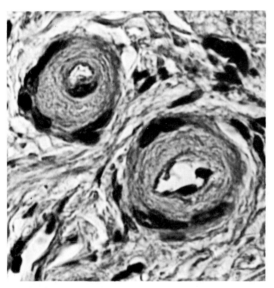

Fig. 11.7 Hyaline arteriolosclerosis of afferent glomerular arteriole in chronic systemic hypertension. The arteriole is not only thickened but also tortuous, and so has been cut twice in cross-section in the same plane. ×1500 (Reproduced, with permission, from R. N. M. MacSween and K. Whaley (Eds.), 1992, *Muir's Textbook of Pathology*, 13th edn, Edward Arnold, London.)

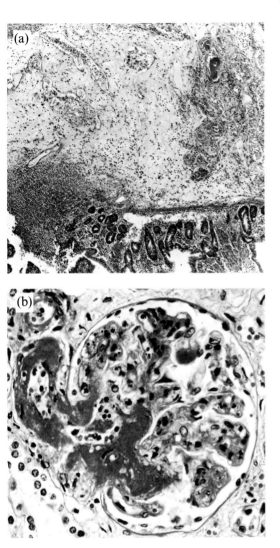

Fig. 11.8 Arteriolar lesions in malignant hypertension. (**a**) Ulceration of the colonic mucosa due to fibrinoid necrosis and thrombosis of arterioles; one such vessel is seen (lower left) in the submucosa. (**b**) Fibrinoid necrosis of a glomerular afferent arteriole and part of the tuft. (Reproduced, with permission, from R. N. M. MacSween and K. Whaley (Eds.), 1992, *Muir's Textbook of Pathology*, 13th edn, Edward Arnold, London.)

Clinical picture

People with high blood pressure have fewer complaints than those with a normal pressure! This means that they will not usually present to their doctor; they have to be sought.

Headache very rarely occurs in hypertensive subjects. It develops only in the patient with very severe elevation of the pressure; this headache will tend to be worse in the morning on waking. The only symptom that is found more frequently in hypertensive subjects than in the normotensive is shortness of breath.

Once the degenerative consequences, or target organ damage, have begun, the symptoms and signs will be determined by the organ affected.

Signs

The signs of essential hypertension will reflect the stage and duration of the disease process. Physical examination will have already excluded the likelihood of secondary hypertension.

The pulse will usually feel forcible. The blood pressure will be elevated. The apex beat will reflect the underlying hypertrophy; it will be sustained or heaving but will not be displaced. A fourth heart sound may develop, reflecting the increased atrial pressure due to decreased compliance of the ventricle secondary to the hypertrophy.

The optic fundi may show changes of hypertension; these need to be differentiated from those associated with arteriosclerosis. Arteriovenous nipping, increased tortuosity and increased light reflex ('copper wiring') are all due to increased thickness of the arterial wall; they may be associated with hypertension but are frequently due to ageing. Copper wiring is also frequently misnamed silver wiring. This latter condition is due to the appearance of a thrombosed artery. The specific appearances of the hypertensive optic fundus are:

1. Irregularity of the arterioles.
2. Cotton wool exudates, which are in fact a cluster of the swollen ends of fragmented axons in an area of oedematous retina. They are not exudates at all! They are caused by ischaemia but will completely resolve with treatment.
3. Flame-shaped haemorrhages reflect further breakdown in the integrity of the vessel wall. Their shape is determined by the nerve fibres coursing towards the disc.
4. Papilloedema, or swelling of the optic disc, may be present with or without haemorrhages and exudates. It probably occurs as a result of general brain oedema due to a breakdown in the autoregulatory control of flow in the presence of a very high pressure (Fig. 11.9).

All of these exudative lesions of the optic fundus may be seen in other conditions such as severe anaemia, a vasculitis such as disseminated lupus erythematosus or uraemia. If these are present in the context of hypertension, it constitutes a medical emergency and the blood pressure needs to be immediately reduced.

Papilloedema itself also occurs in other conditions such as raised intracranial pressure due to a cerebral tumour.

Investigations

Once the persistent elevation of the patient's blood pressure has been confirmed, the question arises as to how far to take investigations. The answer to this

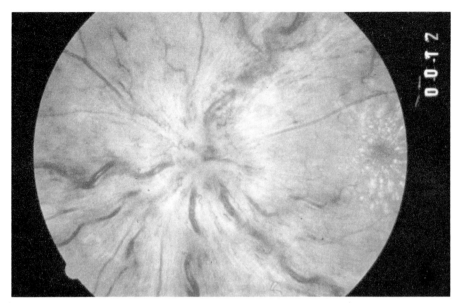

Fig. 11.9 Optic fundus showing papilloedema, exudates and haemorrhage in a patient with accelerated hypertension. (By courtesy of Miss Clare Davey.)

question is likely to be different in the community, where the cause of the hypertension is likely to be essential, compared with hospital practice, where the more difficult or the more extreme cases are seen. There are three possible reasons for performing investigations: firstly to identify the rare patient with a secondary cause; secondly to assess the degree of existing target organ damage; and thirdly to uncover any other disease that requires treatment in its own right (examples of these might be diabetes or anaemia).

First-line investigations that might be performed for a patient presenting in the community are outlined in Table 11.2. If abnormalities are found, further investigations will be required to elucidate the cause of the hypertension or the degree of target organ damage.

Table 11.2 First-line investigations for a patient presenting to the general practitioner

Investigation	Information required
Urine	Microscopy for casts or cells Reagent strips for protein, blood, sugar
Blood	Haemoglobin Urea and electrolytes
ECG	Looking for left ventricular hypertrophy

Prognosis

The prognosis for essential hypertension is very variable. Some of the reasons for the variability are understood. The outcome is related to the interplay between the height of the pressure elevation, the duration of the elevation and, particularly in the case of coronary artery disease, the existence of other risk factors. The risk factors for coronary artery disease (Fig. 11.10) are discussed in Chapter 1. The main factor that influences the mortality and morbidity for cerebrovascular disease, which includes both haemorrhage and thrombosis, is the level of the blood pressure; the prediction of risk can be made on the basis of the diastolic, systolic or mean arterial pressure. The risk increases with increasing levels of blood pressure in all ages and in each sex. There is no sex difference in the incidence. The other factors such as cigarette smoking, hyperlipidaemia and obesity exert little influence on the incidence of cerebrovascular disease (Fig. 11.11).

Treatment

Before treatment can be offered, the patient with hypertension must be identified. The only practical method is screening for the condition. In the UK it has been shown that within a 3-year period most general practitioners will have seen 80–87 per cent of their patients. This figure is much lower in inner city practices. The opportunity therefore exists to screen the population very effectively and at a relatively small additional cost.

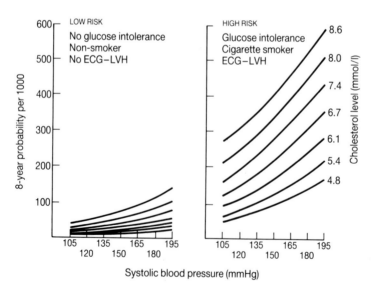

Fig. 11.10 Risk of cardiovascular disease according to systolic blood pressure and serum cholesterol value in otherwise high- and low-risk subjects: 35-year-old men. (Framingham Study, 18-year follow-up.) (Data from W. B. Kannel and T. D. Dawber, 1974, *British Journal of Hospital Medicine,* **7**, 508.)

The treatment of moderate or severe hypertension (phase V diastolic pressure >110 mmHg) is of proven value and reduces the risk of stroke, renal failure and heart failure.

The treatment of mild hypertension (phase V diastolic pressure 100–109 mmHg) is more controversial. The British Hypertension Society has recommended the following management for patients under the age of 80:

1. Those whose diastolic blood pressure averages 100 mmHg or more over 3–4 months will need treatment.
2. Those whose diastolic averages 95–99 mmHg over this interval should not be treated but should be carefully followed up at intervals of 3–6 months.
3. Those whose blood pressure is initially raised but then falls below 95 mmHg should have the blood pressure checked yearly.

Non-drug therapy

There are several important measures to consider before embarking on drug treatment. Weight reduction for the overweight patient will reduce and sometimes 'cure' the hypertension. The reduction in excessive alcohol consumption may have a similar effect. The opportunity exists to advise the patient about other risk factors such as smoking. Advice about a healthy lifestyle will also include guidance about the need for regular exercise, which in itself may help reduce the blood pressure.

Behavioural techniques including biofeedback have been somewhat disparaged in the past by the more conventional clinicians. They can be effective in

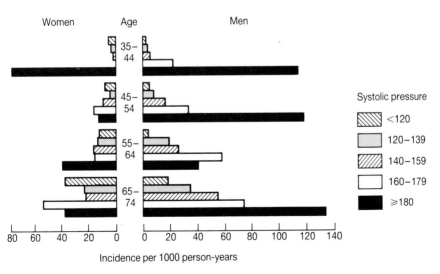

Fig. 11.11 Incidence of all cardiovascular–renal deaths, myocardial infarctions, angina pectoris and cerebrovascular accidents according to systolic pressure, age and sex in Rhondda Fach and Vale of Glamorgan, 1971. (Data from W. E. Miall and R. H. Chinn, 1974, *British Medical Journal*, **3**, 600.)

some patients with mild hypertension and produce prolonged reduction in blood pressure. They are discussed more fully in Chapter 13.

Drug therapy

At the outset it is very important to give the patient some understanding of the condition and to emphasize that drug treatment is unlikely to make them feel any better. The drug treatment is being introduced to prevent problems in the future – a sort of insurance policy! It is also important to emphasize the need for continued follow-up at regular intervals. Unfortunately, one of the major problems in the successful treatment of hypertension is that of patient compliance. It is very convenient, but not very productive, to blame the patient for this unhelpful behaviour! It is hardly surprising that compliance is a real problem with a condition that has no symptoms and which, when treated, is likely to make the patient feel less well than better!

There is now a huge choice of drugs for the treatment of hypertension. The clinician needs to become familiar with the use of two or three drugs and use them correctly. The drugs can be divided into categories by their mode of action (Table 11.3).

Table 11.3   Categories of drugs used in the treatment of hypertension

Drug group	Examples
Diuretics	Hydrochlorothiazide
β-Adrenoceptor blocking drugs	Propranolol, atenolol
α-Adrenoceptor blocking drugs	Phentolamine, phenoxybenzamine
Vasodilators acting on vessel walls	Hydralazine, prazocin, sodium nitroprusside
Drugs acting on central nervous system	Reserpine, methyldopa
Sympathetic blocking agents	Guanethidine, bethanidine
Calcium antagonists	Nifedipine
Angiotensin-converting enzyme inhibitors	Enalapril, captopril, lisinopril

The sympathetic blocking agents are now very little used. They have been superseded by better drugs with fewer side effects.

There have been spectacular advances in the development of new drugs and new classes of drugs for the treatment of hypertension. This has meant that there is no longer any uniformity in the approach to treatment.

Mild hypertension
The British Hypertension Working Party suggest that either a β-adrenergic blocking drug or a diuretic should be used as the initial treatment.

Moderate or severe hypertension
The initial choice lies between a calcium antagonist or a β-adrenoceptor blocking drug. It may be necessary to use a combination of these drugs. An angiotensin-

converting enzyme (ACE) inhibitor may be an alternative but often needs to be used together with a diuretic to achieve its full effect.

Accelerated hypertension
When reducing the pressure from very high levels, the aim should be for a smooth reduction over a few hours rather than a dramatic immediate effect. Bedrest together with the introduction of labetalol, which has both α- and β-blocking effects, may be all that are required. Occasionally, intramuscular or intravenous hydralazine is required and is usually effective.

Hypertension in pregnancy
Thiazide diuretics, methyldopa and β-adrenoceptor blocking drugs have all been used safely and effectively in pregnancy.

Hypertension in aortic dissection
In this condition the blood pressure must be lowered immediately in order to reduce the shearing force on the vessels. Intravenous sodium nitroprusside is the drug of choice and its dosage can be accurately titrated to control the systolic pressure below 100 mmHg.

Further reading

MacSween, R. M. N. and Whaley, K. (Eds.) (1992) *Muir's Textbook of Pathology*, 13th edition. Edward Arnold, London.

Petrie, J. C., O'Brien, E. T., Littler, W. A. and de Swiet, M. (1987) *Recommendations on Blood Pressure Measurement*, British Medical Journal, London.

12

RESUSCITATION

And when Elisha was come into the house, behold, the child was dead, and laid upon his bed. He went in therefore, and shut the door upon them twain, and prayed unto the Lord. And he went up, and lay upon the child and put his mouth upon his mouth, and his eyes upon his eyes, and his hands upon his hands: and he stretched himself upon the child; and the flesh of the child waxed warm. Then he returned, and walked in the house to and fro; and went up, and stretched himself upon him: and the child sneezed seven times, and the child opened his eyes.

2 Kings 4:32–35

Since biblical times, attempts have been made to restore life to the dead or nearly dead individuals. In the eighteenth century it was a common practice to throw unconscious persons over the back of a trotting horse or to roll them over a barrel in an attempt to move air in and out of their chest. A more recent technique used in the early part of the twentieth century was that of exerting pressure on the lower back; this method of artificial respiration forced air from the lungs. These methods were viewed as a means of providing lung ventilation but recent research suggests that circulation of the blood might also have occurred concurrently.

In 1960 the present techniques of external cardiac massage and artificial respiration were developed. This technique of cardiopulmonary resuscitation (CPR) has gained popularity and has been shown to be effective.

The original hypothesis suggested that blood flow from the heart to the periphery occurred during external cardiac compression. This flow was a direct result of compression of the heart between the sternum and the vertebral column (Fig. 12.1). It was assumed that chest compression produced a similar set of circumstances to systole and the blood was squeezed from both ventricles into the great arteries. Retrograde flow was prevented by the closure of the relevant valves. It was suggested that, during the release of chest compression, a situation similar to diastole prevailed. The ventricles were then filled by a suction effect. This concept has been shown to be inconsistent with a number of observations both in animal models and in humans. There is a close correlation between the rise in intrathoracic pressure during chest compression and the apparent magni-

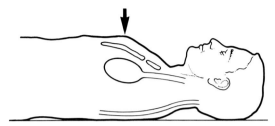

Fig. 12.1 How external cardiac massage will compress the heart between the sternum and the vertebral column.

tude of blood flow and blood pressure in the carotids. The importance of intrathoracic pressure is demonstrated by the observations that, by the continuous early initiation of coughing, patients in ventricular fibrillation can maintain consciousness as long as coughing is continued.

In order for blood flow to occur in a fluid-filled system such as the circulation, a pressure gradient must be present. For a structure to function as a pump, a pressure gradient must be present across the pump. During chest compression a peripheral arteriovenous pressure gradient appears and blood flow occurs as a result (Fig. 12.2). In this system there is no pressure gradient across the heart; the heart therefore cannot be the pump responsible for generating blood flow

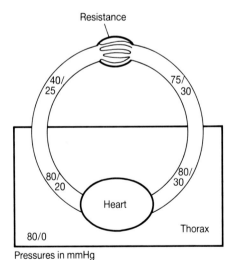

Pressures in mmHg

Fig. 12.2 Representative pressures recorded during external cardiac massage; the pressures are those recorded with compression. There is no significant gradient across the heart. The extrathoracic arterial pressure is similar to the intrathoracic aortic pressure. There is an extrathoracic arteriovenous pressure gradient resulting in forward flow. When the compression is released, intrathoracic pressures fall towards zero and blood flows into the thorax. Retrograde flow into the aorta is limited by the relatively low capacitance and also by the closing of the aortic valve.

during CPR and it is functioning as a passive conduit. When chest pressure is released the intrathoracic pressure falls towards zero and there is venous flow into the right heart and lungs. Retrograde flow into the aorta from the extra-thoracic arteries also occurs but is limited by the relatively low capacitance of the intrathoracic arterial bed and also by the closure of the aortic valve.

It has not yet been possible to draw final conclusions as to the relative importance of external cardiac massage and ventilation during CPR in human beings. However, two-dimensional echocardiographic studies during CPR show that, during chest compression, both the mitral and the aortic valves are open and there is little deformity of the left ventricular chamber cavity.

The current techniques of cardiopulmonary resuscitation have been developed to take cognisance of these factors.

Results of cardiopulmonary resuscitation

In Seattle and its environs in the USA, 30 per cent of patients who develop ventricular fibrillation survive to leave hospital. These results are from perhaps the most sophisticated community-based resuscitation system in the world. The emergency vehicles that rush to the scene of the arrest are staffed by highly trained paramedical staff. An intensive training course for the public has been in operation for some years; within the hospital, doctors and nurses are all well trained. Considerable efforts are being made in the UK to train doctors, nurses and paramedical staff. Several areas of the country now use ambulance staff trained in advanced resuscitation. Attempts are being made to train the community in basic resuscitation, using television programmes backed up by local practical training.

It has been shown that hospital medical and nursing staff in the UK often do not have the skills to perform even basic resuscitation! This is often a very poor reflection on the training programmes in the hospital or medical school. These programmes ought to teach both the factual knowledge necessary and also the practical skills. Resuscitation manikins and simulated cardiac arrests are very valuable. There is a vital need for these skills to be acquired and practised at regular intervals. The inclusion of manikins in qualifying examinations will do a lot to concentrate the mind on the need for learning the practical skills as well as the theory. The requirement to attend a practical revision course at the beginning of every new post will help refresh these skills. With better training it will be possible to improve the success rate of resuscitation within the hospital. It must be emphasized that the prognosis for a patient surviving CPR after a myocardial infarction is the same as for the patient who did not have a cardiac arrest. In other words, the actual development of ventricular fibrillation does not adversely affect the prognosis as long as resuscitation is successful!

The ABC of resuscitation

Resuscitation is the emergency treatment of any condition in which the brain does not receive enough oxygen. At present, ABC stands for Airway, Breathing and Circulation. The American Heart Association suggested in 1985 that ABC should stand for Assess, Breathe and Circulate since this is a more accurate description of what the rescuer should do.

Assess

The first step should be to assess the surroundings and the patient. The surroundings will need to be assessed for such dangers as leaking gas, traffic, falling masonry or electrical wiring. Attention should now be turned to establishing whether the patient is conscious. The patient should be carefully shaked and asked 'Are you all right?'; care must be taken about overvigorous shaking in case there are injuries to the neck (Fig. 12.3).

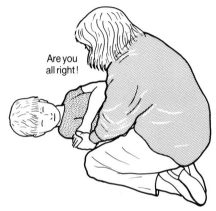

Are you all right!

Fig. 12.3 The patient should be shaked carefully and asked 'Are you all right?'

Airway

Once it is certain that the patient is unconscious, the next step is to ensure that there is a patent airway and the patient can breathe. The chest should be inspected for any respiratory movement and, with the cheek of the rescuer next to the patient's mouth, breath sounds should be listened for and a note made of the feel of any expired air on the cheek.

Airway obstruction

If the patient is not breathing or has difficulty in breathing, there may be an obstruction in the airway. In the unconscious patient the relaxation of the tongue, neck and pharyngeal muscles causes soft tissue obstruction in the supraglottic airway (Fig. 12.4). Patency of the airway can be restored either by extending, but not hyperextending, the neck or by lifting the chin forwards with one hand and pressing the forehead backwards with the heel of the other (Fig. 12.5). Alternatively, the jaw can be thrust upwards by elevating the xygomatic processes.

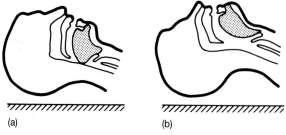

(a)   (b)

Fig. 12.4 (a) Airway obstruction is caused by relaxation of the tongue, neck and pharyngeal muscles. **(b)** Patency of the airway has been restored by correctly extending the neck and lifting the chin forwards.

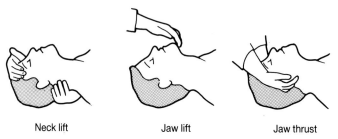

Neck lift   Jaw lift   Jaw thrust

Fig. 12.5 The means by which patency of the airway can be restored. See text for explanation.

The patient who has an adequate circulation and spontaneous respiration but cannot protect the airway is at risk in the supine position. The patient should be turned into the coma or recovery position. This will allow the tongue to fall forwards and fluid can drain out of the mouth rather than down the trachea (Fig. 12.6). Recovery positions vary from a true lateral position to the semiprone. The lower arm can be extended behind the back to prevent a reverse roll. The patient may lie on either side. If there is concern about a spinal injury, the patient needs to be turned into the true lateral recovery position by several people so that rotation of the spine can be prevented.

Vomiting and regurgitation

Vomiting and regurgitation are common problems with an unconscious patient. Vomiting is an active process involving stomach contraction and retrograde propulsion up the oesophagus. Regurgitation is a passive flow of stomach contents up the oesophagus. Sometimes there is a warning that the patient is going to vomit; this will allow time to put the patient into the recovery position or head down (Trendelenburg) tilt and to be prepared for suction or manual removal of the debris from the mouth and pharynx.

Asphyxia

Asphyxia due to the impaction of food or other foreign body in the upper airways is a frightening event and is often mistaken for a heart attack. This 'café coronary'

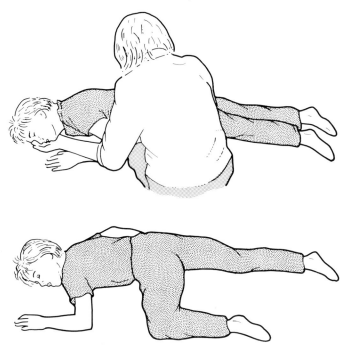

Fig. 12.6 Two recovery, or coma, positions for patients who have adequate circulation and spontaneous respiration but who cannot protect their own airway.

requires urgent action. In the conscious patient, the following manoeuvres should be performed:

1. Manual removal. The victim's mouth should be opened and attempts made to dislodge any obvious foreign object with the finger.
2. Back blows. Several sharp blows with the heel of the hand should be delivered high on the vertebral column between the shoulder blades.
3. Heimlich manoeuvre (Fig. 12.7). While standing immediately behind the victim, a series of sharp thrusts to the upper abdomen should be performed with both hands entwined together. These thrusts can also be used directly in the unconscious supine patient. If administered incorrectly, this manoeuvre can lead to abdominal injury.

Attempts can be made to provoke coughing or vomiting. If these measures are not successful the patient will become unconscious. When supine, further Heimlich thrusts can be performed. If still unsuccessful the ensuing hypoxic arrest will be similar to other causes of arrest and will need to be managed in an identical way. Occasionally, external cardiac massage may clear the obstruction. The next step is to proceed to laryngotomy, which may be life saving. Any strong sharp knife, scissor point or cannula can be used to create an opening in the cricothyroid membrane (Fig. 12.8). This opening must be created in the midline; the membrane is easily identified by running the finger down from the notch on

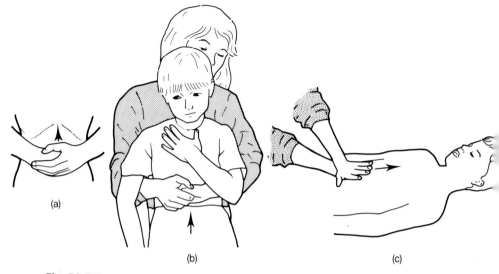

Fig. 12.7 The Heimlich manoeuvre: (**a, b**) in the standing position, and (**c**) in the prone position. See text for details.

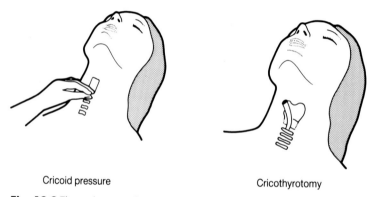

Cricoid pressure   Cricothyrotomy

Fig. 12.8 The technique of cricothyrotomy or laryngotomy. See text for details.

the thyroid cartilage to the bottom of the cartilage. The membrane is between the thyroid and cricoid cartilages and there are no other intervening structures between the skin and the trachea. Once created, the opening will need to be maintained by appropriate means.

Breathing

If no spontaneous respiration is present despite a patent airway, expired air respiration must be started immediately. The 16% oxygen in expired air is more than adequate for the patient's needs. The mouth to mouth technique is the most used and can be applied effectively by relatively unskilled rescuers. An alternative method is mouth-to-nose ventilation.

Expired air ventilation

The 'mouth to mouth' technique (Fig. 12.9) requires the rescuer to take a deep breath, to seal the lips around those of the patient and to pinch the nose of the patient. During the procedure the airway has to be kept patent as described above. The rescuer then breathes out until the chest of the patient is seen to expand. The patient is then allowed to exhale passively. The next breath is given so that the rate of breathing is about 12–16 per minute.

Mouth to nose ventilation has some advantages, which include better head extension with jaw thrust, reduced contact with saliva and vomit, and is more suitable for the rescuer with a small mouth. Its main disadvantage is the introduction of a slightly higher resistance to ventilation.

There may be anxiety in the mind of the rescuer lest the collapsed patient is HIV positive or has AIDS. There is no risk of acquiring the infection by mouth to mouth ventilation; however, it is a reasonable precaution to interpose a handkerchief or paper tissue between the mouth of the rescuer and the patient.

Masks and airways are useful aids if available. The ventilation mask is applied firmly to the patient's face, ensuring an airtight fit. The airway must be kept patent. The rescuer needs to use two hands to ensure the appropriate head extension and jaw position while maintaining an airtight seal; this can prove to be too complicated, particularly for those with small hands, and unsatisfactory ventilation results. Artificial airways can be used to maintain patency. The classic Guedel airway (Fig. 12.10) improves the patency but also often needs supplementary jaw support; unfortunately, it can also stimulate the oropharynx and cause vomiting. A number of ventilation devices are available. One of the most commonly used is the Brook airway which provides some protection for the rescuer by having a non-return valve (Fig. 12.11). The airway is inserted into the patient's mouth, ensuring that the tongue does not cause obstruction. An adequate seal is achieved around the mouth, the nose is again squeezed and the operator blows down the tube. This technique has a number of advantages and is more aesthetic for the operator. It is again vitally important that the adequacy of the airway is checked and maintained.

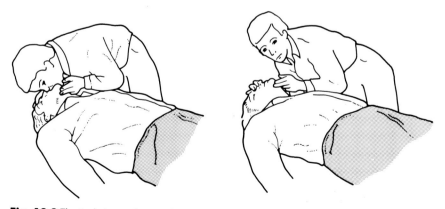

Fig. 12.9 The technique of expired air ventilation. See text for details.

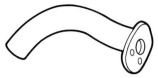

Fig. 12.10 The classic Guedel airway, which can improve the patency of the airway but also often needs supplementary jaw support.

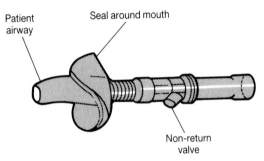

Fig. 12.11 The Brook airway, which provides some protection for the rescuer by having a non-return valve.

Intubation

Endotracheal intubation requires experience and special skills. At the scene of the patient being resuscitated, access to the mouth and trachea may be very difficult and, in contrast to the controlled environment of the anaesthetic room of the operating theatre, intubation may be extremely difficult. It should not be attempted by the inexperienced; there is considerable potential harm that can occur if too much time is expended struggling with the attempted intubation, particularly if the other aspects of the resuscitation stop to allow a still environment. Perfectly adequate ventilation can be achieved by the other methods described above and these can be continued until the skilled intubator arrives.

Circulation

If there is no pulse in a major artery, such as the carotid or femoral artery, the circulation must be established with external cardiac massage which is sometimes called closed cardiac compression. Rapid diagnosis is essential for two main reasons: firstly, permanent cerebral anoxic damage may occur rapidly; secondly, the success of resuscitative measures is related to the rapidity with which they are instituted following the arrest.

External cardiac massage

The landmarks for the performance of good external cardiac massage are important. The pressure must be exerted in the midline over the sternum. The ideal spot on the sternum is at the junction of the upper two-thirds and lower third; alternatively, the hand can be placed two fingers above the xiphisternal junction (Fig. 12.12). The ideal rate of compression is 60 sternal pressures per minute. At least half of each compression/relaxation cycle should be devoted to compression. Because of the curious apparent behaviour of time during cardio-pulmonary resuscitation, it is suggested that a three-syllable phrase is mouthed during the procedure; i.e. one e-le-phant, two e-le-phant, three e-le-phant etc. There should be one inflation for every five compressions. The compressions should not halt to permit ventilation; there is every reason to believe that massage is more effective if the chest is inflated. The resistance to ventilation during compression may necessitate some co-ordination.

The importance of sufficient chest compression cannot be overemphasized. It is actually difficult to gauge; the sternum should be depressed by 4–5 cm. The adequacy of chest compression can be checked by the generation of a palpable femoral or carotid arterial pulse. The ideal position for the rescuer to adopt is one in which the arms can be kept straight and the massage applied by a rocking movement (Fig. 12.13).

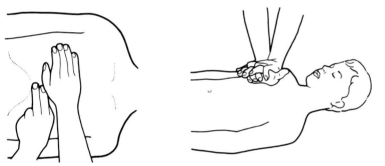

Fig. 12.12 The position of the hands for performing external cardiac massage. See text for full description.

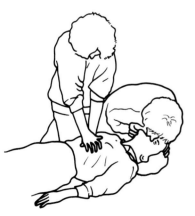

Fig. 12.13 The ideal position for the rescuer to perform external cardiac massage. The arms of the rescuer can be kept straight and the massage applied by a rocking movement.

Organization

When two rescuers are present, one will be responsible for ventilating the lungs and the other for external cardiac massage. When the person performing cardiac massage becomes tired the two rescuers should swap roles. If there is only one rescuer present the division of labour should be 15 compressions followed by 2 inflations. If there are more than two people present it is important that the most experienced rescuer takes charge of the whole procedure and co-ordinates the efforts and subsequent treatment. In a hospital setting too many people can actually impede the smooth running of the procedure; some people will need to be sent away.

Definitive treatment

In some instances the patient will not be attached to a monitor when they collapse. It is recommended that, whenever the defibrillator arrives, a DC shock is given prior to connecting a monitor. The time thus saved before the first shock is given is crucial: if the patient was in ventricular fibrillation the shock may be successful; if asystole was present, no harm will have been done.

Ventricular fibrillation

This is the most common mechanism of cardiac arrest in patients with ischaemic heart disease. Ventricular fibrillation is electrical anarchy within the myocardium (Fig. 12.14). The only reliable treatment for this condition is electrical

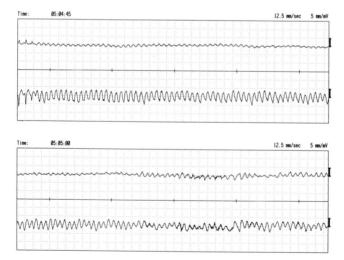

Fig. 12.14 A 24-hour ambulatory recording of two leads (V_5 above and V_1 below) on a patient who died during the recording. The recordings are at 12.5 mm/s and the calibration (on the right) is 5 mm/mV. In the top rhythm strip the first two complexes on the left are the patient's inherent rhythm. The rhythm changes abruptly into a coarse ventricular flutter and then into ventricular fibrillation.

defibrillation. Very occasionally it reverts spontaneously or with a thump on the chest.

DC shock

A large electrical impulse is delivered to the chest, which causes depolarization of all myocardial cells that are not totally refractory. If sufficient cells are depolarized, the fibrillatory waveform of random depolarization is no longer propagated through the myocardium and the normal pacemaker of the heart can once again take control of the heart beat.

Defibrillators either are powered by rechargeable batteries or are mains operated. The equipment allows a variable energy to be stored in the capacitor for subsequent discharge across the chest wall. The ideal position of the two electrode paddles is shown in Fig. 12.15. One paddle should be to the right of the sternum and the other near the apex of the heart. The polarity of the plates does not matter. Good contact of the paddles with the skin is important; a low resistance electrode gel needs to be interposed between the paddle and the skin. Prepacked impregnated sheets are useful and avoid a lot of mess. Alternatively, electrode gel can be squeezed from a tube. It is important that a smear of electrode gel does not connect the two defibrillator paddle positions because shorting can occur across this smear, with resulting burns and inadequate defibrillation.

The correctly placed paddles need to be firmly pressed against the chest wall; before defibrillation, everyone present must separate themselves from the patient or from the bed before the shock is given. The sequence shown in Fig. 12.16 is suggested.

If the ECG shows fine fibrillation waves, defibrillation is often unsuccessful. The administration of intravenous adrenaline (10 ml of 1 in 10000) results in a more vigorous and coarse fibrillation, which is often more responsive. For recurrent defibrillation the administration of intravenous lignocaine (100 mg) followed by repeated defibrillation may increase the likelihood of returning to a stable sinus rhythm. Other useful drugs in this regard are bretylium tosylate (400 mg) and amiodarone which can be used after the sixth shock.

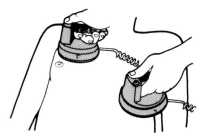

Fig. 12.15 Defibrillation. The ideal position of the two defibrillator paddles on the chest. A low-resistance electrode gel is interposed between each paddle and the chest wall.

1 Basic life support
2 Give first shock: 200 J
3 Check pulse
4 If no pulse, give 15 chest compressions

5 If fibrillation present

↓

Give second shock: 200 J
Check pulse
15 compressions
Read ECG
6 If fibrillation still present

↓

Give third shock: 400 J
Check pulse
15 compressions
Read ECG
7 If fibrillation still present

↓

Give lignocaine

↓

Give fourth shock: 400 J
Check pulse
15 compressions
Read ECG
8 If fibrillation still present

↓

Give adrenaline

↓

Give fifth shock: 400 J
Check pulse
15 compressions
Read ECG
9 If fibrillation still present

↓

Give sodium bicarbonate

↓

Give sixth shock: 400 J

Fig. 12.16 Sequence of steps for electrical defibrillation.

Asystole

Ventricular asystole is the commonest cause of cardiac arrest associated with anaesthesia induction or surgical procedures. Atropine (0.5–1.2 mg) given intravenously can be very effective. If asystole is diagnosed a vigorous blow on the precordium can sometimes restart the heart. If it does not, CPR should be started immediately. Isoprenaline can be a useful drug in this setting.

Ventricular asystole due to complete atrioventricular block with an extremely slow ventricular rate may require temporary pacing. This technique is discussed in Chapter 1. Ventricular asystole due to extensive myocardial damage does not respond to pacing. The calcium antagonist drugs are of no value in the treatment of asystole.

Atrial arrhythmias very rarely cause cardiac arrest unless ventricular function is so bad as to be virtually dependent on atrial systole.

Electromechanical dissociation

In electromechanical dissociation there is evidence of satisfactory electrical activity on the ECG but there is failure of an effective output. It is important to recognize the possible causes of this condition, which are:

1. Hypovolaemia due to severe haemorrhage
2. Pericardial tamponade
3. Tension pneumothorax
4. Pulmonary embolism
5. Myocardial rupture

Signs of these problems should be sought and appropriate treatment instituted. The treatment of pericardial tamponade is considered in Chapter 8. The treatment of pulmonary embolism is dealt with in Chapter 3. The treatment of a tension pneumothorax requires the insertion of a needle or tube into the pleural space on the appropriate side of the chest. Little can be done for myocardial rupture.

Establishment of an intravenous route

If the resuscitation procedure is not immediately successful, a centrally placed intravenous catheter is required. This is inserted while external cardiac compression and ventilation are being continued. The ideal veins to use are the jugular or the subclavian. If the intravenous route cannot be established, drugs can be administered via the endotracheal tube into the bronchial tree.

Other drugs

Sodium bicarbonate
With a protracted arrest a metabolic acidosis is likely to develop. This may adversely affect the likelihood of restoring a normal rhythm. It is important not to give too much sodium bicarbonate because this will result in metabolic alkalosis,

hyperosmolality and impaired release of oxygen to the organs that need it. If the arrest is not immediately successful, sodium bicarbonate (1 mmol/kg) is administered. Half this dose is then repeated approximately every 15 minutes.

Calcium chloride
Calcium chloride enhances the contractile state of the heart. It is useful when there is severe hypotension and electromechanical dissociation that are refractory to adrenaline or isoprenaline.

Summary of definitive treatment

The scheme outlined in Fig. 12.17 is suggested by the Resuscitation Council of the UK.

When to stop

Despite full resuscitation the patient may not regain a spontaneous circulation. The decision to stop performing CPR is influenced by a number of factors and the following guidelines are used:

1. Absence of any electrical activity of the heart
2. Electrical activity that persists without any effective cardiac output
3. Persistent fixed dilated pupils
4. Presence of an incurable or incapacitating disease
5. Delay between collapse and the start of CPR

These guidelines need to be altered in patients with hypothermia, a barbiturate overdose or after drowning. Full recovery can take place in these instances even after several hours of resuscitation.

Post-arrest care

Patients who have been resuscitated successfully usually require monitoring in an intensive care setting. They continue to be prone to cardiac arrhythmias and to haemodynamic and respiratory instability. Ventilatory support on a ventilator may be necessary. The following measures are usually performed:

1. With laryngoscope, check position of endotracheal tube
2. Ensure adequate ventilation and use supplemental oxygen
3. Estimate arterial pH and blood gases
4. Estimate serum potassium
5. Arrange chest x-ray
6. Insert urinary catheter
7. Arrange 12-lead ECG

For the prevention of cerebral oedema the patient is usually hyperventilated, keeping the arterial P_{CO_2} at a level below 4 kPa (30 mmHg) for 24 hours. There is no evidence that steroids have any benefit.

It is important to try to identify the cause of the arrest in order to prevent

CARDIOPULMONARY RESUSCITATION

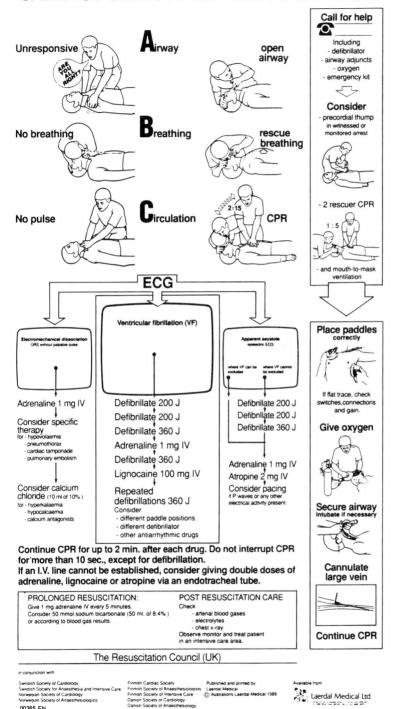

Call for help

Including
- defibrillator
- airway adjuncts
  - oxygen
- emergency kit

Consider
- precordial thump
  in witnessed or
  monitored arrest

- 2 rescuer CPR
  1 : 5

- and mouth-to-mask
  ventilation

Unresponsive — **A**irway — open airway

No breathing — **B**reathing — rescue breathing

No pulse — **C**irculation — 2:15 — CPR

ECG

Electromechanical dissociation QRS without palpable pulse	Ventricular fibrillation (VF)	Apparent asystole isoelectric ECG	
		where VF can be excluded	where VF cannot be excluded

Adrenaline 1 mg IV	Defibrillate 200 J	Defibrillate 200 J	
	Defibrillate 200 J	Defibrillate 200 J	
Consider specific therapy for - hypovolaemia - pneumothorax - cardiac tamponade - pulmonary embolism	Defibrillate 360 J	Defibrillate 360 J	
	Adrenaline 1 mg IV		
	Defibrillate 360 J	Adrenaline 1 mg IV	
	Lignocaine 100 mg IV	Atropine 2 mg IV	
Consider calcium chloride (10 ml of 10%) for - hyperkalaemia - hypocalcaemia - calcium antagonists	Repeated defibrillations 360 J Consider - different paddle positions - different defibrillator - other antiarrhythmic drugs	Consider pacing if P waves or any other electrical activity present	

Place paddles correctly

If flat trace, check switches, connections and gain.

Give oxygen

Secure airway
Intubate if necessary

Cannulate large vein

Continue CPR

Continue CPR for up to 2 min. after each drug. Do not interrupt CPR for more than 10 sec., except for defibrillation.
If an I.V. line cannot be established, consider giving double doses of adrenaline, lignocaine or atropine via an endotracheal tube.

PROLONGED RESUSCITATION:	POST RESUSCITATION CARE
Give 1 mg adrenaline IV every 5 minutes. Consider 50 mmol sodium bicarbonate (50 ml. of 8.4%) or according to blood gas results.	Check - arterial blood gases - electrolytes - chest x-ray Observe monitor and treat patient in an intensive care area.

The Resuscitation Council (UK)

in conjunction with

Swedish Society of Cardiology
Swedish Society for Anaesthesia and Intensive Care
Norwegian Society of Cardiology
Norwegian Society of Anaesthesiologists
00365 EN

Finnish Cardiac Society
Finnish Society of Anaesthesiologists
Finnish Society of Intensive Care
Danish Society of Cardiology
Danish Society of Anaesthesiology

Published and printed by
Laerdal Medical
© illustrations Laerdal Medical 1989

Available from

Laerdal Medical Ltd.

Fig. 12.17 Summary of definitive treatment. (Reproduced by courtesy of the Resuscitation Council of the United Kingdom.)

further episodes. Potential problems that may occur after the arrest include acute renal failure, bowel infarction, infection and sepsis.

Patients who regain consciousness may well have amnesia for the event. They may also develop abnormal behaviour. Both the patient and the family will need advice and appropriate reassurance during the recovery period. After an arrest it is all too easy to forget the needs of other patients who have witnessed the procedure; they will need some help in coping with an alarming experience.

Whom to resuscitate

It is clear that some patients ought not to be resuscitated if they collapse. It is also abundantly clear that the decision about who should and who should not be resuscitated must be made well in advance of an arrest. It is important to emphasize that the decision relates only to the collapse of the patient; care up to that point is entirely normal. The patient with terminal cancer or other serious life-limiting pathology ought to be allowed to die with dignity. The whole cardiac arrest procedure is a very undignified process and not without risk. The decision about who should not be resuscitated must be made at a senior level and should ideally involve not only the medical staff but also the nursing staff. The next of kin or close relatives of the patient can also be included in the decision-making process. Care must be taken to ensure that the responsibility for the final decision about the patient is not perceived to be left with the relative; nevertheless, involvement in the decision is entirely appropriate and to be encouraged. There are occasions when the patient should also be involved in this process; this is not appropriate in some instances. It must always be done in a very sensitive manner.

Drowning and near-drowning

Human beings have been recovered from the water apparently dead after as much as 40 minutes' submersion and yet still make a full recovery. The reasons for this remarkable phenomenon are only partly understood; the theories include the presence of the diving reflex in humans and the protective effect of hypothermia. The diving reflex is present in aquatic mammals but has not yet been shown to be present in man. It enables mammals to shunt blood away from tissues that can metabolize anaerobically and redistribute it to organs such as the heart and brain which have little anaerobic capacity. Slowing of the heart rate also occurs. Cooling of the body prolongs the safe period for which the circulation can be stopped; this is probably the single most important factor in humans, and particularly in children and infants in whom circulatory arrest occurs at a lower temperature than adults and in whom core cooling occurs more quickly.

Whatever the reasons for the remarkable phenomenon, rescuers should continue for at least an hour even though there is no initial sign of life. The techniques of CPR are identical to those described above. At one stage it was taught that the lungs should first be emptied of water by a variety of manoeuvres; this is usually unnecessary because there is little water actually down in the lung itself and much time can be wasted for little return. The large airways can be emptied of water relatively easily.

It is very difficult to continue effective CPR while transporting a patient; CPR is therefore continued until a pulse has been re-established, before starting to move the patient.

Changes can occur in the electrolyte concentrations. Hypernatraemia occurs after salt-water drowning and hyponatraemia after fresh-water drowning. Hypokalaemia develops after either. Acute pulmonary oedema may occur as a result of some aspiration into the lungs. There is usually a warning of this complication, reflected in a falling arterial Po_2. Ventilation of the patient may be required.

Resuscitation of infants and children

Hypoxia is the most common cause of cardiac arrest in infants and children. Ventricular fibrillation and ventricular tachycardia are usually not a primary problem. The other causes of arrest include septicaemia, congenital heart disease and the loss of blood or body fluids such as with gastroenteritis.

The approach to the resuscitation of infants and children is similar to that described above; there are, however, some important differences, which will be emphasized below.

Airway

Opening the airway involves tilting the head and supporting the lower jaw (Fig. 12.18a). Care must be taken to avoid overextending the neck and causing the soft trachea to obstruct. Pressure ought not to be applied to the soft tissues in the floor of the mouth as this will force the tongue to obstruct the airway.

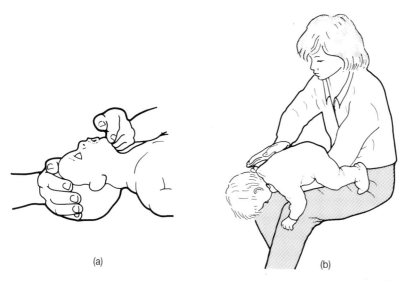

(a)   (b)

Fig. 12.18 (a) The position necessary to open the airway in an infant or young child. **(b)** The position that can be adopted to relieve obstruction caused by a foreign body in an infant or young child.

The small infant is an obligatory nose breather, so the patency of the nasal passage must be checked.

Obstruction

This may be caused by vomit or by a foreign body. Careful removal is essential; rough handling can make the situation worse. Inverting the child and applying back blows is an effective and safe way of clearing the obstruction (Fig. 12.18b). The Heimlich manoeuvre (abdominal thrust) can be used in older children.

Infectious diseases of the upper airway can cause respiratory obstruction. Croup is a term used when there is inspiratory stridor. Breathing humidified air may help this condition but inexperienced further measures may lead to a rapid worsening of the condition. The child will need to be moved to a hospital to be cared for by an expert team with the necessary equipment.

Breathing

Expired air ventilation must be started immediately if the child is not breathing. With the airway held open the rescuer should cover the infant's mouth and nose with his mouth and breathe gently into the infant until the chest is seen to rise. The appropriate volume can be judged by the observation of the chest movement. Ventilation can be increased by raising the rate but the volume should not be changed. The rate of breathing should be in the order of 15–30 breaths per minute according to the size of the infant: the smaller, the faster.

Circulation

The circulation is assessed by feeling the brachial pulse, which is easier than the carotid in the small child or infant. A bradycardia may accompany the hypoxia and will improve as the latter is treated.

If there is no adequate pulse, external cardiac massage must be started. The site of compression is the same as in an adult. The method of compression depends on the size of the patient. A small baby is best managed using both hands encircling the chest; the sternum is compressed by both thumbs and support is supplied by the interlaced fingers behind the back. In a larger subject two fingers can apply the pressure, and in a larger child the heel of the hand can be used (Fig. 12.19).

The rate and pressure will also depend on the size of the subject. The pressure requires to generate a peripheral pulse and will need to be modified accordingly. A rate of about 100 per minute is required. A ratio of 5 compressions to 1 ventilation is the ideal for small children and infants.

Advanced life support

The use of equipment for advanced life support is full of difficulties. A wide range of equipment must be available to correspond with the various sizes of child. The rescuer must also be skilled enough to be able to use the equipment effectively.

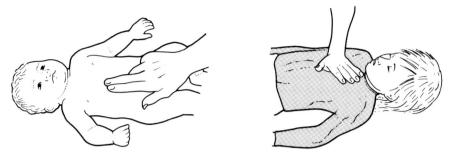

Fig. 12.19 The technique of external cardiac massage in (**a**)an infant or (**b**) a young child.

The paediatric airway must be of the appropriate size. Both oropharyngeal and nasopharyngeal airways are available in different sizes. In intubation is required, it must be performed by a person with the appropriate skills. If defibrillation is required, small paediatric paddles are necessary. The energy level can be calculated on the basis of 2 J/kg body weight. Intravenous access is one of the main difficulties with a paediatric arrest; the choice of cannula and its siting are matters of personal preference. Knowledge of the fluid requirements and the drug dosages for the size of child is crucial. Alternative routes by which to give drugs include the endotracheal tube or a needle inserted into the bone marrow.

The maintenance of the child's temperature is important during the arrest procedure. Care after successful resuscitation is similar in principle to the care of the adult.

Further reading

Evans, T. R. (Ed.) (1986) *ABC of Resuscitation*. British Medial Journal, London.

13

<hr>

PSYCHOLOGICAL ASPECTS OF CARDIOVASCULAR DISEASE

Cardiovascular disorders remain the major cause of death in the industrialized world. Considerable success has been achieved in reducing death due to infectious diseases; for example, we have recently witnessed the eradication of smallpox with preventative and environmental measures. In contrast, little progress has been made in the prevention or cure of cardiovascular disorders, largely because their aetiology is poorly understood. There is increasing evidence of the need to abandon the unidimensional, biological models for cardiovascular diseases. Instead it is necessary to take into account social, behavioural, emotional and personality factors. In a number of cardiovascular disorders the influence of psychological factors on the genesis and aetiology is well documented. Recent research has improved our understanding of the ways in which psychological conditions may interact with physiological regulatory mechanisms, leading to new approaches to treatment or prevention.

Coronary artery disease

The aetiology of coronary artery disease is multifactorial. Most of the accepted predisposing risk factors have been discussed in Chapter 1. There are major limitations to this rather narrow approach to the identification of those at particular risk. Firstly, a high proportion of patients who develop coronary artery disease do not have treatable risk factors; secondly, a large proportion of patients with risk factors do not develop the disease. Psychosocial characteristics are important and can be overlooked in this era of the 'high technology' approach to disease.

Two approaches have been taken to assess the psychosocial factors: the first has been to attempt to identify a particular behaviour pattern; the second has been to identify potentially stressful situations that may increase the risk of coronary artery disease.

Type A behaviour pattern

Clinical observation of patients in the late 1950s led cardiologists to describe a 'coronary-prone behaviour pattern'. The features of this type A behaviour include excessive competitiveness, sense of being under time pressure, sustained aggression and easily provoked hostility. These people are impatient, constantly alert and often intensely committed to achieving goals. People who do not display these characteristics and act in a more relaxed and deliberate manner are labelled type B. Type A behaviour is not strictly a personality-type although it is often called type A personality. Type A behaviour is generally regarded as pattern or response style, rather than as a fixed personality trait or attribute. The type A characteristics are not present all the time but emerge only with appropriate challenges. It was first shown to be an independent risk factor for coronary artery disease in 1975 and achieved widespread acceptance in North America over the next few years. The hostility component is a very potent risk factor.

Longitudinal studies in the USA have demonstrated that people categorized as having type A behaviour pattern, on the basis of a behavioural personality test, have more than twice the incidence of coronary artery disease than have those diagnosed as type B. The type A behaviour pattern appears to play an independent and statistically proven role, and occurs in both men and women and in various cultures. Depending on the method of assessment, the type A behaviour pattern is independent of other common emotional or personality variables and of social class. European epidemiological studies have not shown quite the same close link with type A behaviour and coronary artery disease. Type A behaviour pattern does not appear to be a feature of Japanese society; perhaps this is because the culture is characterized by a high degree of social support whilst individual competitiveness is discouraged in favour of, or loyalty to, the organization.

Stressful life events

Stressful life events have been shown to be associated with an increased likelihood of illness. Such events include bereavement, divorce or separation, moving house or the birth of a child. The life events can be weighted according to their relative stress. The relative weighting can be measured in life change units (Table 13.1).

Bereavement has been studied extensively. Widowers aged 55 and over have been shown to have an increased mortality, largely from cardio- and cerebro-vascular disease, and especially coronary thombosis, during the first 6 months following bereavement. After a year the mortality rate returns to that usually expected. In a survey of 903 bereaved relatives in a semi-rural area of Wales, 4.8 per cent had died within a year, compared with 0.6 per cent in a non-bereaved comparison group. There is an increased consultation rate for both psychiatric and physical conditions in the first 6 months of bereavement, but the classic psychosomatic illnesses show no increase.

Complementary to research on particular events such as bereavement, at-

Table 13.1   Some life change events, ranked in descending order of perceived importance

Health	Work
Recent illness (in bed for 1 week, or hospitalization)	Recently out of work
	Recently fired from work
Change in heavy physical work or exercise	Change to new type of work
	Change in work responsibilities
Change in sleeping habits	Troubles with boss
Change in eating habits	Work going well

Home and family	Personal and social
Concern over health of a family member	Death of spouse
	Divorce
Recently married	Held in jail
Separation from spouse due to marital problems	Sexual difficulties
	Death of a close relative
Gaining a new family member	Death of a close friend
Separation from spouse due to work	Unpaid bills leading to threatened legal action
Engaged to be married	
Son or daughter leaving home	Change in personal habits
Troubles with in-laws	
Change to a new residence	
Vacation	

tempts have been made to estimate the amount of stress brought about by events that occur in everyday life. The results have tended to be interesting but confusing. The occurrence of a myocardial infarct or sudden death in connection with a traumatic life event is a common observation in clinical practice. The family doctor will recognize this coincidence more frequently perhaps than the hospital specialist. Chronic or acute conflicts, strains or dissatisfactions at work, particularly conflicts with bosses and co-workers, stand out among the events preceding myocardial infarction. There is a higher incidence of coronary artery disease in this group with prolonged work, family or financial problems. Among the men who have such problems, the incidence of coronary artery disease is higher when their wives were reported as being cold or indifferent, than among those with the same problems who described their wives as showing them love and giving them support.

Patients with a myocardial infarct have gone through more life changes in the year prior to their attack, both at work and in family situations, than have controls. Although a major stressful life event can immediately precede the development of a myocardial infarct or sudden death, it is often a relatively minor stress that precipitates the event. This minor stress will often occur in the context of increased emotional vulnerability which can be associated with chronic depression, fatigue, frustration or disappointment. This 'life setting' that appears to be conducive to illness was described by Engel in 1968 as 'the giving-up–given-up complex'. Examination of the life setting in which patients fall ill has revealed that the presenting illness is preceded by a period of psychological disturbance during which the patient feels unable to cope. This has five psychological characteristics:

1. A feeling of giving up, experienced as helplessness or hopelessness
2. A depreciated image of the self
3. A sense of loss of gratification from relationships or roles in life
4. A feeling of disruption of the sense of continuity between past, present and future
5. Reactivation of memories of earlier periods of giving up

This state may reflect the temporary failure of the mental coping mechanisms, with consequent activation of the neurally regulated biological emergency patterns. It is a contributory factor to the development of the disease but is not propounded as a cause of the disease.

The social network

The social network and prevailing mores may have very important influences on the effects of coronary prone behaviour. Social networks are becoming increasingly recognized as being of central importance in influencing the ways in which psychosocial factors affect the health of an individual. The relationships between social networks, social support, isolation, social integration and mortality are now being studied extensively.

Coronary artery disease is more common in wealthy countries than in poor countries. Paradoxically, it is the poorer groups who are most at risk in the wealthy countries. This arose in the 1950s, when the mortality from cardiovascular disease in working class men rose more steeply and overtook the mortality in the middle and upper classes. The reasons for this change are not completely understood. Only a small component can be accounted for by smoking habits, which have become relatively more common in working class men and women. The effect of the accumulation of job strains and status insecurity in the lower classes has been shown to be more important. It has been suggested that those in the lower socioeconomic groups are less well able to cope successfully with adversity because they have less money, knowledge and social contacts than those in the middle and upper classes.

Psychobiological mechanisms

There are several potential pathways by which psychosocial factors can damage the arteries and the heart. Stress has been shown to raise the serum cholesterol level. The reverse has also been shown; behaviour modification and relaxation exercises can reduce the serum cholesterol level. It is well established that normal people may develop transient rises in blood pressure in response to threatening life events. Yoga and biofeedback techniques have been used successfully in the treatment of elevated blood pressure. Excessive liberation of catecholamines under conditions of arousal, aggression, anxiety and stress may be harmful. Individuals with type A behaviour respond to stimuli with a heightened and prolonged neuroendocrine and sympathetic nervous system activation. These levels persist for a time after the stimulus has ceased, in contrast to those individuals with type B behaviour. There are other theoretical links mediated through the haemostatic pathways; platelet aggregation and fibrinolytic activity, together with fibrinogen levels may be adversely altered in stressful states and could be one of the links between stress and coronary artery disease.

The reaction of the circulation to emotion has been studied much less intensely than has the reaction to exercise. In those researches that have been performed, it has invariably been found that both normal individuals and patients with coronary artery disease respond to emotional arousal with as marked rises in blood pressure, pulse rate or cardiac output as during the performance of heavy work.

The use of psychophysiological and psychobiological techniques in the investigation of cardiovascular disease has increased in the last 10 years. Hypotheses that relate behaviour and emotion to the aetiology and prognosis of cardiovascular disease have stimulated medical and behavioural scientists to explore the cardiovascular and neuroendocrine responses to psychological stimuli. Most of the research has concentrated on the acute experimental situation. Methods of assessing reactivity in everyday life are now being developed. There are many uncertainties about the tests or tasks that should be presented, which physiological variables should be measured and how the responses should be analysed. The problem is further compounded when psychophysiological test procedures are applied to clinical groups that differ either in haemodynamic status or in the drugs that they are taking. There are also complex methodological issues involved in dealing with the vexed problem of adaptation: cardiovascular and neuroendocrine responses frequently diminish with repeated stimuli. The degree of adaptation varies with the nature of the task as well as with the physiological variable being monitored. The relevance of gender and the menstrual cycle to tests in women is also important; the female sex hormones may influence the autoregulatory adjustments.

The interrelationships that exist between the conventional risk factors, the genetic make-up, the behaviour and personality characteristics together with the cardiovascular, neuroendocrine and haemostatic responsiveness are extremely complex. Tremendous advances in research have been made in the various disciplines and also between disciplines. The scene would appear to be set for the development of a much fuller understanding of the complexities of these interrelationships and how they might contribute to the development of coronary artery disease and its complications.

The development of behavioural methods for managing coronary artery disease

The classic biological risk factors, such as cholesterol level, and the more obvious psychological factors can be altered by procedures based on the principles and methods of psychology. There is limited but encouraging evidence that such alterations reduce the likelihood of cardiovascular disease.

The effects of stress management can last for at least 4 years. The best results have been obtained in studies in which the relaxation training is live rather than taped, the patients are encouraged to practise regularly at home and there is an explicit effort to teach the patients to apply the techniques to manage stress in daily life. There are a number of relaxation techniques; these include breathing exercises, progressive muscle relaxation, yogic relaxation posture called Shavanson and several meditative techniques such as Zen, yoga, sufism and Christian prayer. These are all known to be stress reducing and produce a similar physiological response and state of altered consciousness. A biofeedback instrument can sometimes be used to teach relaxation; this will measure and display some physiological function. The person connected to the instrument tries to alter that function in the desired direction by a self-induced change in the subjective state. For instance, galvanic skin resistance with auditory feedback may enable the person to relax the tone of the muscles; as the tone relaxes, so the auditory signal becomes fainter. The sensitivity is then increased and the subject has to relax more deeply before the signals will stop, and so on.

Intervention to alter type A behaviour can, after a myocardial infarction, reduce the likelihood of a further recurrence by 50 per cent compared with a control group. This is a larger reduction than has been achieved with any drug intervention! The participants who showed substantial change in their type A behaviour at the end of 1 year, were four times less likely to have a myocardial infarction in the subsequent 2 years.

The likelihood that simpler, quicker, cheaper and more effective interventions can reduce the risk of recurrence of myocardial infarction is supported by an interesting attempt to deal with stress in the year following an infarction; in this study, patients in an intervention group were regularly contacted by phone and a questionnaire about general health was administered. If symptoms of stress were detected, the patient was visited by a nurse counsellor who took whatever action seemed appropriate.

It is important to remember some common defence or self-preservation mechanisms that are used by both healthy individuals and unwell patients. If they are not recognized and dealt with appropriately by the attendant doctor, the problems may become increasingly detrimental to the subject. Denial is a very common defence reaction to situations of stress. Denial is defined in this context as the conscious or unconscious repudiation of part or all of the totally available meaning of an event in order to allay fear, anxiety or other threatening effects. Displacement may be another form of denial: subjects convince themselves that the pain or discomfort is caused by indigestion or some other 'safer' symptom. Rationalization is yet another means by which the serious symptom of chest pain can be denied; for example, a patient may subconsciously argue that this cannot be pain from the heart 'because I'm too young'.

Psychophysiological aspects of essential hypertension

Sociocultural factors

Blood pressure levels are lower in groups or societies that are based on firm tradition and stable social structures. In societies in which traditions are disintegrating or those in transition such as the southern US Black society in the late 1950s, blood pressure in the population rises. Citizens living in the higher crime and lower socioeconomic part of a city have a higher level of blood pressure than those living in the part with low crime rates. There is less hypertension among rural than urban Zulus; of the latter, more of those who cling to traditional cultural practices and are unable to adapt to the demands of urban living become hypertensive.

Animal models provide further evidence. The manipulation of the social hierarchy of an animal species provides evidence for implicating social and behavioural factors in pathophysiological processes. Socially deprived mice, for instance, when introduced into an established colony with their own hierarchy, develop an increased incidence of hypertension, myocardial fibrosis and renal failure. The aggressive and submissive behaviours are associated with increased secretion of catecholamines or corticosteroids. When the new social roles are established the increased neuroendocrine activity ceases.

Psychological factors

Life changes and traumatic life events have been associated with the onset of sustained hypertension and with a shift from the mild to the accelerated form. In addition, specific personality traits have been implicated as contributory to the development of hypertension. The hypertensive personality may be described as an individual who frequently manifests inhibited and poorly expressed rage and anger. Yet outwardly the hypertensive person manifests a desire to please and a wish to be liked. It is possible that these traits derive from early experience with individuals on whom the person depended and towards whom anger and hostility could not be expressed, because of the real or imagined threat of loss of love. The desire to please and be approved of by authority figures combined with a rebellious unconscious posture is felt to be characteristic of many individuals with essential hypertension.

The measurement of an individual's physiological changes when under a psychological stress is a promising means of identifying people with an enhanced vulnerability to this type of stress. Normotensive air traffic controllers who subsequently become hypertensive for example, show greater reactivity and larger blood pressure responses on the job than do their peers who remain normotensive. The individual's physiological response to mental provocation does have discriminating and predictive value and may provide useful additional information in the detection, prevention and management of cardiovascular disorders.

Much of the initial work in cardiovascular psychophysiology was restricted to observations of the ways in which psychological processes affect heart rate and blood pressure. The ability to measure the baroreflex sensitivity has broadened the approach. Subjects with an elevated blood pressure have a reduced baro-reflex sensitivity. The explanations of this loss of sensitivity have varied: some have argued that it is a direct loss of sensitivity whilst others have suggested a resetting to a higher threshold. A more comprehensive hypothesis about the pathophysiology of essential hypertension suggests an interaction between elevated blood pressure and the pain regulatory mechanisms. Activation of the baroreceptor reflex arc results in central inhibitory effects that reduce the aversion to noxious stimulation and hence reinforce blood pressure elevation.

Under frequent stressful conditions, hypertension could develop through conditioning, with the baroreceptors adapting their sensitivity to the ensuing pressor responses. There are several examples that appear to lend support to this hypothesis. For instance, it has been found that workers at the Volvo factory in Sweden had a positive correlation between hearing loss and blood pressure. The prolonged exposure to a stressful stimulus, in this instance the noise, may cause repeated rises in blood pressure, leading to a circulatory adaptation and a permanent rise in blood pressure. The direct consequence of these environmental events is a central state of discomfort or aversiveness. In a conventional scheme there is a pathway that translates central aversiveness into a peripheral physiological response or symptom. For hypertension this is usually thought to be some combination of humoral or neural mechanism which eventually has an effect on the blood pressure. There may be an additional mechanism which depends on instrumental learning of blood pressure and an intrinsic baroreceptor-mediated reinforcement mechanism (Fig. 13.1). A substantial body of work has now accumulated which indicates that baroreceptor stimulation has many of the properties commonly associated with certain behavioural reinforcers; in particular, its action resembles that of addictive drugs.

The effect of baroreceptor stimulation is to ameliorate anxiety or reduce the aversiveness of noxious stimuli. If baroreceptor stimulation is an effective reinforcer, and blood pressure elevation a learnable response, since the inevitable consequence of blood pressure elevation is stimulation of the baroreceptors, elevation of blood pressure could be expected to more or less automatically trigger the baroreceptor reinforcement mechanisms. In the presence of noxious stimuli or anxiety the patient may learn to elevate blood pressure as a way of self-stimulating the baroreceptors and consequently reducing the aversiveness of the situation.

Under the baroreceptor reinforcement hypothesis a number of definable factors, such as behavioural and genetic, interact to produce hypertension as the emergent problem.

The development of behavioural methods for managing essential hypertension

This has been one of the great successes in behavioural medicine. Research has moved beyond the stage of the simple demonstration of the effects of behavioural interventions in the laboratory. Many different groups have now shown the beneficial effects of behavioural programmes on the ambulatory blood pressure and have shown that the lowered blood pressure can persist for months or years. Many of these studies are based on the assumption that stress is involved in the aetiology of hypertension; the behavioural approach can include programmes to help develop coping skills in everyday life, biofeedback techniques, psychotherapeutic intervention and stress management training. Successful blood pressure reductions are associated with improved coping skills and alteration in the ways in which patients view their social and physical environment. It is possible that some of the benefit is associated with the alterations in patterns of

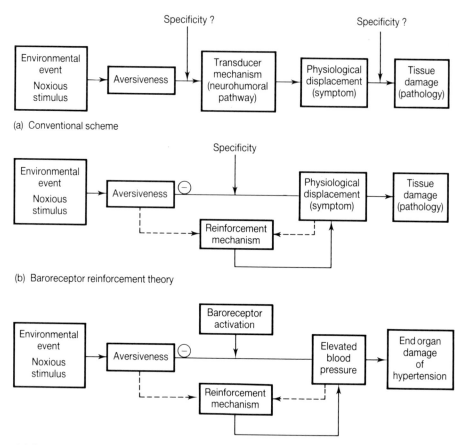

Fig. 13.1 Outline of the pathogenesis of psychosomatic disease: (**a**) the conventional scheme; (**b**) the baroreceptor reinforcement theory and (**c**) the baroreceptor reinforcement theory of essential hypertension. The first two blocks in (**a**) and (**b**) are identical; a disturbing event produces a central state of aversiveness. In (**a**) this state, acting through an innate pathway, produces a symptom. In (**b**), the instrumental or learning model, the central state of aversiveness need not have a direct effect on the symptom; the symptom must, though, reduce the level of aversiveness. This reduction in aversiveness is a reinforcing stimulus that rewards and strengthens the symptom. In (**c**) is illustrated the instrumental learning scheme of hypertension.

harmful behaviour, rather than the relaxation-based behavioural therapy itself.

It is clearly important to be able to identify those people who are most likely to benefit from any particular approach and to tailor the therapy appropriately. Certain psychological characteristics can be identified that are important in predicting outcome. Behavioural therapies can be administered by trained personnel without medical or psychological qualifications. They can be integrated with both the general advice and encouragement to adopt a healthy lifestyle and to give up smoking, as well as with the pharmacological approaches to management.

Cardiac arrhythmias

Psychosocial stress has been known for many hundreds of years to be a risk factor for sudden cardiac death. Poets and authors throughout history have recognized the links between the heart, the emotions and death. Almost 2000 years ago, Celsus described how emotional states could influence the heart. More recently, John Hunter (1728–1793), a very distinguished surgeon and surgeon general to the King, commented 'my life is in the hands of any rascal who chooses to annoy or tease me'. He knew that he had heart disease which is now recognized as angina. His prediction was proved correct when, at a board meeting at St George's Hospital, a colleague made some disparaging remarks about him and precipitated his rapid death. Voodoo deaths are another example of such a link between psychological stress and death. Surprisingly little attention has been paid to the connection between psychological stress and arrhythmias, in contrast to the huge interest in the effect of drug treatment on the rhythm of the heart. It is unwise to extrapolate the results of animal research too quickly to the human. However, it is of considerable interest that, in some animals, defined stressor events must be present for coronary artery occlusion to result in ventricular fibrillation! Moreover, this evoked ventricular fibrillation in stressed animals can be prevented by learned adaption to the stressor or blockade of the frontocortical projections to the brain-stem cardiovascular nuclei or the intracerebral (but not intravenous) injection of propranolol.

Patients with heart disease and a lot of ectopic activity have been shown to have an exaggerated cerebral response to a benign stimulus. This exaggerated response is manifested by a characteristic waveform in the electroencephalogram (EEG). These findings raise the possibility that the primary trigger and/or cause of unexpected sudden death may be related to cerebral noradrenergic over-reaction. This transmits a pattern of dual autonomic output to the heart, which increases its vulnerability to arrhythmias. The location of this cerebral dysfunction appears to be in the frontal lobes. In humans there is also some evidence that psychological stress can lower the threshold for ventricular fibrillation.

Mitral valve prolapse

The association of mitral valve prolapse (discussed in Chapter 4) and panic attacks has been described for a number of years. There have been a profusion of papers linking these symptoms to the underlying prolapsing valve; associated abnormal hormonal changes have also been described. The possible links between panic disorder and mitral valve prolapse have been overemphasized. If they exist, they are small and not specific to the mitral valve prolapse and are of no clinical help or significance.

The link with neurotic behaviour is more likely to be through weight loss; mitral valve prolapse occurs in patients with anorexia and in those with weight loss due to other conditions.

Panic disorder and hyperventilation

Panic disorder

Among psychiatric conditions, symptoms of panic disorder comprise one of the commonest reasons for which people seek professional help. At the beginning of the disorder the patients present not to psychiatrists or psychologists, but to primary care doctors, physicians or accident and emergency departments. Cardiovascular complaints number among the patients' most frequent and distressing symptoms. Indeed, many sufferers have intense fear that they may sustain a heart attack during a panic episode.

Panic attacks are discrete episodes of intense fear or discomfort with symptoms such as dyspnoea, palpitation, chest pain, faintness, sweating, hot flushes or chills, feelings of unreality, or fear of dying or going crazy. Panic attacks have a sudden onset and can occur unpredictably. The attacks usually last minutes, sometimes hours but never days. After a panic attack the sufferer may be drained physically and emotionally and will often have apprehension of a further attack. Many patients may develop phobic avoidance behaviour. Interest in this condition as a separate entity is very recent although Sigmund Freud described the phenomenon in 1895.

Cardiovascular manifestations of anxiety have been known in the medical and psychological sciences for a long time. Over the last 100 years clinical descriptions of patients with a variety of diagnoses (Table 13.2) have borne many similarities to the diagnostic criteria for panic attacks. Interest in these conditions is always stimulated in times of war when some young men become incapacitated by functional cardiac symptoms. In times of peace similar syndromes are described, but mostly in women. There is still a lot of controversy about the aetiology of this condition. It is of interest that many of the current research ideas, such as the relationship with hyperventilation, blood acid–base balance or exercise intolerance, were already mentioned in the literature of nineteenth and early twentieth centuries!

Table 13.2 Syndromes that have been described which have features similar to panic disorder and which may be associated with hyperventilation

Neurasthenia	Irritable heart
Anxiety neurosis	Cardiac neurosis
Soldier's heart	Effort syndrome
Neurocirculatory asthenia	Da Costa's syndrome
Hyperkinetic heart syndrome	Vasoregulatory asthenia
Nervous heart complaint	

Hyperventilation

The lack of satisfactory or widely accepted criteria for the definition and diagnosis of hyperventilation has hindered the understanding of the pathophysiological and psychopathological processes involved. Some have even expressed doubt about the existence of such a disorder. Although it was a commonly diagnosed disorder between the two world wars, most of the modern standard textbooks of medicine do not even mention it.

The term 'hyperventilation syndrome' was first used in 1937 to describe the spontaneous occurrence of prolonged hyperventilation related to anxiety, in the absence of ascertainable organic disease. Subsequent investigation of this syndrome by physicians, psychiatrists and psychologists has led to a profusion of descriptive accounts but very little consensus. An extraordinary array of terms have been used in which hyperventilation is now considered to play a part (see Table 13.2).

Hyperventilation is a physiological term that implies the breathing in excess of metabolic requirements and cannot be present without hypocapnia (Table 13.3).

Table 13.3 Some causes of hypocapnia

Physiological	Pyrexia
	High altitude
Organic	Asthma
	Pulmonary embolus
	Heart failure
	Severe pain
	CNS lesions
Drugs	Aspirin
Psychiatric	Anxiety
	Panic
	Depression
Idiopathic	Chronic hyperventilation

The symptoms of hypocapnia and hyperventilation are varied and not specific. Tetany is rare, and tingling around the lips occurs occasionally. Atypical chest pain and dyspnoea are common presentations; these can sometimes be associated with ST segment changes on the resting or ambulatory ECG. The dyspnoea can manifest itself as air hunger or an inability to take a satisfying breath. The more common symptoms and the suggested mechanisms are shown in Table 13.4.

The diagnosis of hyperventilation can be difficult, as can finding the evidence of a causal link with the symptoms. Measurement of end-tidal P_{CO_2} at rest and after a variety of stressors sometimes produces helpful information. The diagnosis is not an end in itself; the next step is to discover the aetiological factors, which may be multiple. A careful, full history will often begin to unravel the relevant complex interactions between different organic and psychosocial factors, which may explain the precipitation and persistence of the symptoms. It is important not to miss previously undiagnosed asthma, which can have many similarities to hyperventilation and panic attacks.

The treatment of panic disorder or hyperventilation can be considered in several stages. The first step is to exclude any underlying organic disease as the

Table 13.4   Some symptoms and their possible mechanisms associated with hyperventilation

System	Symptom	Possible mechanism
Cardiac	Left-sided chest pain Central chest pain Palpitation	Spasm/fatigue of intercostal muscles Coronary artery spasm Paroxysmal arrhythmia
CNS	Dizziness, syncope	Cerebral vasoconstriction
Respiratory	Sighing/air hunger	Enhanced proprioception from intercostal muscles
Gastrointestinal	Dry mouth Retrosternal pain	Mouth breathing Increase in oesophageal contractility
Psychiatric	Poor concentration Panic, anxiety	Cerebral vasoconstriction Any hyperventilation-induced symptom can induce panic if interpreted in a catastrophic fashion
General	Weakness, listlessness	Increase in sympathetic nervous system activity

cause of the symptoms; the patient needs to be appropriately reassured. This can often be given in the form of full and detailed explanations of the problem. Occasionally the patient will need to be persuaded by provocative tests that the symptoms really are related to the explained mechanism. Many patients respond to counselling over some months; this may involve explanations and reattribution of symptoms. Some may need exercises that are designed to enhance the voluntary control of breathing. Drugs have a very limited role and are best avoided in most patients.

Further reading

Elbert, T., Langosch, W., Steptoe, A. and Vaitl, D. (Eds.) (1988) *Behavioural Medicine in Cardiovascular Disorders.* John Wiley, Chichester.

INDEX